Epidemiology for Public Health Practice
Third Edition

Robert H. Friis, PhD
Professor and Chair
Department of Health Science
California State University, Long Beach
Long Beach, California

Thomas A. Sellers, PhD, MPH
Associate Center Director
H. Lee Moffitt Cancer Center and Research Institute
University of South Florida
Tampa, Florida

JONES AND BARTLETT PUBLISHERS
Sudbury, Massachusetts
BOSTON   TORONTO   LONDON   SINGAPORE

World Headquarters
Jones and Bartlett Publishers
40 Tall Pine Drive
Sudbury, MA 01776
978-443-5000
info@jbpub.com
www.jbpub.com

Jones and Bartlett Publishers Canada
2406 Nikanna Road
Mississauga, ON L5C 2W6
CANADA

Jones and Bartlett Publishers International
Barb House, Barb Mews
London W6 7PA
UK

Library of Congress Cataloging-in-Publication Data
Friis, Robert H.
    Epidemiology for public health practice /Robert H. Friis, Thomas A. Sellers.—3rd ed.
        p. ; cm.
    Includes bibliographical references and index.
    ISBN 0-7637-3170-6
        1. Epidemiology. 2. Public health personnel. I. Sellers, Thomas A. II. Title.
    [DNLM: 1. Epidemiology. 2. Public Health. WA 105 F912e 2003]
RA651.F686 2003
614.4—dc21

                                                                        2003054996

Production Credits
Publisher: Michael Brown
Production Manager: Amy Rose
Manufacturing Buyer: Therese Bräuer
Associate Editor: Chambers Moore
Associate Production Editor: Karen C. Ferreira
Associate Marketing Manager: Joy Stark-Vancs
Manufacturing and Inventory Coordinator: Amy Bacus
Text Design: Paw Print Media
Cover Design: Brianna Donahue
Composition: Dartmouth Publishing, Inc.
Printing and Binding: Courier Westford
Cover Printing: Courier Westford

Printed in the United States of America

07 06 05 04   10 9 8 7 6 5 4 3 2

Table of Contents

Preface

My interest in epidemiology began during the 1960s when, as an undergraduate student at the University of California at Berkeley and a graduate student at Columbia University, I observed the student revolts and activism that occurred during that era. Student unrest was, I believed, a phenomenon that occurred in large groups and could be explained by a theoretical framework, perhaps one that would include such concepts as alienation or anomie. I became interested in studying the distribution of these psychologic states in student populations. Unknowingly, I had embarked upon epidemiologic research. I find epidemiology to be a field that has great personal appeal, because it is capable of affecting the health of large groups of people through improvements in social conditions and environmental modifications.

My formal training in epidemiology began at the Institute for Social Research of the University of Michigan, where I spent two years as a postdoctoral fellow. My first professional position in epidemiology was as an assistant professor in the Division of Epidemiology at the School of Public Health, Columbia University. As a fledgling professor, I found epidemiology to be a fascinating discipline, and began to develop this textbook from my early teaching experiences. I concluded that there was a need for a textbook that would be oriented toward the beginning practitioner in the field, would provide coverage of a wide range of topics, and would emphasize the social and behavioral foundations of epidemiology, as well as the medical model. This textbook has evolved from my early teaching experience at Columbia, as well as later teaching and research positions at Albert Einstein College of Medicine, Brooklyn College, the University of California at Irvine, and the California State University system. Practical experience in epidemiology, as an epidemiologist in a local health department in Orange County, California, is also reflected in the book.

I welcome comments and suggestions from our readers. Please e-mail me at rfriis@csulb.edu.

—Robert H. Friis

Like many others now reading this book, I had absolutely no idea what epidemiology was before I took my first required class in it at Tulane University School of Public Health and Tropical Medicine. What I discovered was a method to combine my training in nutrition and interest in health with an aptitude for math and analytical reasoning. This led to a change in majors and ultimately a PhD in epidemiology.

My first faculty appointment was at the University of Minnesota School of Public Health. Before I knew it, I was assigned to teach the introduction to epidemiology course during the winter quarter. This was the time of year when only nonmajors enrolled. I quickly learned, as had my predecessors before me, that my teaching and learning styles were quite different from those of my students. Moreover, most of the textbooks available at that time were geared toward epidemiology majors. For nine years I studied learning styles (and even co-developed and co-taught a graduate course on teaching) and experimented to find new ways to present the fundamentals of epidemiology in a nontechnical, nontheoretical, intuitive manner. This text reflects these learning experiences.

—*Thomas A. Sellers*

Acknowledgments

First, I express my gratitude to my teachers and colleagues at the settings where I have worked during the past three decades. Their insights and suggestions have helped me clarify my thinking about epidemiology. Among these individuals are Dr. Sidney Cobb and Dr. John R. P. French, Jr., who were my postdoctoral supervisors at the University of Michigan's Institute for Social Research. Dr. Mervyn Susser was responsible for offering me my first professional employment in epidemiology at the School of Public Health, Columbia University. He and Dr. Zena Stein helped me to increase greatly my fund of knowledge about research and teaching in the field. Professor Anna Gelman provided me with many practical ideas regarding how to teach epidemiology. Dr. Stephen A. Richardson also contributed to my knowledge about epidemiologic research. Finally, Dr. Jeremiah Tilles, Associate Dean, California College of Medicine, University of California at Irvine, provided extremely valuable instruction regarding the epidemiology of infectious diseases.

I also thank students in my epidemiology classes who contributed their suggestions and read early drafts of the first edition. The comments of anonymous reviewers were particularly helpful in revising the manuscript. Jonathan Horowitz, former instructor in Health Science at California State University, Long Beach, spent a great deal of time reviewing several chapters of a very early version of the text, and I acknowledge his contributions. Sherry Stock, a former student in medical sociology at Long Beach, typed the first draft and provided much additional valuable assistance in securing bibliographic research materials. Dr. Yee-Lean Lee, Associate Professor, Infectious Disease Division, Department of Medicine, University of California at Irvine, reviewed and commented on the chapter dealing with the epidemiology of infectious diseases. Also, Dr. Harold Hunter, Professor of Health Care Administration, California State University, Long Beach, reviewed several chapters of the manuscript. Finally, my wife, Carol

Friis, typed the final version of the manuscript and made helpful comments. Without her support and assistance, completion of the text would not have been possible.

For the second edition of the text, I again thank my epidemiology students, who continued to provide much useful feedback. Graduate students Janelle Yamashita, Cindy Bayliss, and Jocelin Sabado were extremely helpful in conducting literature searches and in preparing the text. Sharon Jean assisted with typing the manuscript.

With respect to the third edition, I would like to thank students at my home university and at other universities who provided many worthwhile suggestions for enhancement of the text. I am also grateful for the informal feedback I have received from faculty members (across the United States and in several foreign countries) who have adopted this text in their courses. California State University graduate student Ibtisam Khoury conducted background research, provided ideas for clarification of complex concepts, and helped to develop several new tables. Faculty members Dr. Javier Lopez-Zetina and Dr. Dennis Fisher, housed at the same university, reviewed several of the chapters. Dr. Ezra Levy aided in the development of some of the new figures included in the text. Critiques from anonymous reviewers also were instrumental in development of the third edition. Once again, I am deeply indebted to my wife, Carol Friis, who assisted with editing and typing the manuscript. Without her keen eye, writing this book would have been a much more difficult task.

R.H.F.

I have been most fortunate to have received training and guidance from a significant number of individuals. First and foremost, I thank Dr. Dorothy Clemmer, who taught me my first course in epidemiology at Tulane University School of Public Health and Tropical Medicine. Her enthusiasm and support helped me to "see the light." The early years of my education included mentorship with Dr. Gerald Berenson and Dr. Robert C. Elston. Both have been extremely influential in my practical and theoretical understanding of this discipline. Dr. J. Michael Sprafka was a great supporter and colleague for those first precarious episodes of teaching. I owe many thanks to the numerous bright and challenging public health students at the University of Minnesota for their support, encouragement, and patience while I experimented with methods of presentation to find out what worked best for "nonmajors." Finally, I acknowledge my father, Gene R. Sellers, who has published many fine textbooks and gave me the courage to attempt this project; my loving wife, Barbara, for her understanding and enduring belief in me; and my two sons, Jamison Thomas and Ryan Austin, who are my inspiration and loves of my life.

For the third edition I'd like to acknowledge the contributions of several former colleagues at the Mayo Clinic who unknowingly or unwittingly provided inspiration for some of the new examples used. These include L. Joseph Melton, III, MD, a phenomenal epidemiologist with uncanny insight and ability to cut to the chase on any perceived complex problem; Steven Jacobsen, MD, PhD, a selfless leader with excellent perspective on work/life balance, who taught me a lot about clinical epidemiology; James R. Cerhan, MD, PhD, a creative and tireless investigator with outstanding organizational skills, incredible integrity, and a wry sense of humor; and Celine Vachon, PhD, an energetic young investigator who is just beginning to realize her true potential and who will certainly be the origin of many of the examples in the next edition of this book.

T.A.S.

About the Authors

Robert H. Friis, PhD, is a Professor of Health Science and Chair of the Department of Health Science at California State University, Long Beach, and Director of the CSULB-VAMC, Long Beach, Joint Studies Institute. He is also Clinical Professor of Community and Environmental Medicine at University of California, Irvine. Previously, he was an Associate Clinical Professor in the Department of Medicine, Department of Neurology, and School of Social Ecology, University of California, Irvine. His entire professional career has been devoted to the field of epidemiology. He has conducted research and taught epidemiology and related subjects for more than three decades at universities in New York City and in Southern California. In addition to previous employment in a local health department as an epidemiologist, he has conducted research and published and presented numerous papers related to mental health, chronic disease, disability, minority health, and psychosocial epidemiology. Dr. Friis has been principal investigator or co-investigator on grants and contracts from University of California's Tobacco-Related Disease Research Program, from the National Institutes of Health, and from other agencies for research on geriatric health, depression in Hispanic populations, and nursing home infections. His research interests have led him to conduct research in Mexico City and European countries. He has been a visiting professor at the Center for Nutrition and Toxicology, Karolinska Institute, Stockholm, Sweden; the Max Planck Institute, Munich, Germany; and Dresden Technical University, also in Germany. He reviews articles for scientific journals, including *International Migration Review* and *Social Science and Medicine*. Dr. Friis is a member of the Society for Epidemiologic Research and the American Public Health Association. Among his awards have been a postdoctoral fellowship for study at the Institute for Social Research, University of Michigan, and the Achievement Award for Scholarly and Creative Activity from California State University, Long Beach. His biography is listed in *Who's Who in America*.

Thomas A. Sellers, PhD, MPH, is Associate Center Director, H. Lee Moffitt Cancer Center and Research Institute, University of South Florida. Previously, he was a Professor of Epidemiology in the Department of Health Sciences Research at the Mayo Clinic and the Deputy Director of the Mayo Clinic Cancer Center. He was an Associate Professor at the University of Minnesota School of Public Health, where he taught the Introduction to Epidemiology course to non-majors for nine years. His primary research interests include understanding the etiology of common adult cancers, such as breast, lung, and ovarian cancer; he has published more than 150 scientific articles and book chapters. Most of his research employs the methods of genetic epidemiology and involves investigation of gene-environment interactions. Dr. Sellers has published widely in a number of scientific journals, and has reviewed articles for the *New England Journal of Medicine, Journal of the American Medical Association, American Journal of Epidemiology, Epidemiology, Cancer Research,* and many others. He is a founding member of the International Genetic Epidemiology Society and is also a member of the Society for Epidemiologic Research, the American Society for Human Genetics, the American Association for Cancer Research, and the American Society for Preventive Oncology. Dr. Sellers has been an invited member of Advisory Committees to the National Cancer Institute, has provided invited lectures all over the world, and has served on numerous grant review panels.

Introduction

Epidemiology is an exciting and rewarding field! Evidence of the importance of epidemiology to society comes from the incessant flow of media reports on flare-ups of new diseases, outbreaks of illness on cruise ships, and, even more ominous, the intentional spread of pathogenic microorganisms through acts of bioterrorism. One of the difficult tasks for the authors has been to incorporate with sufficient breadth and depth all of the fascinating components of this discipline. Since the publication of the first and second editions, epidemiologic researchers have continued to develop an even greater wealth of findings that have won the attention of the popular media, as well as space in professional journals. Indeed, it has been a challenge to select information from all of the excellent research that has been published within the past few years, as well as during the entire history of the field. For example, some of these recent discoveries relate to continuing advances in genetics and molecular biology, recognition of emerging infections, and the growing use of the Internet. As a result, the second edition introduced several enhancements: a new chapter on molecular and genetic epidemiology, a new chapter on experimental epidemiology, material on epidemiology web sites, and updated charts and tables throughout the text. The third edition incorporates a new chapter on cohort designs, a glossary, and expanded coverage of ecologic and case-control study designs. We also have included new material on the role of epidemiology in policy-making, epidemiology and geographic information systems, and the definition of race used in Census 2000. A new Appendix A provides an extended guide to critiquing published research studies in public health and epidemiology. Several new tables summarize unadjusted measures of morbidity and mortality, contrast different types of observational study designs, and compare observational versus intervention study designs.

We intend the audience for the textbook to be beginning public health master's degree students, undergraduate and graduate health education and social ecology students, undergraduate medical students, nursing students, residents in primary care medicine, and applicants who are preparing for medical board examinations. These students are similar to those with whom both authors have worked over the years. Students from the social and behavioral sciences have also found epidemiology to be a useful tool in medical sociology and behavioral medicine. The authors have included study questions and exercises at the end of each chapter; this material would be helpful to review for board examinations. Appendix B contains an expanded answer set to selected problems.

Each chapter begins with a list of learning objectives and an outline to help focus the reader's attention to key points. Some of the major issues and examples are highlighted in text boxes and tables. Chapter 1, which defines epidemiology and provides a historical background for the discipline, is complemented by Chapter 2, which provides examples of practical applications of epidemiology, as well as a discussion of causal inference. While examples of epidemiologic statistical techniques are interspersed throughout the book, Chapter 3 focuses on the "nuts and bolts" of measures of morbidity and mortality. Chapters 4 through 11 deal with the important topics of descriptive epidemiology, data sources, study designs, measures of effect, data interpretation, and screening. Chapters 12 through 15 focus on four content areas in epidemiology: infectious diseases, occupational and environmental health, molecular and genetic epidemiology, and psychosocial epidemiology. This text provides a thorough grounding in the key areas of methodology, causality, and the complex issues that surround chronic and infectious disease investigations. The authors assume that the reader will have had some familiarity with introductory biostatistics, although the text is intelligible to those who do not have such familiarity.

CHAPTER 1

The History and Scope of Epidemiology

LEARNING OBJECTIVES

By the end of this chapter the reader will be able to:

- define the term *epidemiology*
- define the components of epidemiology (determinants, distribution, morbidity, and mortality)
- name and describe characteristics of the epidemiologic approach
- discuss the importance of Hippocrates' hypothesis and how it differed from the common beliefs of the time
- discuss Graunt's contributions to biostatistics and how they affected modern epidemiology
- explain what is meant by the term *natural experiments,* and give at least one example

CHAPTER OUTLINE

Introduction

Epidemiologic speculations and research findings often blaze across media headlines and arouse public hysteria. Some of the questions raised by media reports include: "What is more dangerous: vaccination against smallpox or infection with the disease itself through a terrorist attack?" "Is Ebola virus a danger to the general public?" "Should I give up eating fatty foods?" "Is it safe to drink coffee or alcoholic beverages?" "Will chemicals in the environment cause cancer?" "Is it safe to consume tap water from public drinking supplies or should one purchase bottled water?"

Take the example of tap water consumption and its potential linkages to human birth outcomes (Exhibit 1-1). Epidemiologic research suggested that tap water consumption might endanger pregnant women by causing spontaneous abortions. Panicked citizens besieged public health officials with their concerns about the safety of the water supply. A flurry of reports and an acerbic public debate ensued for several weeks.

Epidemiologic research methods are a powerful tool for studying health. Exhibit 1-1 raises several issues that are typical of many epidemiologic research studies:

- When there is a linkage or association between a factor (such as contaminants in water) and a health outcome, does this observation mean that the factor is a cause of disease?
- If there is an association, does the amount of disease vary according to the amount of exposure to the factor?
- Based on the observation of such an association, what practical steps should individuals and public health departments take?
- Do the findings from an epidemiologic study merit panic or a measured response?
- How applicable are the findings to settings other than the one in which the research was conducted?

In this chapter as well as in later chapters of this book we will answer the foregoing questions. We will discuss the stages that are necessary to unravel mysteries about diseases, such as those due to chemical exposure problems or those for which the cause is entirely unknown.

Epidemiology is a discipline that describes, quantifies, and postulates causal mechanisms for health phenomena in populations. The study of tap water and spontaneous abortions illustrated some of the classic methods of epidemiology—

EXHIBIT 1-1

Findings That Link Tap Water to Miscarriages Evoke Panic

Los Angeles Area Residents Urged To Show Prudence

"Reacting to a new study that suggests a possible link between drinking tap water and miscarriages by pregnant women in their first trimester, Los Angeles officials said Tuesday that the city's water often contains amounts of the suspect contaminants exceeding the levels that have triggered concern. But the officials advised prudence rather than panic."[1]

During early 1998, the media reported a possible association between use of tap water from public drinking water supplies and increased risk of miscarriages. Physicians were besieged by calls from anxious patients and some young expectant couples agonized over how they would pay the cost of bottled water.

Epidemiologists Shanna H. Swan, Kirsten Waller, and colleagues, affiliated with California's Department of Health Services, published findings on potential reproductive health effects of drinking water use.[2] With increasing industrialization, urbanization, and population growth, some residential water supplies may carry dangerous pollution levels. Industrial solvents and chemicals as well as household pesticides may leach into aquifers or contaminate ground water that is used in tap water. Even when the public water supply is free from these sources of pollution, potentially dangerous chemicals may also be released when the chlorine used to sanitize the water and kill microbial agents reacts with organic materials in the water supply. The resulting end products are known as trihalomethanes (THM). The abbreviation TTHM is used to denote total trihalomethanes.

The investigators noted that TTHMs are found in nearly all US drinking water supplies. TTHMs, which include chemicals such as chloroform, have possible associations with reproductive abnormalities in animal studies. Human exposure to TTHMs may be related to adverse pregnancy outcomes, such as spontaneous abortions.

In their research, Swan, Waller, and colleagues addressed the specific issue of whether use of tap water was associated with adverse pregnancy outcomes in humans. The investigators' previous research (based on

continues

EXHIBIT 1-1 *continued*

retrospective studies) reported an association between spontaneous abortion rates and use of tap water in comparison to bottled water among pregnant women in a single California county. In subsequent research (a prospective study), they followed pregnant women who resided in three California regions, two in the north (regions I and II) and one in the south (region III), served by the Kaiser Permanente Medical Care Program. The respective regions were served by ground water mixed with surface water or either primarily surface or ground water. A total of 5,342 pregnant women completed interviews during the first trimester of their pregnancy. Information was collected on a range of topics, including medical history, lifestyle and psychosocial factors, and water consumption practices during the week beginning with the last menstrual period and the week before the interview. For example, information regarding use of cold tap water, heated tap water, noncarbonated bottled water, and carbonated water was assessed. Water consumption was quantitated in glasses per day. Finally, pregnancy outcomes were ascertained from various sources that included review of medical and vital records and telephone interviews.

The study demonstrated that spontaneous abortion rates were slightly different from one region to another, ranging from 9.2% to 10.1%. In region I only, consumption of cold tap water in comparison to none was associated with the occurrence of spontaneous abortions. High levels of tap water consumption were even more strongly related to the rate of spontaneous abortions. High consumption levels of bottled water in comparison to tap water seemed to be associated with a reduced rate of spontaneous abortions. Type of water consumption did not alter the risk of spontaneous abortion in the other two regions studied. Further research showed that one type of TTHM (bromodichloromethane) found in cold tap water was associated with spontaneous abortions.[3] ∎

first, making a descriptive statement and then following up with a more carefully controlled study. It also illustrated the method of quantification—in this example, assessing the outcome of the study (spontaneous abortions) as well as measuring the exposure variable (consumption of tap water). There also was careful attention to the selection of the study sample (the population) and their characteristics. It hypothesized a causal mechanism (i.e., the role of trihalomethanes (THM) in the public water supply). All of these features are hallmarks of epidemiologic research.

Epidemiology Defined

The word *epidemiology* derives from *epidemic,* a term that provides an immediate clue to its subject matter. Epidemiology originates from the Greek words *epi* (upon) + *demos* (people) + *logy* (study of). Although some conceptions of epidemiology are quite narrow, the authors, in suggesting a broadened scope for epidemiology, propose the following definition:

> **Epidemiology is concerned with the distribution and determinants of health and diseases, morbidity, injuries, disability, and mortality in populations. The key aspects of this definition are determinants, distribution, population, and health phenomena (e.g., morbidity and mortality).**

Determinants

Determinants are factors or events that are capable of bringing about a change in health. Some examples are specific biologic agents (e.g., bacteria) that are associated with infectious diseases or chemical agents that may act as carcinogens. Other potential determinants for changes in health may include less specific factors, such as stress or adverse lifestyle patterns (lack of exercise or a diet high in saturated fats). The following four vignettes illustrate the concern of epidemiology with disease determinants. Considering the steps taken to explore the health effects of public water supplies, contemplate the position of an epidemiologist once again. Imagine a possible scenario for describing, quantifying, and identifying the determinants for each of the vignettes.

Case 1: Intentional Dissemination of Bacteria that Cause Anthrax

On September 11, 2001, the United States experienced the worst terrorist attack in its history. As the nation sought to deal with this tragedy, it would face a second wave of terrorism—this time, in the form of a biological attack. The suspicion of anthrax in a patient by an astute infectious disease clinician along with capable clinical and public health laboratory staff in Florida would lead to the discovery that *Bacillus anthracis*

continues

CASE 1 *continued*

spores had been intentionally distributed through the postal system, causing 22 cases of anthrax, including 5 deaths, and forever changing the realm of public health.[4]

The popular press has been filled with reports of anthrax exposure since September 11th [2001]. Usually a disease that strikes mostly livestock and wild animals, it has become a household word since its use as a weapon of terror. The most severe form of the disease results from inhalation of *Bacillus anthracis* spores, which are engulfed or phagocytised by macrophages in the lung. Phagocytosis of bacteria by macrophages is a normal and effective method of the innate immune system to fight the spread of infection. However, in the case of anthrax, the bacteria survive phagocytosis, reproduce within the cells, and use the macrophages as a transport mechanism to invade lymph nodes and eventually the blood-stream, leading to widespread infection, disease, and death.[5]

Since October 3, 2001, [Centers for Disease Control and Prevention] CDC and state and local public health authorities have been investigating cases of bioterrorism-related anthrax. . . . [As of October 31, 2001,] A total of 21 cases (16 confirmed and five suspected) of bioterrorism-related anthrax have been reported among persons who worked in the District of Columbia, Florida, New Jersey, and New York City. . . .[6]

Florida: To date, the investigation in Florida has identified two con-firmed inhalational cases.[6] The index case of inhalational anthrax in October 2001 was in a man who lived and worked in Florida. However, during the 3 days before illness onset, he had traveled through North Carolina, raising the possibility that exposure to *Bacillus anthracis* spores could have occurred there. On October 4, concurrent investigations were initiated in Florida and North Carolina to identify the naturally occurring or bioterrorism-related source of his exposure. In less than a week, investiga-tors isolated *B. anthracis* from the patient's place of employment in Florida. . . . However, the history of travel to North Carolina had already resulted in a substantial public health effort in that state.[7]

On October 4, 2001, the Palm Beach County Health Department (PBCHD), the Florida State Department of Health (FSDOH), and CDC reported a case of anthrax in a 63-year-old resident of Florida. The patient

continues

CASE 1 *continued*

was hospitalized with the respiratory form of anthrax and subsequently died. PBCHD, FSDOH, and CDC initiated an epidemiologic investigation and public health surveillance to identify how infection with *Bacillus anthracis* occurred and to identify other infections. An environmental investigation identified one sample taken from the patient's workplace (America Media Inc. [AMI], Boca Raton, Florida) as positive for anthrax. *B. anthracis* also was identified in one nasal sample from another worker in the same building, which suggests exposure.[8]

New York: To date, the investigations in New York City have identified one confirmed inhalational case and six (three confirmed and three suspected) cutaneous anthrax cases; . . . The six cutaneous cases were associated with four media companies (A-D); the most recent suspected cutaneous case is associated with company D. The most recent confirmed inhalational case is not directly associated with any media company or with mail handling. No cases among postal workers have been identified.[6]

The most recent suspected cutaneous case occurred in a 34-year-old man who worked in the mail room of company D who might have handled a letter postmarked September 18, which the patient handled during October 12-15 and subsequently was found to contain *B. anthracis*. . . .

The inhalational anthrax case occurred in a 61-year-old woman who worked in the stockroom of a hospital in Manhattan. The patient became ill on October 25 with malaise and myalgias. During the next several days, she had shortness of breath, chest discomfort, and a productive cough with blood-tinged sputum. She reported no fever, chills, or night sweats. She presented to an emergency department on October 28 in respiratory distress. Her temperature was 102° F (39° C), and she was admitted to the intensive care unit and required mechanical ventilation. . . . The patient died on October 31.[6]

New Jersey: To date, investigations in New Jersey and Pennsylvania have identified seven (five confirmed and two suspected) anthrax cases. . . cutaneous disease was confirmed in two patients, and inhalational anthrax was confirmed in two patients, one of whom was previously classified as a suspected case-patient. Five patients worked in New Jersey at one of two postal facilities. Although no specific contaminated letter was

continues

CASE 1 *continued*

implicated in these cases, contaminated letters destined for both New York City and the District of Columbia passed through at least one of the postal facilities in New Jersey. Inhalational anthrax was confirmed in a 56-year-old female postal worker who initially was classified as a suspected case-patient . . . .[6]

On October 13, a 54-year-old Delaware resident who worked as a mail sorter at a New Jersey postal processing and distributing center developed a painless lesion on the dorsum of his left hand. . . . On October 15, a 43-year-old female postal worker who worked at a facility in which anthrax cases have been documented developed fever, headache, chills, and shortness of breath. . . .[6]

On October 17, a 51-year-old woman developed a large pimple on her forehead with erythema and swelling. On October 18, the lesion enlarged, was slightly painful, nonpruritic, and drained a small amount of yellowish fluid. . . . [Seeking medical care, the patient was hospitalized.] The patient improved and was discharged on October 27. . . The patient worked as a bookkeeper and reported receiving no unusual or powder-containing mail at home or work. She had made no visits to any post offices in several months.[6]

District of Columbia: To date, investigations in the District of Columbia, Maryland, and Virginia have confirmed inhalational anthrax in four persons who worked at one postal facility in the District of Columbia. An additional case of inhalational anthrax has been confirmed in a 59-year-old postal worker in a U.S. State Department mail sorting facility that receives mail from the District of Columbia postal facility associated with the previous four cases.[6]

Connecticut: The source of exposure for the case of inhalational anthrax in a 94-year-old woman who lived in Oxford, CT, remains unknown. Multiple environmental samples collected from all places (e.g., the patient's home, church, voting place, restaurants, and cars in which she traveled) the patient was known to have visited during the 60 days preceding illness onset were negative for *B. anthracis* by culture. Nasal swab specimens were negative from 16 persons epidemiologically linked to the case (e.g., persons who worked in the home and assisted with shopping).[9]

continues

CASE 1 *continued*

Environmental sampling was performed at the postal processing and distribution center in Wallingford, CT, which serves the towns of Oxford and Seymour, and identified *B. anthracis* spores in three high-speed mail sorters. This facility receives mail from several postal distribution facilities known to have been contaminated by *B. anthracis* spores, including the postal center in Hamilton, NJ, which was the origination site for envelopes containing *B. anthracis* powder that were addressed to two U.S. senators. . . . No record of mail to the CT case-patient processed at Hamilton was found, and no *B anthracis* spores have been recovered from envelopes found at her home.[9] ■

Case 2: Outbreak of Fear

When a 36-year-old lab technician known as Kinfumu checked into the general hospital in Kikwit, Zaire, . . . complaining of diarrhea and a fever, anyone could have mistaken his illness for the dysentery that was plaguing the city. Nurses, doctors, and nuns did what they could to help the young man. They soon saw that his disease wasn't just dysentery. Blood began oozing from every orifice in his body. Within four days he was dead. By then the illness had all but liquefied his internal organs.

That was just the beginning. The day Kinfumu died, a nurse and a nun who had cared for him fell ill. The nun was evacuated to another town 70 miles to the west where she died—but not until the contagion had spread to at least three of her fellow nuns. Two have since died. In Kikwit, the disease raged through the ranks of the hospital's staff. Inhabitants of the city began fleeing to neighboring villages. Some of the fugitives carried the deadly illness with them. Terrified health officials in Kikwit sent an urgent message to the World Health Organization. The Geneva-based group summoned expert help from around the globe: a team of experienced virus hunters . . . composed of tropical-medicine specialists, microbiologists and other researchers. They grabbed their lab equipment and their bubble suits and clambered aboard transport planes headed for Kikwit.[10] ■

Case 3: Fear on Seventh Avenue

On normal workdays, the streets of New York City's garment district are lively canyons bustling with honking trucks, scurrying buyers and sweating rack boys pushing carts loaded with suits, coats and dresses. But last week a tense new atmosphere was evident. Sanitation trucks cruised the side streets off Seventh Avenue flushing pools of stagnant water from the gutters and spraying out disinfectant. Teams of health officers drained water towers on building roofs. Air conditioners fell silent for inspection, and several chilling signs appeared on 35th Street: "The New York City Department of Health has been advised of possible causes of Legionnaires' disease in this building." By the weekend, there were six cases of the mysterious disease, 73 more suspected and two deaths. . . . In the New York City outbreak, three brothers were the first victims. Carlisle, Gilbert, and Joseph Leggette developed the fever, muscle aches, and chest congestion that make the disease resemble pneumonia. Joseph and Gilbert recovered; Carlisle did not. "He just got sick and about a week later he was dead," said John Leggette, a fourth brother who warily returned to his own job in the garment district last week. "I'm scared," he said. "But what can you do?"[11] ■

Case 4: Red Spots on Airline Flight Attendants

From January 1 to March 10, 1980, Eastern Airlines (EAL) received 190 reports of episodes of red spots appearing on the skin of flight attendants (FAs) during various flights. . . . Complaints of symptoms accompanying the spots were rare, but some FAs expressed concern that the spots were caused by bleeding through the skin and might indicate a serious health hazard. On March 12, investigators from CDC [Centers for Disease Control and Prevention] traveled to Miami to assist in the investigation. . . . No evidence of damage to underlying skin was noted on these examinations, nor was any noted by consultant dermatologists who examined affected FAs after the spots had disappeared. Chemical tests on clinical specimens for the presence of blood were negative.

continues

CASE 4 *continued*

Airline personnel had investigated the ventilation systems, cleaning materials and procedures, and other environmental factors on affected aircraft. Airflow patterns and cabin temperatures, pressures, and relative humidity were found to be normal. Cleaning materials and routines had been changed, but cases continued to occur. Written reports by FAs of 132 cases occurring in January and February showed that 91 different FAs had been affected, 68 once and 23 several times. Of these cases, 119 (90%) had occurred on a single type of aircraft. Of the 119 cases from implicated aircraft, 96% occurred on north- or south-bound flights between the New York City and Miami metropolitan areas, flights that are partially over water. Only rarely was a case reported from the same airplane when flying transcontinental or other east-west routes.[12] ■

Health departments, the Centers for Disease Control and Prevention (CDC) in Atlanta, and epidemiologic researchers frequently confront a problem that has no clear determinants or etiologic basis. The methods and findings of epidemiologic studies may direct one to, or suggest, particular causal mechanisms underlying health-related events or conditions, such as the four examples cited earlier in the vignettes: anthrax, the suspected outbreak of Ebola virus, Legionnaires' disease, and red spots on airline flight attendants. Read the following solution to clear up the mystery of Case 4.

Solution to Case 4: Red Spots

The investigation then concentrated on defining the clinical picture more clearly. An Eastern Airlines (EAL) physician, a consultant dermatologist, and a physician from the National Institute for Occupational Safety and Health (NIOSH) rode on implicated flights on March 14 and examined three new cases considered by the EAL physician and other flight attendants (FAs) to be typical cases. Although the spots observed consisted of red liquid, they did not resemble blood. To identify potential environmental sources of red-colored material, investigators observed the standard activities of FAs on board implicated flights. At the beginning of each flight FAs routinely demonstrated the use of life vests, required in emer-

continues

SOLUTION TO CASE 4 *continued*

gency landings over water. Because the vests used for demonstration were not actually functional they were marked in bright red ink with the words "Demo Only." When the vests were demonstrated, the red ink areas came into close contact with the face, neck, and hands of the demonstrator. Noting that on some vests the red ink rubbed or flaked off easily, investigators used red material from the vests to elicit the typical clinical picture on themselves. On preliminary chemical analyses, material in clinical specimens of red spots obtained from cases was found to match red-ink specimens from demonstration vests. On March 15 and 16, EAL removed all demonstration model life vests from all its aircraft and instructed FAs to use the standard, functional, passenger-model vests for demonstration purposes. The airline will continue to request reports of cases to verify the effectiveness of this action. Although all demonstration vests were obtained from the same manufacturer, the vests removed from specific aircraft were noted to vary somewhat in the color of fabric and in the color and texture of red ink, suggesting that many different production lots may have been in use simultaneously on any given aircraft.[12] ■

Distribution

Frequency of disease occurrence may vary from one population group to another. For example, hypertension may be more common among young African American men than among young white men. Mortality from coronary heart disease may vary between Hispanics and non-Hispanics.[13] Such variations in disease frequency illustrate how disease may have different distributions depending upon the underlying characteristics of the populations being studied.

Population

Epidemiology examines disease occurrence among population groups rather than among individuals. Lilienfeld[14] noted that this focus is a widely accepted feature of epidemiology. For this reason, epidemiology is often referred to as "population medicine." The epidemiologic and clinical descriptions of a disease are quite different as a result. Note the different descriptions of toxic shock syndrome (TSS), a condition that showed sharp increases during 1980 in comparison to the immediately previous years. TSS is a severe illness that in the 1980 outbreak was found to be associated with vaginal tampon use. The clinical description of TSS would include specific signs and symptoms, such as high fever, headache, malaise, and other more dramatic symptoms, such as vomiting and profuse watery diarrhea. The epidemiologic description would indicate which age groups would be most likely to be affected, time trends, geographic trends, and other variables that affect the distribution of TSS. A second example is myocardial infarction (MI). A clinical description of MI (heart attack) would list specific signs and symptoms, such as chest pain, heart rate, nausea, and other individual characteristics of the patient. The epidemiologic description of the same condition would indicate which age groups would be most likely to be affected, seasonal trends in heart attack rates, geographic variations in frequency, and other characteristics of persons associated with the frequency of heart attack in populations.

Referring again to the vignettes, one may note that the problem that plagued Kinfumu in case 2 was recognized as a particularly acute problem for epidemiology when similar complaints from other patients were discovered and the disease began to spread. If more than one person complains about a health problem, the health practitioner may develop the suspicion that some widespread exposure rather than something unique to an individual is occurring. The clinical observation might suggest further epidemiologic investigation of the problem.

Health Phenomena

As indicated in the definition, epidemiology is used to investigate many different kinds of health outcomes. These range from infectious diseases to chronic disease, and various states of health, such as disability, injury, limitation of activity, and mortality.[15] Other health outcomes have included positive functioning of the individual and active life expectancy as well as health-related events, including mental disorders, suicide, substance abuse, and injury. Epidemiology's concern with positive states of health is illustrated by research into active life expectancy among geriatric populations. This research seeks to determine the factors associated with optimal mental and physical functioning as well as enhanced quality of life and ultimately aims to limit disability in later life.

Morbidity and Mortality

Two other terms central to epidemiology are *morbidity* and *mortality*. The former, morbidity, designates illness, whereas the latter, mortality, refers to death. Note that most measures of morbidity and mortality are defined for specific types of morbidity or causes of death.

Aims and Levels

The preceding sections hint at the complete scope of epidemiology. As the basic method of public health, epidemiology is concerned with efforts to describe, explain, predict, and control.

- To *describe* the health status of populations means to enumerate the cases of disease, to obtain relative frequencies of the disease within subgroups, and to discover important trends in the occurrence of disease.
- To *explain* the etiology of disease means to discover causal factors as well as to discover modes of transmission.
- To *predict* the occurrence of disease is to estimate the actual number of cases that will develop as well as to identify the distribution within populations. Such information is crucial to planning interventions and allocation of health care resources.
- To *control* the distribution of disease, the epidemiologic approach is used to prevent the occurrence of new cases of disease, to eradicate existing cases, and to prolong the lives of those with the disease.

The implication of these aims is that epidemiology has two different goals. One is improved understanding of the natural history of disease and the factors that influence its distribution. With the knowledge that is obtained from such efforts, one can then proceed to accomplish the second goal: intervention.

Foundations of Epidemiology

Epidemiology Is Interdisciplinary

Epidemiology is an interdisciplinary field that draws from biostatistics and the social and behavioral sciences as well as from the medically related fields of toxicology, pathology, virology, genetics, microbiology, and clinical medicine. Terris[5] pointed out that epidemiology is an extraordinarily rich and complex science that derives techniques and methodologies from many disciplines. He wrote that epidemiology "must draw upon and synthesize knowledge from the biological sciences of man and of his parasites, from the numerous sciences of the physical environment, and from the sciences concerned with human society."[16(p203)]

To elaborate, some of the contributions of microbiology include information about specific disease agents, including their morphology and modes of transmission. The investigations of anthrax, Legionnaires' disease, TSS, and infant botulism (a condition linked to ingestion of spores, often found in honey, that cause botulism) utilized microbiologic techniques to identify possible infectious agents. When the infectious agent is a virus, the expertise of a virologist may be required. Clinical medicine is involved in the diagnosis of the patient's state of health, that is, defining whether the patient has a particular disease or condition. A pathologist's expertise may help differentiate between normal and diseased tissue. From our previous examples, clinical medicine diagnosed the individuals' symptoms or signs of ill health. Astute physicians and nurses may suggest epidemiologic research on the basis of clinical observations. Toxicology is concerned with the presence and health effects of chemical agents, particularly those found in the environment and the workplace. Regarding hazardous waste sites, toxicologic knowledge helps determine the presence of noxious chemical agents and whether the health effects observed are consistent with the known effects of exposure to toxic agents. When responses to exogenous agents vary from person to person, geneticists may become part of the team. Social and behavioral sciences elucidate the role of race, social class, education, cultural group membership, and behavioral practices in health-related phenomena. Social and behavioral science disciplines, that is, sociology and psychology, are devoted respectively to the development of social theory and the study of behavior. The special concern of social epidemiologic approaches is the study of social conditions and disease processes.[17] Furthermore, much of the methodology on sampling, measurement, questionnaire development, design, and delivery, and methods of group comparison are borrowed from the social sciences. Finally, the field of biostatistics is critical to the evaluation of epidemiologic data, especially when one is trying to separate chance from meaningful observations. Epidemiology profits from the interdisciplinary approach because the causality of a particular disease in a population may involve the interaction of multiple factors. The contributions of many disciplines help unravel the factors associated with a particular disease.

Methods and Procedures

Population research is empirical and requires quantification of relevant factors. Quantification refers to the translation of qualitative impressions into numbers. Qualitative sources of information about disease may be, in illustration, a physician's observations derived through medical practice about the types of people among whom a disease seems to be common. Epidemiologists enumerate cases of disease to objectify subjective impressions. Quantification is a central activity of epidemiology; the standard epidemiologic measures often require counting the number of cases of disease and examining their distribution according to demographic variables, such as age, sex, race, and other variables, such as exposure category and clinical features. The following quotation illustrates a summary of the characteristics of 51 suspected cases of severe acute respiratory syndrome (SARS) that were reported to the CDC as of early 2003:

The Language of Quantification
Severe Acute Respiratory Syndrome (SARS) in the United States

As of March 26, [2003] CDC has received 51 reports of suspected SARS cases from 21 states . . ., identified using the CDC updated interim case definition. [Refer to Table [1-1.]. . . . The first suspected case was identified on March 15, in a man aged 53 years who traveled to Singapore and became ill on March 10. Four clusters of suspected cases have been identified, three of which involved a traveler who had visited Southeast Asia (including Guangdong province, Hong Kong, or Vietnam) and a single family contact. One of these clusters involved suspected cases in patients L and M . . . who had stayed together at hotel M during March 1–6, when other hotel guests were symptomatic. Patient L became sick on March 13 after returning to the United States. His wife, patient M, became ill several days after the onset of her husband's symptoms, suggesting secondary transmission. Three patients in the United States with suspected SARS (patients I, L, and M) reported staying at hotel M when other persons staying in the hotel were symptomatic. The fourth cluster began with a suspected case in a person who traveled in Guangdong province and Hong Kong. Two [health care workers] subsequently became ill at the U.S. hospital where this patient was admitted.[18(p244)] ■

Epidemiologists sometimes present quantified information as graphs and tables that illustrate pictorially the frequency of disease. Quantification enables the epidemiologist to investigate the sources of variation of a disease by time, place, and person: When did the case occur? Where was it located? Who was affected?

We will offer many examples of quantification throughout this text. Table 1-1 reports the characteristics of SARS cases in selected locations in 2003.

Table 1-1. Exposure Category, Clinical Features, and Demographics of Reported Severe Acute Respiratory Syndrome (SARS) Cases* —Selected Locations, 2003

Category	HONG KONG No.	(%)	VIETNAM No.	(%)	THAILAND No.	(%)	TAIWAN No.	(%)	UNITED STATES No.	(%)
Total cases †	290 § (As of 3/25/03-S/P)	(100)	59 (As of 3/24/03-P)	(100)	4 (As of 3/23/03-S/P)	(100)	6 (As of 3/25/03-S)	(100)	51 § (As of 3/25/03-P)	(100)
Exposure										
Health-care worker	134	(46)	37	(63)	1	(25)	0		2	(4)
Close contact ¶	156	**	NA ††		0		2	(33)	5	(10)
Clinical features										
Ever hospitalized	290	(100) §	59	(100)	4	(100)	6	(100)	20 §	(39)
Pneumonia	286	(99)	NA		3	(75)	6	(100)	14	(27)
Ever ventilated	NA		5	(9)	1	(25)	2	(33)	1	(2)
Dead	10	(4) §	2	(3)	0		0		0 §	
Demographics										
Age	NA NA		Median: 38 yrs (range: 18–66 yrs)		Median: 38 yrs (range: 1–49 yrs)		Median: 53 yrs (range: 25–64 yrs)		Median: 42 yrs (range: 8 mos–78 yrs)	
Sex §§										
Female	Approximately 50%		37	(63)	1	(25)	3	(50)	26	(51)
Male	Approximately 50%		22	(37)	3	(75)	3	(50)	25	(49)

* Locations used different SARS case definitions. † S = Suspected case; P = Probable case; U = Unknown.

§ One U.S. resident (Patient B) was hospitalized in Vietnam and died in Hong Kong before he could return to the United States. He is counted as a Hong Kong case.

¶ Person having cared for, lived with, or had direct contact with respiratory secretions and body fluids of a person with SARS.

** Of the 290 SARS patients in Hong Kong, most of the remaining 156 patients are believed to be close contacts.

†† Not Available.

§§ Only percentages were reported for sex data.

Source: Centers for Disease Control and Prevention. Update: Outbreak of severe acute respiratory syndrome—worldwide, 2003. *Morb Mortal Wkly Rep* 2003;52:244.

Other key methods for the graphic presentation of data are the use of pie charts, bar charts, and line graphs. See Figure 1-1 for an example of each type. Figure 1-1 illustrates a pie chart (A, fatal occupational injuries in the United States); a bar chart (B, firearm injury death rates); and a line graph (C, motor vehicle traffic death rates). Epidemiologists use these types of graphs to describe characteristics of data, such as subgroup differences and time trends.[19]

Use of Special Vocabulary

Epidemiology employs a unique vocabulary of terms to describe the frequency of occurrence of disease. These terms are presented in Chapters 3 and 4. A different collection of terms is used in reference to the array of study designs available to epidemiologists. Chapters 6, 7, and 8 define and characterize these study approaches. Finally, special terms have been developed to convey the results and to aid in the interpretation of epidemiologic investigations. These are defined and illustrated in Chapter 10.

Dorland's Illustrated Medical Dictionary defines the word *epidemic* as "attacking many people at the same time, widely diffused and rapidly spreading." More precisely, an epidemic refers to an excessive occurrence of a disease: "Most current definitions [of epidemic] stress the concept of excessive prevalence as its basic implication in both lay and professional usage."[20(p2)] The following passage illustrates this notion by defining an epidemic as:

> The occurrence in a community or region of cases of an illness (or an outbreak) clearly in excess of expectancy. The number of cases indicating presence of an epidemic will vary according to the infectious agent, size and type of population exposed, previous experience or lack of exposure to the disease, and time and place of occurrence; epidemicity is thus relative to usual frequency of the disease in the same area, among the specified population, at the same season of the year. A single case of a communicable disease long absent from a population or the first invasion by a disease not previously recognized in that area requires immediate reporting and epidemiologic investigation; two cases of such a disease associated in time and place are sufficient evidence of transmission to be considered an epidemic.[21(p499)]

In current thinking, an epidemic is not confined to infectious diseases. Take, for example, the Love Canal incident that generated spirited public debate and media attention during the late 1970s. Love Canal was a toxic waste disposal site located in Niagara Falls, New York. It was the location for burial of thousands of chemical-filled drums deposited by the Hooker Chemicals & Plastics Corp. Eventually, the waste disposal site was covered and converted into a housing tract. Subsequently,

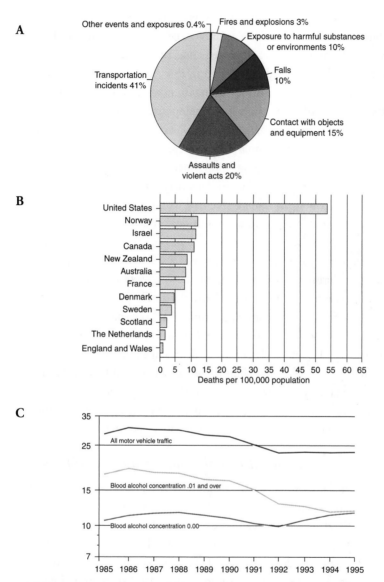

FIGURE 1-1 (**A,** Pie chart) Percentage distribution of fatal occupational injuries, according to event: United States, 1994–1995. (**B,** Bar graph) Firearm injury death rates among males 15–24 years of age for selected countries and selected years, 1992–1995. (**C,** Line graph) Motor vehicle traffic death rates by alcohol involvement among persons 15–34 years of age: United States, 1985–1995. *Source:* Reprinted from LA Fingerhut and M Warner, *Injury Chartbook. Health, United States, 1996–97,* 1997. National Center for Health Statistics.

residents of the area reported several different types of health effects, including mis-carriages, birth defects, and mental retardation. The Love Canal site was the focus of extensive health effects studies and epidemiologic research.

By referring to the case studies reported in this text, you will see additional examples—red spots among airline flight attendants and toxic shock syn-drome—that illustrate two instances in which epidemiologic methodology was employed to study noninfectious conditions. Toxic shock syndrome and red spots among airline flight attendants both represented apparent epidemics because the usual or expected rate was nil. Epidemiologic methods also are used to investigate occupationally associated illness (e.g., brown lung disease among textile workers and asbestosis among shipyard workers), environmental health hazards (e.g., toxic chemicals and air pollution), and disease associated with lifestyle (e.g., accidents, ischemic heart disease, and certain forms of cancer).

Related to the term epidemic is the term *pandemic,* which refers to an epidemic on a worldwide scale; during a pandemic, large numbers of persons may be affected and a disease may cross international borders. Examples are flu pandemics, such as the pandemic of 1918 and more recent flu pandemics that occur periodically. The term *endemic* is used to characterize a disease that is habitually present in a particular geo-graphical region. To illustrate, malaria is endemic in some tropical areas of Asia and cholera is endemic to less developed countries where sanitation is lacking. Previously, during the 19th century, cholera was endemic to Western countries, such as England and the Unted States. However, cholera is no longer endemic to these two countries because of the introduction of sanitation and other public health measures.

Methods for Ascertainment of Epidemic Frequency of Disease

The CDC and vital statistics departments of state and local governments collect surveillance data on a continuing basis to determine whether an epidemic is tak-ing place. The word *surveillance* can be defined as the systematic collection of data pertaining to the occurrence of specific diseases, the analysis and interpreta-tion of these data, and the dissemination of consolidated and processed informa-tion to contributors to the surveillance program and other interested persons. For example, if 500 heart attack deaths are reported in an upstate New York community during a particular year, this information by itself would be insuffi-cient to justify the assertion that an epidemic of heart attacks has occurred. The usual frequency of heart attacks would need to be determined in the same com-munity at some prior time, and the size, age, and sex distribution of the popula-tion would need to be known. A second example is shown in Figure 1-2 for influenza and pneumonia deaths.

FIGURE 1-2 Weekly pneumonia and influenza (P&I) mortality as a percentage of all deaths in 122 cities—United States, January 3, 1993–April 5, 1997. Source: Reprinted from Influenza Activity, MMWR, Vol 46, p 327, 1997, Centers for Disease Control and Prevention.

Figure 1-2 exhibits weekly pneumonia and influenza deaths in the United States from winter 1993 to spring 1997. It demonstrates that the flu has an underlying seasonal baseline, reflected in its cyclic seasonal increases and declines in mortality. The lower line denotes the usual number of deaths to be expected from pneumonia-influenza during each week of the year. An upper parallel line indicates the frequency of disease at the epidemic threshold, that is, the minimum number of deaths that would support the conclusion that an epidemic was under way. Figure 1-2 demonstrates that pneumonia-influenza deaths exceeded the epidemic threshold early in each of the years shown with the exception of 1995.

Historical Antecedents of Epidemiology

To put the discipline in proper perspective, we now outline some of the historical trends that led to the development of epidemiology. It may be said that epidemiology began with the Greeks, who in their concern for the ancient epidemics and deadly toll of diseases, attributed disease causality to environmental factors. Early causal explanations for epidemics included various events, such as the wrath of the gods, the breakdown of religious beliefs and morality, the influence of weather, and "bad air." Much later, during the late Renaissance, pioneer biostatisticians quantified morbidity and mortality trends. Often cited as another major development is John Snow's investigations of London cholera outbreaks, reported in *Snow on Cholera.*[22] A contemporary of Snow, William Farr, promoted innovative uses of vital statistics data. During the 19th century, early microbiologists formalized the germ theory of disease, which attributed diseases to specific organisms. Each of the stages in the genesis of epidemiology is discussed in turn below.

The Environment as a Factor in Disease Causation

The following account of a deadly disease by Thucydides records, in detail, the ravages produced by the disease[23]; such graphic descriptions of major epidemics in history indicate this early author's concern with the causality of these remarkable phenomena:

> Many who were in perfect health, all in a moment, and without apparent reason, were seized with violent heats in the head and with redness and inflammation of the eyes. Internally the throat and the tongue were quickly suffused with blood, and the breath became unnatural and fetid. There followed sneezing and

a hoarseness; in a short time the disorder, accompanied by a violent cough, reached the chest; then fastening lower down, it would move the stomach and bring on all the vomits of bile to which physicians have ever given names; and they were very distressing. An ineffectual retching producing violent convulsions attacked most of the sufferers; some as soon as the previous symptoms had abated, others not until long afterwards. The body externally was not so very hot to the touch, nor yet pale; it was of a livid color inclining to red, and breaking out in pustules and ulcers. But the internal fever was intense; the sufferers could not bear to have on them even the finest linen garment; they insisted on being naked, and there was nothing which they longed for more eagerly than to throw themselves into cold water. . . . While the disease was at its height, the body, instead of wasting away, held out amid these sufferings in a marvelous manner, and either they died on the seventh or ninth day, not of weakness, for their strength was not exhausted, but of internal fever, which was the end of most; or, if they survived, then the disease descended into the bowels and there produced violent ulceration; severe diarrhea at the same time set in, and at a later stage caused exhaustion, which finally with a few exceptions carried them off.[23(p21)]

Hippocrates, in *On Airs, Waters, and Places*,[24] gave birth in about 400 BC to the idea that disease might be associated with the physical environment; his thinking represented a movement away from supernatural explanations of disease causation to a rational account of the origin of humankind's illnesses. Note in the following passage his reference to climate and physical environment:

Whoever wishes to investigate medicine properly should proceed thus: in the first place to consider the seasons of the year, and what effects each of them produces (for they are not at all alike, but differ much from themselves in regard to their changes). Then the winds, the hot and the cold, especially such as are common to all countries, and then such as are peculiar to each locality. We must also consider the qualities of the waters, for as they differ from one another in taste and weight, so also do they differ much in their qualities. In the same manner, when one comes into a city to which he is a stranger, he ought to consider its situation, how it lies as to the winds and the rising of the sun; for its influence is not the same whether it lies to the north or the south, to the rising or to the setting sun. These things one ought to consider most attentively, and concerning the waters which the inhabitants use, whether they be marshy and soft, or hard, and running from elevated and rocky situations, and then if saltish and unfit for cooking; and the ground, whether it be naked and deficient in water, or wooded and well watered, and whether it lies in a hollow, confined situation, or is elevated and cold; and the mode in which the inhabitants live, and what are their pursuits, whether they are fond of drinking and eating to excess, and given to indolence, or are fond of exercise and labor, and not given to excess in eating and drinking.[24(pp156-157)]

Use of Mortality Counts

John Graunt, in 1662, published *Natural and Political Observations Made upon the Bills of Mortality.*[25] This work recorded descriptive characteristics of birth and death data, including seasonal variations, infant mortality, and excess male over female differences in mortality. Graunt's work made a fundamental contribution by discovering regularities in medical and social phenomena. He is said to be the first to employ quantitative methods in describing population vital statistics by organizing mortality data in a mortality table and has been referred to as the Columbus of statistics. Graunt's procedures allowed the discovery of trends in births and deaths due to specific causes. Although his conclusions were sometimes erroneous, his development of statistical methods was highly important.[26]

Concerning sex differences in death rates, Graunt wrote:

> *Of the difference between the numbers of Males and Females.* The next Observation is, That there be more *Males than Females.* . . . There have been Buried from the year 1628, to the year 1662, *exclusive,* 209436 *Males,* and but 190474 *Females:* but it will be objected, That in *London* it may be indeed so, though otherwise elsewhere; because *London* is the great Stage and Shop of business, wherein the *Masculine Sex* bears the greatest part. But we Answer, That there have been also *Christened* within the same time 139782 *Males,* and but 130866 *Females,* and that the Country-Accounts are consonant enough to those of *London* upon this matter.[25(p44)]

Figure 1-3 shows the 10 leading causes of mortality from the Yearly Mortality Bill for 1632.

Use of Natural Experiments

Snow investigated a cholera epidemic that occurred during the mid-19th century in Broad Street, Golden Square, London. Snow's work, a classic study that linked the cholera epidemic to contaminated water supplies, is noteworthy because it utilized many of the features of epidemiologic inquiry: a spot map of cases and tabulation of fatal attacks and deaths. Through the application of his keen powers of observation and inference, he developed the hypothesis that contaminated water might be associated with outbreaks of cholera. He made several observations that others had not previously made. One observation was that cholera was associated with water from one of two water supplies that served the Golden Square district of London.[27] Broad Street was served by two separate water companies, the Lambeth Company and the Southwark and Vauxhall Company. Lilienfeld and Lilienfeld[28] wrote:

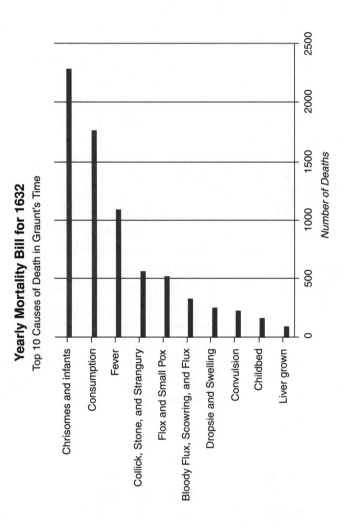

FIGURE 1-3 Leading causes of death in Graunt's time. Data from *Natural and Political Observations, Mentioned in a Following Index, and Made Upon the Bills of Mortality* by J Graunt, p. 8, Second Edition, London: Tho. Roycroft, 1662.

In London, several water companies were responsible for supplying water to different parts of the city. In 1849, Snow noted that the cholera rates were particularly high in those areas of London that were supplied by the Lambeth Company and the Southwark and Vauxhall Company, both of whom obtained their water from the Thames River at a point heavily polluted with sewage.[28(p36)]

Snow's account of the outbreak of 1849 is found in Exhibit 1-2.

Between 1849 and 1854 the Lambeth Company had its source of water relocated to a less contaminated part of the Thames. In 1854, another epidemic of cholera occurred. This epidemic was in an area that consisted of two-thirds of London's resident population south of the Thames and was being served by both companies. In this area, the two companies had their water mains laid out in an interpenetrating manner, so that houses on the same street were receiving their water from different sources.[28]

This was a naturally occurring situation, a "natural experiment," if you will, because in 1849 all residents received contaminated water from the two water companies. After 1849, the Lambeth Company used less contaminated water by relocating its water supply. Snow demonstrated that a disproportionate number of residents who contracted cholera in the 1854 outbreak used water from one water company, which received polluted water, in comparison with the other company, which used relatively unpolluted water.

Snow's methodology maintains contemporary relevance. His methods utilized logical organization of observations, a natural experiment, and a quantitative approach.[28] All these methods are hallmarks of present-day epidemiologic inquiry. Note that it is possible to visit the site of the pump that figured so prominently in Snow's investigation of cholera; a London public house on the original site of the pump has been named in Snow's honor. A replica of the pump is located nearby. Refer to Exhibit 1-3 for pictures and a reproduction of the text on the base of the replica.

Another epidemiologic study, occurring during the mid-19th century, also used sophisticated epidemiologic methods. Ignaz Semmelweis,[29] in his position as a clinical assistant in obstetrics and gynecology at a Vienna hospital, observed that women in the maternity wards were dying at high rates from puerperal fever. In 1840, when the medical education system changed, he found a much higher mortality rate among the women on the teaching wards for medical students and physicians than on the teaching wards for midwives. He postulated that medical students and physicians had contaminated their hands during autopsies. As a result, they transmitted infections while attending women in the maternity wards.[30] When the practice of handwashing with chlorinated solutions was

EXHIBIT 1-2

Snow on Cholera

The most terrible outbreak of cholera which ever occurred in this kingdom, is probably that which took place in Broad Street, Golden Square, and the adjoining streets, a few weeks ago. Within two hundred and fifty yards of the spot where Cambridge Street joins Broad Street, there were upwards of five hundred fatal attacks of cholera in ten days. The mortality in this limited area probably equals any that was ever caused in this country, even by the plague; and it was much more sudden, as the greater number of cases terminated in a few hours. The mortality would undoubtedly have been much greater had it not been for the flight of the population. Persons in furnished lodgings left first, then other lodgers went away, leaving their furniture to be sent for when they could meet with a place to put it in. Many houses were closed altogether, owing to the death of the proprietors; and, in a great number of instances, the tradesmen who remained had sent away their families: so that in less than six days from the commencement of the outbreak, the most afflicted streets were deserted by more than three-quarters of their inhabitants.

There were a few cases of cholera in the neighbourhood of Broad Street, Golden Square, in the latter part of August; and the so-called outbreak, which commenced in the night between the 31st August and the 1st September, was, as in all similar instances, only a violent increase of the malady. As soon as I became acquainted with the situation and extent of this irruption of cholera, I suspected some contamination of the water of the much-frequented street-pump in Broad Street, near the end of Cambridge Street; but on examining the water, on the evening of the 3rd September, I found so little impurity in it of an organic nature, that I hesitated to come to a conclusion. Further inquiry, however, showed me that there was no other circumstance or agent common to the circumscribed locality in which this sudden increase of cholera occurred, and not extending beyond it, except the water of the above mentioned pump. I found, moreover, that the water varied, during the next two days, in the amount of organic impurity, visible to the naked eye, on close inspection, in the form of small white, flocculent particles; and I concluded that, at the commencement of the outbreak, it might possibly have been still more impure.

continues

EXHIBIT 1-2 *continued*

The deaths which occurred during this fatal outbreak of cholera are indicated in the accompanying map [Figure 1-4], as far as I could ascertain them. . . . The dotted line on the map surrounds the sub-districts of Golden Square, St. James's, and Berwick Street, St. James's, together with the adjoining portion of the sub-district of St. Anne, Soho, extending from Wardour Street to Dean Street, and a small part of the sub-district of St. James's Square enclosed by Marylebone Street, Titchfield Street, Great Windmill Street, and Brewer Street. All the deaths from cholera which were registered in the six weeks from 19th August to 30th September within this locality, as well as those of persons removed into Middlesex Hospital, are shown in the map by a black line in the situation of the house in which it occurred, or in which the fatal attack was contracted. . . . The pump in Broad Street is indicated on the map, as well as all the surrounding pumps to which the public had access at the time. It requires to be stated that the water of the pump in Marlborough Street, at the end of Carnaby Street, was so impure that many people avoided using it. And I found that the persons who died near this pump in the beginning of September, had water from the Broad Street pump. With regard to the pump in Rupert Street, it will be noticed that some streets which are near to it on the map, are in fact a good way removed, on account of the circuitous road to it. These circumstances being taken into account, it will be observed that the deaths either very much diminished, or ceased altogether at every point where it becomes decidedly nearer to send to another pump than to the one in Broad Street. It may also be noticed that the deaths are most numerous near to the pump where the water could be more readily obtained. . . . The greatest number of attacks in any one day occurred on the 1st of September, immediately after the outbreak commenced. The following day the attacks fell from one hundred and forty-three to one hundred and sixteen, and the day afterwards to fifty-four. . . . The fresh attacks continued to become less numerous every day. On September the 8th—the day when the handle of the pump was removed—there were twelve attacks; on the 9th, eleven; on the 10th, five; on the 11th, five; on the 12th, only one; and after this time, there were never more than four attacks on one day. During the decline of the epidemic the deaths were more numerous than the attacks, owing to the decrease of many persons who had lingered for several days in consecutive fever [Figure 1-5]. ■

Source: Reprinted from *Snow on Cholera* by J Snow, pp 38–51, Harvard University Press © 1965.

FIGURE 1-4 Cholera deaths in neighborhood of Broad Street, August 19th to September 30, 1849. *Source:* Reprinted from *Snow on Cholera* by J Snow, Map 1, Harvard University Press, © 1965.

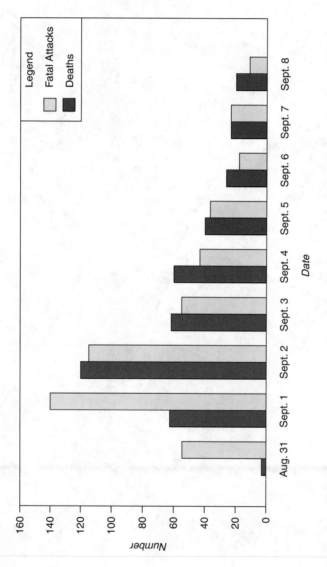

FIGURE 1-5   The 1849 cholera outbreak in Golden Square district, London. Fatal attacks and deaths, August 31–September 8. *Source:* Data from *Snow on Cholera*, by J Snow, p 49, Harvard Universtiy Press, © 1965.

introduced, the death rate for puerperal fever in the wards for medical students and physicians dropped to a rate equal to that in the wards for midwives.

William Farr

A contemporary of John Snow, William Farr in 1839 assumed the post of "Compiler of Abstracts" at the General Register Office, located in England. Farr held this position for 40 years. Some of Farr's contributions to public health and epidemiology included the development of a more sophisticated system for codifying medical conditions than was previously in use. Farr's classification scheme, which departed from a narrow medical view, provided the foundation for the International Statistical Classification of Diseases (ICD) in use today. Also noteworthy is the fact that Farr used data such as census data to study occupational mortality in England. In addition, he explored the possible linkage between mortality rates and population density, showing that both the average number of deaths and births per 1,000 living persons increased with population density (defined as number of persons per square mile). Because of the excess of births over deaths in all except the most crowded areas, the population tended to increase in the less crowded areas. With respect to deaths in high mortality districts, such as Liverpool, which had a mortality rate more than 22 per 1,000 greater than that experienced in healthier districts, he attributed mortality to factors such as ". . . impurities of water, pernicious dirts, floating dusts, zynotic contagions, [and] crowdings in lodgings, . . ."[31(p90)]. The healthier districts had ". . . a salubrious soil, and supply the inhabitants with water generally free from organic impurities."[31(pp90-91)].

Identification of Specific Agents of Disease

In the late 1800s, Koch espoused the concept that diseases are caused by specific living organisms. His epoch-making study, *Die Aetiologie der Tuberkulose,* was published in 1882. This breakthrough made possible greater refinement of the classification of disease by specific causal organisms.[32] Previously, the grouping together of diseases according to grosser classifications had hampered their epidemiologic study.

King[33] noted that Koch's postulates are usually formatted as follows:

1. The microorganism must be observed in every case of the disease.
2. It must be isolated and grown in pure culture.
3. The pure culture must, when inoculated into a susceptible animal, reproduce the disease.
4. The microorganism must be observed in, and recovered from, the experimentally diseased animal.[33]

EXHIBIT 1-3

A Visit to the Broad Street Pump and the Sir John Snow Public House, Located at 39 Broadwick Street, London, England W1F9QJ

FIGURE 1-7: Picture of John Snow.

Figure 1-7 shows John Snow. Figure 1-8 displays a replica of the Broad Street pump, and Figure 1-9 presents a picture of the John Snow Pub. Broad Street has been renamed Broadview Street. The following section is reprinted from a plaque at the base of the replica. The plaque describes "The Soho Cholera Epidemic":

"Dr. John Snow (1813-1858), a noted anaesthesiologist, lived near the focus of the 1854 Soho cholera epidemic, which centered on Broad Street, as Broadwick Street was then called. In September of that year alone, over 500 people died in Soho from the disease. Snow had studied cholera in the 1848-9 epidemic in Southwark and Wandsworth. His theory that polluted drinking water was the [source] of transmission of the disease [was] confirmed when he mapped cholera deaths in Soho with the source of the victims' drinking water. He found that they were concentrated on the Broad Street public water pump. His theory initially met with some disbelief but

continues

EXHIBIT 1-3 *continued*

such was his conviction that he had the pump handle removed to prevent its further use. Soon afterwards the outbreak ended. The original pump is believed to have been situated outside the nearby 'Sir John Snow Public House.'"

FIGURE 1-8: A replica of the Broad Street Pump near its approximate original location. *Source*: Robert Friis.

FIGURE 1-9: The John Snow Pub named in honor of the British Anesthesiologist. *Source:* Robert Friis.

King noted, "What Koch accomplished, in brief, was to demonstrate for the first time in any human disease a strict relation between a micro-organism and a disease."[33(p351)] This specification of the causal disease organism provided a definite criterion for the identification of a disease, rather than the vague standards Koch's predecessors and contemporaries had employed.

Increasing awareness of the role of microbial agents in the causation of human illness, the germ theory of disease, eventually reached the public health community. One method to limit the spread of infectious disease was through the use of cartoons published in the popular media. Figure 1-6 suggested that skirts that trail on the ground (in fashion around the turn of the 20th century) could bring deadly germs into the household.[34]

Other Significant Historical Developments

We mention as other developments the work of Alexander Langmuir, Wade Hampton Frost, and Joseph Goldberger. Langmuir, regarded as the father of infectious disease epidemiology, established in 1949 the epidemiology section of the federal agency presently called the Centers for Disease Control and Prevention. This section later came to be known as the Epidemiologic Intelligence Service (EIS), which celebrated its 50th anniversary in 2001 and is discussed later in this chapter. Frost, who held the first professorship of epidemiology in the United States beginning in 1930 at Johns Hopkins University, advocated the use of quantitative methods to illuminate public health problems, although his concept of epidemiology tended to be restricted narrowly to the study of infectious diseases. (Frost's seminal work on cohort analysis is covered in Chapter 7.) Finally, Goldberger's discovery of the cure for pellagra, a nutritional deficiency disease characterized by the so-called three Ds (dermatitis, diarrhea, and dementia), led to reductions in the occurrence of the disease, which had gained attention in the early 1900s.

Recent Applications of Epidemiology

Epidemiologic activity has exploded during the past several decades.[35] For example, the ongoing Framingham Heart Study, begun in 1949, is one of the pioneering research investigations of risk factors for coronary heart disease.[36] Another development, occurring after World War II, was research on the association between smoking and lung cancer.[37] An example is the work of Doll and Peto,[38] based on a fascinating study of British physicians. The computer and powerful

FIGURE 1-6   Samuel D. Erhart, "The Trailing Skirt: Death Loves A Shining Mark," *Puck,* August 8, 1900 (original in color). *Source:* Reprinted with permission from B Hansen, The Image and Advocacy of Public Health in American Caricature and Cartoons from 1860 to 1900, *American Journal of Public Health,* Vol 87, No 11, p 1805, © 1997, American Public Health Association.

statistical software have aided the proliferation of epidemiologic research studies. Popular interest in epidemiologic findings is also intense. Almost every day now, one encounters media reports of epidemiologic research into such diverse health concerns as acquired immune deficiency syndrome (AIDS), chemical spills, breast cancer screening, and the health effects of second-hand cigarette smoke. Table 1-2 reports triumphs in epidemiology; these are examples in which epidemiologists have identified risk factors for cancer, heart disease, infectious diseases, and many other conditions. While many of the terms used in the table have not yet been discussed in this book, later sections of the text will cover some of them. Additional examples of applications of epidemiology are provided below.

Infectious Diseases in the Community

Infectious disease epidemiology, one of the most familiar types of epidemiology, investigates the occurrence of epidemics of infectious and communicable diseases. Examples are studying diseases caused by bacteria, viruses, and microbiologic agents; tracking down the cause of food-borne illness; and investigating new diseases, such as SARS, that apparently have an infectious origin. An illustration is the use of epidemiologic methods to attempt to eradicate, when possible, polio, measles, smallpox, and other communicable diseases. Another example is outbreaks of infectious diseases in hospitals (nosocomial infections). More information about this topic is presented in Chapter 12. The role of the Epidemiologic Intelligence Service in investigating disease outbreaks is defined as follows:

> The Epidemiologic Intelligence Service (EIS) is a corps of disease detectives who work for the Centers for Disease Control (CDC) in Atlanta, Georgia. The EIS consists of approximately 65 physicians, nurses, and other public health experts who are on call 24 hours a day for two years. Up to 3,000 disease outbreaks occur each year in the United States. EIS officers may be responsible for tracking down unusual disease outbreaks in the U.S., as well as in foreign countries. For example, an outbreak of cholera in Guinea-Bissau, Africa, was linked to the body of a dockworker, smuggled home for burial. About half of the participants at a funeral feast for the deceased later developed cholera. Other investigative work has included: measles outbreaks, hepatitis in a day care center, tuberculosis in New York City, and Lyme disease in Connecticut. The CDC monitors a wide range of health conditions that include influenza epidemics, chronic diseases, such as heart disease, and AIDS.[39]

Health and the Environment

Occupational exposure, air pollution, contaminated drinking water, accidental injuries, and other environmental agents may affect human health. Occupational

Table 1-2 Triumphs in Epidemiology

Risk Factor Categories	Disease	Risk Factors	Direction
Alcohol	esophageal cancer	alcohol (interaction with smoking)	IR
Viruses	liver cancer	hepatitis B virus	IR
	Burkitt's lymphoma	Epstein Barr virus	IR
	Kaposi's sarcoma	Herpes simplex virus type B	IR
	cervical cancer	something transmitted sexually (human papilloma virus)	IR
	nasopharyngeal carcinoma	Epstein Barr virus	IR
	yellow fever	"something transmitted by mosquitos" (Flavivirus)	IR
	new variant (nv) Creutzfeldt-Jacob Disease	prions (interaction with genotype)	IR
Bacteria	cholera	"something in water" (*Vibrio cholera*)	IR
	peptic ulcer	*Helicobactor pylori*	IR
	puerperal fever	"something on doctor's hands" (group B *Streptococcus*)	IR
Nutrition	pellagra	"something in bread" (niacin)	P
	neural tube defects	folic acid, folate	P
	oral clefts	folic acid	P
Occupation	lung cancer	asbestos (interaction with smoking)	IR
	bladder cancer	aniline dye	IR
	mesothelioma	asbestos	IR
	lung cancer	asbestos (interaction with smoking)	IR
	angiosarcoma	vinyl chloride	IR
	infertility (male)	DBCP	IR
	nasal cancer	nickel smelting	IR
	lung cancer	"something in uranium mines" (interaction with smoking)	IR
Environment	dental caries	fluoride	P
	cancer	arsenic	IR
Drugs/ Devices	myocardial infarction	aspirin	P
	micoagthnia	iso-retinene during pregnancy	IR
	pelvic inflammatory disease	Dalkon Shield IUD	IR
	septic abortion	Dalkon Shield IUD	IR
Hormones	clear cell adenocarcinoma of the vagina	diethylstilbestrol prenatally	IR
	venous thromboembolism	combined estrogen/progestin (oral contraceptives)	IR
	venous thromboembolism	post-menopausal estrogen	IR
	ovarian cancer	oral contraceptives	P
	endometrial cancer	combined estrogen/progestin	P
	endometrial cancer	oral contraceptives— post-menopausal estrogen	IR
	iron deficiency anemia	oral contraceptives	P
	benign breast disease	oral contraceptives	P
	myocardial infarction	oral contraceptives (interaction with smoking)	IR
	ischemic stroke	oral contraceptives (interaction with hypertension; modified by dose)	IR

continues

Table 1-2 *continued*

Risk Factor Categories	Disease	Risk Factors	Direction
Genetics	breast cancer	"something genetic" (BRCA1, BRCA2 mutations)	IR
	ovarian cancer	"something genetic" (BRCA2 mutations)	IR
	colon cancer	"something genetic" (APC1 mutations)	IR
Miscellaneous	toxic shock syndrome	super absorbent tampons	IR
	SIDS	prone sleep position	IR
	Reyes syndrome	aspirin (interaction with infection)	IR
Smoking	lung cancer	smoking	IR
	coronary disease	smoking	IR
	hemorrhagic stroke	smoking	IR
	ischemic stroke	smoking	IR
	abdominal aortic aneurism	smoking	IR
	peripheral vascular disease	smoking	IR
	Parkinson's disease	smoking	P
	ulcerative colitis	smoking	P
	laryngeal cancer	smoking	IR
	intrauterine growth retardation	smoking during pregnancy	IR
	toxemia/pre-eclampsia	smoking during pregnancy	P

Abbreviations: IR, increased risk; P, protective. (See Chapters 3, 6, and 7.)

Source: Compiled by Diane Petitti. Adapted with permission from *The Epidemiology Monitor*, October 2001, p 6.

and environmental epidemiology address the occurrence and distribution of conditions, such as dust diseases, occupational dermatoses, or diseases linked to harmful physical energy, such as ionizing radiation from X-ray machines or other sources. Many of the diseases studied by environmental epidemiologists have agent factors and manifestations similar to those in occupational epidemiology, for example, the role of pesticides in causing environmentally associated illness. Injury control epidemiology studies risk factors associated with motor vehicle accidents, bicycle injuries, trauma, and evaluation of seat belt use. Study results may suggest preventive measures by modifying the environment. Reproductive and perinatal epidemiology investigates environmental and occupational exposures and reproduction. Related health outcomes are sudden infant death syndrome, epidemiology of neonatal brain hemorrhage, early pregnancy, and methodologic issues in drug epidemiology. Chapter 13 covers environmental and occupational epidemiology.

Chronic Disease, Lifestyle, and Health Promotion

An example of such a topic is the role of exercise, diet, smoking, and alcohol consumption in physical health outcomes, such as coronary heart disease, arthritis, diabetes, and cancer. Hypothesized risk factors studied include the antecedent variables within the person's psychosocial environment that may be associated with health and disease. To illustrate, there have been studies of stress as a risk factor for hypertension, ulcers, colitis, heart disease, and cancer. A related area involves epidemiologic studies of personality factors and disease, exemplified by the type A personality and its potential link to heart disease. More information about this topic is presented in Chapters 4 and 15.

Psychologic and Social Factors in Health

Stress, social support, and socioeconomic status may affect mental health and physical illnesses, such as arthritis, peptic ulcer, and essential hypertension. Psychiatric epidemiology is concerned with the distribution and determinants of mental illness. Examples are the definition and measurement of mental illness, social factors and mental illness, and urban and rural differences in frequency of mental illness. Major research studies have investigated the epidemiology of depressive symptomatology. Also studied are factors that affect the distribution of mental retardation, including certain genetic syndromes. Social, cultural, and demographic factors (socioeconomic status, gender, employment, marital status, and race) are considered correlates of mental health status. Chapter 15 considers this area in more detail.

Molecular and Genetic Epidemiology

Genetic epidemiology studies the distribution of genetically associated diseases among the population. For example, research on the genetic bases for disease hypothesized possible inherited susceptibility to severe alcoholism[40] and to breast and ovarian cancer.[41] Molecular epidemiology applies the techniques of molecular biology to epidemiologic studies. An illustration is the use of genetic and molecular markers, including deoxyribonucleic acid (DNA) typing, to examine their influence upon behavioral outcomes and host susceptibility to disease. An overview of molecular and genetic epidemiology is provided in Chapter 14.

Conclusion

Epidemiology is the study of the distribution and determinants of diseases, states of health, disability, morbidity, and mortality in the population. Epidemiology, which examines disease occurrence in the population rather than in the individual, is sometimes called population medicine. Several examples demonstrated that the etiologic bases of disease and health conditions in the population are often unknown. Epidemiology is used as a tool to suggest factors associated with occurrence of disease.

Three aspects characterize the epidemiologic approach. The first is quantification (e.g., counting of cases of disease and construction of tables that show variation of disease by time, place, and person). The second is use of special vocabulary (e.g., epidemic and epidemic frequency of disease). The third is an interdisciplinary composition (drawing from microbiology, biostatistics, social and behavioral sciences, and clinical medicine).

The historical antecedents of epidemiology began with Hippocrates, who implicated the environment as a factor in disease causation. Second, Graunt, one of the biostatistics pioneers, compiled vital statistics in the mid-1600s. Third, Snow used natural experiments to track a cholera outbreak in Golden Square, London. Finally, Koch's postulates advanced the theory of specific disease agents. At present, epidemiology is relevant to many kinds of health problems found in the community.

Study Questions and Exercises

1. Using your own words, give a definition of epidemiology. Before reading Chapter 1, what were your impressions regarding the scope of epidemiology? Based on the material presented in this chapter, what topics does epidemiology cover? That is, to what extent does epidemiology focus exclusively upon the study of infectious diseases or upon other types of diseases and conditions?

2. How would the clinical and epidemiologic descriptions of a disease differ, and how would they be similar?

3. To what extent does epidemiology rely on medical disciplines for its content, and to what extent does it draw upon other disciplines? Explain the statement that epidemiology is interdisciplinary.

4. Describe the significance for epidemiology of the following historical developments:

a. associating the environment with disease causality
b. use of vital statistics
c. use of natural experiments
d. identification of specific agents of disease
5. Explain what is meant by the following components of the definition of epidemiology:
a. determinants
b. distribution
c. morbidity and mortality
6. The following questions pertain to the term epidemic.
a. What is meant by an epidemic? Give a definition in your own words.
b. Describe a scenario in which only one or two cases of disease may represent an epidemic.
c. What is the purpose of surveillance?
d. Give an example of a disease that has cyclic patterns.
e. What is the epidemic threshold for a disease? In what sense is the epidemic threshold a statistical concept?
7. Epidemiologic research and findings often receive dramatic media coverage. Find an article in a media source (e.g., *The New York Times*) on a topic related to epidemiology. In a one-page essay, summarize the findings and discuss how the article illustrates the approach of epidemiology to the study of diseases (health conditions) in populations.
8. What is the definition of a natural experiment? Can you identify any recent examples of natural experiments? To what extent might changes in legislation to limit smoking in public places or to increase the speed limit on highways be considered natural experiments?
9. Review Exhibit 1-2, Snow on Cholera. What do you believe was the purpose of each of the following observations by Snow?
a. "small white flocculent particles" in the water from the Broad Street pump
b. the location of cholera deaths as shown in Figure 1-4
c. people who died avoided the pump in Marlborogh Street and instead had the water from the Broad Street pump
d. "the greatest number of attacks in any one day occurred on the 1st of September, . . ."
e. "On September 8th—the day when the handle of the pump was removed . . . " To what extent do you think removing the pump handle was effective in stopping the disease outbreak?

10. How does quantification support the accomplishment of the four aims of epidemiology?

11. How did Koch's postulates contribute to the advancement of epidemiology? To what extent is identification of specific agent factors a prerequisite for tracking down the causes of disease outbreaks?

References

1. Newton J, Maugh TH II. Water officials suggest prudence, not panic. *Los Angeles Times*. February 11, 1998, p 1.

2. Swan SH, Waller K, Hopkins B, et al. A prospective study of spontaneous abortion: Relation to amount and source of drinking water consumed in early pregnancy. *Epidemiology*. 1998;2:126–133.

3. Waller K, Swan SH, DeLorenze G, Hopkins B. Trihalomethanes in drinking water and spontaneous abortion. *Epidemiology*. 1998;9:134–140.

4. Hughes JM, Gerberding JL. Anthrax bioterrorism: Lessons learned and future directions. *Emerg Infect Dis* [serial online]. 2002;8(10):1–4. Available at: *http://www.cdc.gov/ncidod/EID/vo18no10/02–0466.htm*. Accessed October 22, 2002.

5. Karin M. Anthrax invades and evades the immune system to cause widespread infection. *Environmental Health News, Highlights in Environmental Health Sciences Research, 2002 Highlights*. Division of Extramural Research and Training, National Institute of Environmental Health Sciences. 200:1–2. Available at *http://www.niehs.nih.gov/dert/profiles/hilites/2002/anthrax.htm*. Accessed September 25, 2002.

6. Centers for Disease Control and Prevention. Update: Investigation of bioterrorism-related anthrax and interim guidelines for clinical evaluation of persons with possible anthrax. *MMWR Morb Mortal Weekly Rep*. 2001;50:941–948.

7. Maillard J-M, Fischer M, McKee KT Jr, Turner LF, Cline JS. First case of bioterrorism-related inhalational anthrax, Florida, 2001: North Carolina investigation. *Emerg Infect Dis* [serial online]. 2002;8(10). Available at *http://www.cdc.gov/ncidod/EID/vol8no10/02-0389.htm*. Accessed January 29, 2003.

8. Centers for Disease Control and Prevention. Ongoing investigation of anthrax—Florida, October 2001. *MMWR Morb Mortal Weekly Rep*. 2001;50:877.

9. Centers for Disease Control and Prevention Update: investigation of bioterrorism-related anthrax—Connecticut, 2001. *MMWR Morb Mortal Weekly Rep*. 2001;50:1077–1079.

10. Mathews T, Lee ED. Outbreak of fear. *Newsweek*. 1995; May 22:48, 50.

11. Fear on Seventh Ave. *Newsweek*. 1978; September 18:30.

12. Centers for Disease Control and Prevention. Red spots on airline flight attendants. *MMWR Morb Mortal Weekly Rep*. 1980;29:141.

13. Friis RH, Nanjundappa G, Prendergast T, Welsh M. Hispanic coronary heart disease mortality and risk in Orange County, California. *Public Health Rep*. 1981;96:418–422.

14. Lilienfeld DE. Definitions of epidemiology. *Am J Epidemiol*. 1978;107:87–90.

15. Mausner JS, Kramer S. *Epidemiology: An Introductory Text*. 2nd ed. Philadelphia: Saunders; 1985.

16. Terris M. The epidemiologic tradition. *Public Health Rep*. 1979;94:203–209.

17. Syme SL. Behavioral factors associated with the etiology of physical disease: a social epidemiological approach. *Am J Public Health.* 1974;64:1043–1045.
18. Centers for Disease Control and Prevention. Update: Outbreak of severe acute respiratory syndrome—worldwide, 2003. *MMWR Morb Mortal Weekly Rep.* 2003;52:244
19. Fingerhut LA, Warner M. *Injury Chartbook. Health, United States, 1996–97.* Hyattsville, MD: National Center for Health Statistics. 1997.
20. MacMahon B, Pugh TF. *Epidemiology Principles and Methods.* Boston: Little, Brown; 1970.
21. Benenson AS. *Control of Communicable Diseases in Man.* Washington, DC: American Public Health Association; 1990.
22. Snow J. *Snow on Cholera.* Cambridge, MA: Harvard University Press; 1965.
23. Marks G, Beatty WK. *Epidemics.* New York: Scribner's; 1976.
24. Hippocrates. *On Airs, Waters, and Places.* In: Adams F, ed. *The Genuine Works of Hippocrates.* New York: Wood; 1886.
25. Graunt J. *Natural and Political Observations, Mentioned in a Following Index, and Made Upon the Bills of Mortality,* Second Edition. London: Tho. Roycroft, 1662.
26. Kargon R. John Graunt, Francis Bacon, and the Royal Society: the reception of statistics. *J Hist Med.* 1963;October:337–348.
27. Enterline PE. Epidemiology: "nothing more than common sense?" *Occup Health Saf.* 1979;January/February:45–47.
28. Lilienfeld AM, Lilienfeld DE. *Foundations of Epidemiology.* 2nd ed. New York: Oxford University Press; 1980.
29. Semmelweis IP, Murphy FB, trans. *The Etiology, the Concept and Prophylaxis of Childbed Fever* (1861). *Med Classics.* 1941;5:350–773.
30. Iffy L, Kaminetzky HA, Maidman JE, et al. Control of perinatal infection by traditional preventive measures. *Obstet Gynecol.* 1979;54:403–411.
31. Whitehead M. William Farr's legacy to the study of inequalities in health. *Bull World Health Organ.* 2000;78(1):86–96.
32. Susser M. *Causal Thinking in the Health Sciences.* New York: Oxford University Press; 1973.
33. King LS. Dr Koch's postulates. *J Hist Med.* Autumn 1952:350–361.
34. Hansen B. The image and advocacy of public health in American caricature and cartoons from 1860 to 1900. *Am J Public Health.* 1997;87:1798–1807.
35. Rothman KJ. *Modern Epidemiology.* Boston: Little, Brown; 1986.
36. Kannell WB, Abbott RD. Incidence and prognosis of unrecognized myocardial infarction: an update on the Framingham study. *N Engl J Med.* 1984;311: 1144–1147.
37. Monson RR. *Occupational Epidemiology.* Boca Raton, FL: CRC Press; 1990.
38. Doll R, Peto R. Mortality in relation to smoking: 20 years' observation on male British doctors. *Br Med J.* 1976;2:1525–1536.
39. Jaret P. The disease detectives. *National Geogr Mag.* 1991;January:116–140.
40. Blum K, Noble EP, Sheridan PJ, et al. Association of the A1 allele of the D2 dopamine receptor gene with severe alcoholism. *Alcohol.* 1991;8:409–416.
41. Biesecker BB, Boehnke M, Calzone K, et al. Genetic counseling for families with inherited susceptibility to breast cancer and ovarian cancer. *JAMA.* 1993;269:1970–1974.

CHAPTER 2

Practical Applications of Epidemiology

LEARNING OBJECTIVES

By the end of this chapter the reader will be able to:

- discuss uses and applications of epidemiology
- define the influence of population dynamics on community health
- state how epidemiology may be used for operations research
- discuss the clinical applications of epidemiology
- cite causal mechanisms from the epidemiologic perspective

CHAPTER OUTLINE

Introduction

This chapter provides a broad overview of the range of applications of the epidemiologic approach. As the basic method of public health, epidemiology touches many aspects of the health sciences (see Exhibit 2-1 for a statement of seven uses of epidemiology.[1]) Among its applications, epidemiology is used to help define the full clinical picture of a disease. By describing the occurrence of disease in the community, epidemiology helps health services personnel and administrators plan for allocation of resources. Once such services are implemented, the epidemiologic approach can help evaluate their function and utility. The first part of this chapter considers these types of applications.

The second part of the chapter focuses on applications of epidemiology that are relevant to disease etiology. The causes of many diseases remain unknown; epidemiologists in research universities and federal and private agencies continue to search for clues as to the nature of disease. The knowledge that is acquired through such research may be helpful in efforts to prevent the occurrence of disease. Results of these types of epidemiologic studies are often quite newsworthy. A 1990 editorial in the *New England Journal of Medicine* was devoted to the issue of the growing number of epidemiologic studies being reported in the journal.[2] Among the key reasons for the proliferation of these studies were, first, that they concentrate on associations between diseases and possible lifestyle factors, such as a habit, type of behavior, or some element of the diet, that presumably can be changed. Consequently, "The reports are . . . often of great interest to the popular media and the public, as well as to physicians interested in preventive medicine."[2(p823)] A second reason is that the major diseases that are predominant in American society are "chronic, degenerative diseases that probably have several contributing causes, some of which have to do with life style, operating over long periods."[2(p823)] The editorial pointed out:

> It is usually very difficult to investigate such risk factors through experimental (or interventional) studies. In some cases it is impractical and in some it is unethical. For example, researchers cannot expose half of a group of children to lead for 10 years to compare their IQs 20 years later with those of the unexposed children. We must therefore rely on epidemiologic (or observational) studies.[2(p823)]

Because of the increasingly important role that epidemiology plays in clinical decision making, this chapter also touches on some of the important considerations of this application. Finally, a few words of caution are presented on limitations of epidemiology in determining the cause of disease. To permit a fuller understanding of these issues, there is coverage of the general concept of causality.

EXHIBIT 2-1

Seven Uses of Epidemiology

The epidemiological method is the only way of asking some questions in medicine, one way of asking others, and no way at all to ask many. Several *uses of epidemiology* have been described:

1. To study the *history of the health of populations,* and of the rise and fall of diseases and changes in their character. Useful projections into the future may be possible.

2. To *diagnose the health of the community* and the condition of the people, to measure the true dimensions and distribution of ill-health in terms of incidence, prevalence, disability and mortality; to set health problems in perspective and define their relative importance; to identify groups needing special attention. Ways of life change, and with them the community's health; new measurements for monitoring them must therefore constantly be sought.

3. To study the *working of health services* with a view to their improvement. Operational research translates knowledge of (changing) community health and expectations in terms of needs for services and measure [sic] how these are met. The success of services delivered in reaching stated norms, and the effects on community health—and its needs—have to be appraised, in relation to resources. Such knowledge may be applied in action research pioneering better services, and in drawing up plans for the future. Timely information on health and health services is itself a key service requiring much study and experiment. Today, information is required at many levels, from the local district to the international.

4. To estimate from the group experience what are the *individual* risks on average of disease, accident and defect, and the *chances* of avoiding them.

5. To *identify syndromes* by describing the distribution and association of clinical phenomena in the population.

continues

EXHIBIT 2-1 *continued*

6. To *complete the clinical picture* of chronic diseases and describe their *natural history*: by including in due proportion all kinds of patients, wherever they present, together with the undemanding and the symptomless cases who do not present and whose needs may be as great; by following the course of remission and relapse, adjustment and disability in defined populations. Follow-up of cohorts is necessary to detect early sub-clinical and perhaps reversible disease and to discover precursor abnormalities during the pathogenesis which may offer opportunities for prevention.

7. To *search for causes* of health and disease by computing the experience of groups defined by their composition, inheritance and experience, their behaviour and environments. To confirm particular causes of the chronic diseases and the patterns of multiple causes, describing their mode of operation singly and together, and to assess their importance in terms of the relative risks of those exposed. Postulated causes will often be tested in naturally occurring *experiments of opportunity* and sometimes by *planned experiments*. ■

Source: Reprinted from *Uses of Epidemiology*, 3rd ed, by JN Morris, pp 262–263, © 1975, with permission of Elsevier.

Applications for the Assessment of the Health Status of Populations and Delivery of Health Services

As noted by Morris,[1] principal uses of epidemiology under this category include the history of the health of populations, diagnosis of the health of the community, and the working of health services.

The Historical Use of Epidemiology—Study of Past and Future Trends in Health and Illness

An example of the historical use of epidemiology is the study of changes in disease frequency over time (secular trends). The illnesses that afflict humanity, with certain exceptions, have shown dramatic changes in industrialized nations from the beginning of modern medicine to the present day. In general, chronic conditions have replaced acute infectious diseases as the major causes of morbidity and mortality in contemporary industrialized societies.

Figure 2-1 identifies the top 10 causes of death for two contrasting years: 1900 and 1996. The data show that influenza moved from top position in 1900 to sixth in 1996; diseases of the heart became the leading cause of death, and the overall death rate from all causes declined drastically during this period of about one century.

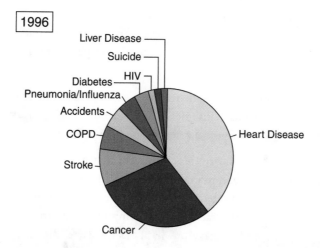

FIGURE 2-1 Leading causes of mortality, 1900 and 1996. *Source:* Data from SJ Ventura, et al, Statistical Abstract of the United States: 1957, p 69, U.S. Bureau of the Census; and Annual Summary of Births, Marriages, Divorces, and Deaths, United States, 1992, Monthly Vital Statistics Report, Vol 41, No 13, pp 20-22, 1993, National Center for Health Statistics.

The leading causes of death over decades of time have shown marked changes (Fig. 2-2). In determining the reasons for these trends, one must take into account certain conditions that may affect the reliability of observed changes. According to MacMahon and Pugh, these are "variation in diagnosis, reporting, case fatality, or some other circumstance other than a true change of incidence."[3(p159)] Specific examples are as follows:

- *Lack of comparability over time due to altered diagnostic criteria.* The diagnostic criteria used in a later time period reflect new knowledge about disease; some categories of disease used in earlier eras may be omitted altogether. The diagnostic criteria may be more precise at a later time; for instance, considerable information has been obtained over three-quarters of a century about the chronic diseases. In some cases, when changes in diagnostic procedures are due to known alterations in diagnostic coding systems, the changes will be abrupt and readily identifiable.
- *Aging of the general population.* As the population ages as a result of reduced impact of infectious diseases, improved medical care, and a decline in the death rate, there may be greater uncertainty about the precise cause of death. Also, there may be inaccurate assignment of the underlying cause of death when older individuals are affected by chronic disease because multiple organ systems may fail simultaneously.
- *Changes in the fatal course of the condition.* Such changes would be reflected over the long run in decreases in the number of people with disease who actually die of it.

Despite the factors that reduce the reliability of observed changes in morbidity and mortality, four trends in disorders may be identified[4]: disappearing, residual, persisting, and new epidemic disorders. These are defined as follows:

- Disappearing disorders are those disorders that were formerly common sources of morbidity and mortality in developed countries but that at present have nearly disappeared in their epidemic form. Under this category are smallpox (currently eradicated), poliomyelitis, and other diseases that have been brought under control by means of immunizations, improvement in sanitary conditions, and the use of antibiotics.
- Residual disorders are diseases for which the key contributing factors are largely known but specific methods of control have not been effectively implemented. The sexually transmitted diseases, perinatal and infant mortality among the economically disadvantaged, and health problems associated with use of tobacco and alcohol are examples.

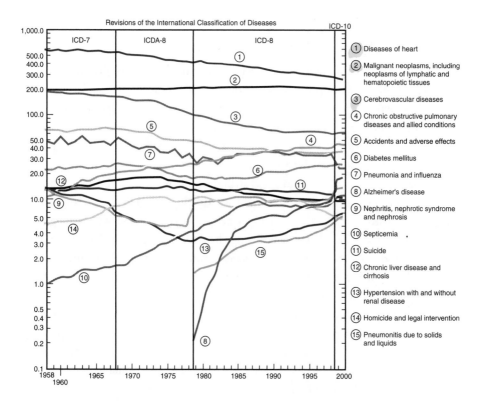

FIGURE 2-2 Age-adjusted death rates for the 15 leading causes of death in the United States from 1960 to 2000. *Source:* Miniño AM, Arias E, Kochanek KD, Murphy SL, Smith BL. Deaths: Final data for 2000. *National Vital Statistics Reports* (vol 50 no 15). Hyattsville, MD: National Center for Health Statistics; 2002.

- Persisting disorders are diseases that remain common because an effective method of prevention or cure evades discovery. Some forms of cancer and mental disorders are representative of this category.
- New epidemic disorders are diseases that are increasing markedly in frequency in comparison with previous time periods. The reader may surmise that examples of these are lung cancer, and, most recently, acquired immune deficiency syndrome. The emergence of new epidemics of diseases may be a result of the increased life expectancy of the population,

new environmental exposures, or changes in lifestyle, diet, and other practices associated with contemporary life.

Predictions about the Future

The study of population dynamics in relation to sources of morbidity and mortality reveals much about possible future trends in the health of a population. A population pyramid represents the age and sex composition of the population of an area or country at a point in time.[5] By examining the distribution of a population by age and sex, one may view the impact of acute conditions as well as the quality of medical care available to a population.

Figure 2-3 shows the age and sex distribution of the population of a more developed and a less developed region. The less developed region has a triangular population distribution with fewer older people in comparison with younger people. Infections take a heavy toll during the childhood years as a result of a constellation of factors associated with poverty and deprivation: poor nutrition, lack of education and potable water, and unavailability of basic immunizations, antibiotics, and sewage disposal and treatment.

Developed (industrialized) societies manifest a more rectangular distribution of the population. Characteristically, there are more older individuals in comparison with a less developed area, approximately equal numbers of individuals at each age grouping except the very oldest age groups, and more older women than men. Because of reduced mortality due to infectious diseases and improved medical care in comparison with a less developed region, residents of developed countries enjoy greater life expectancy. With continuing advances in medical care, one may predict that there will be an increasingly aging population in developed countries. The U.S. Bureau of the Census estimates that about one-fifth the U.S. population in 2030 will be 65 years of age and older. There will be a need for health services that affect aging and all its associated dimensions. Specifically, to give one illustration, programs in the major chronic diseases, both preventive care in the early years and direct care in the older years, will need to be expanded.

Populations Dynamics and Epidemiology

As the population pyramid portends, population characteristics are related to the pattern of health problems found in the community. Three factors affect the size of populations: births, deaths (see Chapt. 3), and migration.[5] When these factors do not contribute to net increases or decreases in the number of persons, the population is in equilibrium. A fixed population adds no new members and,

FIGURE 2-3 Sex-age structure of the population in less developed and more developed regions, 1970 and 2000. *Source:* Reprinted from *The Population Debate: Dimensions and Perspectives* by the United Nations, p 195, © 1974. The United Nations is the author of the original material.

consequently, decreases in size as a result of deaths only; a dynamic population is one that adds new members through migration and births or loses members through emigration and deaths.[6] A population is in steady state when the number of members exiting equals the number entering. The term *demographic transition* refers to the historical shift from high birth and death rates found in agrarian societies to much lower birth and death rates found in developed countries.[5] Decline in the death rate has been attributed in part to improvement in general hygienic and social conditions. Industrialization and urbanization contribute to a decline in the birth rate. Both industrialization and urbanization have led to environmental contamination, concentration of social and health problems in the urban core areas of the United States, and out-migration of inner city residents to the suburbs.

The Health of the Community

This section describes two applications of epidemiology that pertain to the health of the community. First, we will highlight epidemiology as a descriptive tool and second we will cover the potential role of epidemiology in policy evaluation. Epidemiology is a tool that may be used to describe the overall health of a particular community. The resulting description may then provide a key to the types of problems that require attention and also to the need for specific health services. A complete epidemiologic description would include indices of health as well as indicators of the psychosocial milieu of the community. A representative list of variables that might be covered in a description of the health of the community is given in Exhibit 2-2.

A more thorough review of how the set of variables given in Exhibit 2-2 would affect the health of the community is given in Chapter 4. One example is the relationship between age and sex composition and typical health problems. If the community consists primarily of senior citizens (as in a retirement community), health problems related to aging would tend to predominate. Because of the longer life expectancy of women, an older population would tend to have a majority of elderly women, who might have unique health needs. In contrast, a younger community might be more concerned with immunizations against infectious diseases and sexually transmitted diseases or prevention of accidental death and injury.

Exhibit 2-2 lists socioeconomic status (a variable comprising income level, educational attainment, and type of occupation) as a descriptive variable for the health of the community. The socioeconomic characteristics of the community relate in part to the availability of health and social services and ability to pay for

EXHIBIT 2-2

Descriptive Variables for the Health of the Community

Demographic and social variables:
- Age and sex distribution
- Socioeconomic status
- Family structure, including marital status and number of single-parent families
- Racial, ethnic, and religious composition

Variables related to community infrastructure:
- Availability of social and health services
- Quality of housing stock
- Social stability (residential mobility)

Health-related outcome variables*:
- Homicide and suicide rates
- Infant mortality rate
- Mortality from selected conditions (cause specific)
- Magnitude of chronic and infectious diseases
- Alcoholism and drug abuse rates
- Teenage pregnancy rates
- Birth rate

*Definitions of some of these terms are given in Chapter 3.

health care services (refer to Chapt. 4 for an additional discussion of socioeconomic status). The wealthier communities, because of their greater tax resources, may provide a greater range of social and health-related services, which may be more conveniently located than in less affluent areas. Low-income residents may utilize, as their primary source of medical care, public health services, which may be less up to date and more difficult to reach by public transportation. Socioeconomic status also relates to community environmental aspects, such as the quality of housing stock. Some low socioeconomic status communities tend to be overcrowded and are more likely to have associated unsanitary conditions, which obviously are linked to ill health and transmission of infectious diseases. By definition, low socioeconomic status is associated also with low education levels.

Individuals who have low education levels may be less aware of dietary and exercise habits that promote good health than more highly educated persons. The less affluent urban communities of some parts of the United States also are experiencing an out-migration of the younger residents, leaving a majority of older and indigent individuals. It should be pointed out, however, that some of the newer communities, such as those in the Sunbelt of the southern United States, are characterized also by a high degree of residential mobility and lack of social stability. The constant shifting of residents may contribute to a sense of alienation and lack of social connectedness in the community, which in turn may be associated with an increased incidence of mental health problems.

The racial, ethnic, and religious composition of the community affects the health status of its members because certain health problems may be more common in one racial or ethnic group than in another, for example sickle cell anemia among African Americans or Tay-Sachs disease among persons of Eastern European Jewish extraction. Religious practices also may affect health, a case in point being abstinence from alcohol consumption and tobacco products among the Mormons. Thus the health of the community may be determined to some extent by racial, ethnic, and religious factors.

Measures of disease frequency are a barometer of community health needs. An elevated infant mortality rate may reflect inadequate prenatal care, inadequate maternal diet, or a deficit of relevant social and health services. Alienation within the community may produce increased suicide rates and also elevated rates of alcoholism and substance abuse. A resurgence of infectious diseases, such as measles and tuberculosis, may reflect the failure of immunization and community infectious disease surveillance programs. Increases in the occurrence of pregnancies, births, and sexually transmitted diseases among teenagers may suggest the need for appropriate education and counseling services targeted to this age group. Finally, firearm death rates are an indicator of the health of the community. Figure 2-4 portrays firearm and motor vehicle death rates for the South Atlantic states in the United States during 1990–91. According to data reported for these years, Washington, D.C., led all other areas in firearm mortality, with a death rate of approximately 120 per 100,000 population.

Using epidemiology to describe the health of the community relates to Goal 2, "Eliminate Health Disparities" of *Healthy People 2010*. Goal 2 strives ". . . to eliminate health disparities among segments of the population, including differences that occur by gender, race or ethnicity, education or income, disability, geographic location, or sexual orientation."[7(p5 of 16)] Health disparities have been defined as ". . . differences in the incidence, prevalence, mortality, and burden of diseases

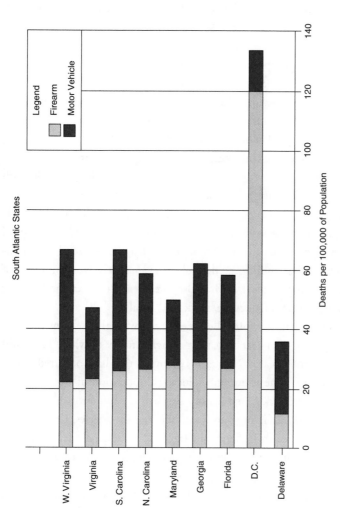

FIGURE 2-4 Firearm and motor vehicle death rates for persons 15–34 years of age, South Atlantic states, United States, 1990–1991. Source: Data from L Fingerhut, C Jones, and D Marduc, Firearm and Motor Vehicle Injury Mortality—Variations by State, Race and Ethnicity, United States, 1990–91, and from National Center for Health Statistics, *Vital and Health Statistics*, No 242, January 1994.

and other adverse health conditions that exist among specific population groups in the United States."[8(p1 of 3)] Six areas are the focus of the U.S. Department of Health and Human Services: infant mortality, cancer screening and management, cardiovascular disease, diabetes, HIV infection/AIDS, and immunizations.

For example, consider infant mortality, which as noted previously is an indicator of the health of the community. While the infant mortality rate in the U.S. has trended downward, it is 24th (based on 1996 data) in comparison to other developed nations. Within the U.S., African-American infants have approximately two times the rate for white infants (14.2 per 1,000 vs. 6.0 per 1,000 in 1996). Similarly, other groups, such as American Indians and Hispanics, have higher infant mortality rates than whites. When epidemiology is used to study the health of the community, this discipline can identify geographic areas that have elevated rates of infant mortality (as well as other adverse health conditions) and assist in identifying risk factors for these elevated rates.

Regarding the health of the community, epidemiology is not only a descriptive tool, but also plays a role in policy evaluation. As Ibrahim has pointed out, "Health planning and policy formulation in the ideal sense should apply to total communities and employ a centralized process, which facilitates an overview of the whole rather than selected health problems."[9(p4)] Samet and Lee wrote: "The findings of epidemiologic research figure prominently in nearly all aspects of developing policies to safeguard the public's health. Epidemiologic evidence receives consideration at the national and even global levels, while also directly and indirectly influencing individual decisions concerning lifestyle, work, and family."[10(pS1)]

Legislators and government officials are charged with the responsibility of enacting laws, enforcing them, and creating policies, many of which have substantial impacts on public health. Numerous examples that have occurred in distant and recent history come to mind, including fluoridation of water, helmet protection for motorcycle riders, mandatory seat belt use in motor vehicles, and requiring automobile manufacturers to install air bags in vehicles. Other examples of laws that impact health are shown in Table 2-1. The remainder of this section will advocate for an increasing role for epidemiologists in informing the policy-making process.

The question arises as to whether such policies merely satisfy public whim, appease well-meaning interest groups or do, in fact, have an established scientific rationale and documented efficacy. The term *evidence-based decisions,* applied to public health policies, implies the enactment of laws that have empirical support for their need as well as for their effectiveness.

Table 2-1 Examples of Laws and Ordinances That Affect Public Health

---

Tobacco control policies
    Smokefree Bars Law (California, U.S.)
    Prohibition of smoking in commercial aircraft
    Prohibition of smoking in airports, U.S., Germany, England, Spain, and other countries
Drug treatment systems for non-prescription drugs, such as cocaine and heroin
Needle distribution programs for prevention of needle sharing among intravenous drug users
Law to regulate amount of particulate matter emitted from automobiles
Removal of high fat and high sugar content foods from vending machines in schools

---

Support for the involvement of epidemiologists in public health policy-making has been advocated strongly.[11] Epidemiologists have an important role to play in the development of evidence-based decisions because of their expertise in studying about risks associated with certain exposures and their familiarity with findings based on human subjects.[12] A clear illustration of epidemiologists' involvement in risk assessment arises in the determination of dose-response relationships in environmental health studies. (This issue will be discussed in more detail in Chapt. 13.)

Further, in their traditional activities, epidemiologists participate in policy-making related to education, research, and publication of manuscripts.[11] Expertise in these areas can be applied readily to other policy arenas. Matanoski pointed out that ". . . epidemiologists can predict future risks based on current trends and knowledge of changing risk factors in the population. Planning for future needs and setting goals to meet these needs will require population-based thinking, for which epidemiologists are well trained."[12(p.541)]

The issue of policy development, which is extremely complex, encompasses several phases known as the policy cycle. These phases include examination of population health, assessment of potential interventions, alternative policy choices, policy implementation, and policy evaluation[13] (see Fig. 2-5 for a diagram of factors that influence policy decision-making). As you can see from Figure 2-5, an epidemiologist might be able to provide input into a number of phases of decision-making, for example those phases that pertain to scientific fact (human health), interpretation of science, cost/benefit analysis, and risk assessment. Refer to the case study (Exhibit 2-3) in which we describe an applied epidemiologic study (conducted by Robert Friis and Julia Lee) to evaluate responses to the Smokefree Bars Law in the U.S. state of California.

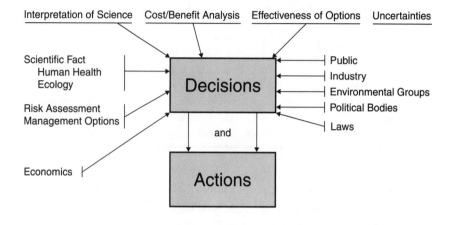

FIGURE 2-5 Factors influencing policy decision-making. *Source*: Reprinted with permission from Matanoski GM. Conflicts between two cultures: Implications for epidemiologic researchers in communicating with policy-makers. Am J Epidemiol. 2001. 154(12 Suppl):S37. Reprinted by permission of Oxford University Press.

EXHIBIT 2-3

Case Study: Using Epidemiologic Methods to Conduct a Policy Evaluation of the Smokefree Bars Law

This research project investigated a community's response to the California Smokefree Bars (SFB) Law, a change in tobacco control policy that was implemented as Assembly Bill (AB) 3037 on January 1, 1998. The SFB Law removed the exemption for bars, taverns, and lounges that had been included in AB 13, the 1995 Workplace Safety Law. AB13/3037 banned smoking in all bars through-out the state (with some exemptions for bars with no employees). For our epidemiologic research, the SFB Law was viewed as a natural experiment, with its form and timing under the control of the California State Legislature.

Tobacco control policy in the form of laws and local ordinances is occurring with increasing frequency as part of the anti-tobacco efforts to reduce the deleterious first- and secondhand health effects of cigarette

continues

EXHIBIT 2-3 *continued*

smoke. Secondhand smoke has documented harmful health consequences (from which customers and workers in alcohol-serving establishments need protection), including cancer, emphysema and other lung disorders, and heart disease. The effects of policies to reduce exposure to second-hand smoke need to be investigated to understand their potential to effect health-related changes in population groups and to suggest recommendations regarding their efficacy.

Our policy analysis of the response to the SFB Law was conducted within Long Beach, which is the fifth-largest city (population, 460,000) in the state of California and the second largest in Los Angeles County, the county in which Long Beach is located. Of particular pertinence is the fact that Long Beach has a distinguished record of local tobacco control. In September of 1994, Long Beach was one of 22 cities in the state that were recognized for protecting the health of its residents through strong tobacco control policies. The Long Beach Smoking Ordinance, enacted in 1991, prohibited smoking in all enclosed work-places and public places. In 1993, the Long Beach City Council strengthened the ordinance by prohibiting smoking in all restaurants and restaurant/bar combinations. Additionally, Long Beach is one of the few cities in the state with its own Health Department, a key factor for the positive community response to both local and statewide tobacco control. Over the years, a very active Tobacco Education Program within the city's Health Department has worked closely with the City to educate the citizens regarding anti-tobacco concerns and also to implement various tobacco control policies.

In order to determine the response to the California SFB Law, we directed our efforts to gathering data from five different perspectives: bar personnel; residents; economic data from the restaurant business; compliance at the bars; and print media. The study was conducted over a four-year period (July 1998-June 2002). Trained interviewers were sent to a sample of alcohol-serving establishments, e.g., restaurant bars and stand-alone bars.

Observations of compliance at Long Beach bars showed a continuing decrease in the proportion of bars with inside ashtrays; no restaurant bars in the sample had ashtrays during Fall 2000 or Spring 2001. Inside

continues

EXHIBIT 2-3 *continued*

smoking increased only for stand-alone bars during Fall 2000, and then decreased in Spring 2001. No inside smoking was observed in any restaurant bars in either Fall 2000 or Spring 2001. Outside smoking continued to increase during the third year. The extent of the smell of smoke was significantly higher in stand-alone bars than in restaurant-bars, whether measured during daytime or early evening hours during Fall 2000 and Spring 2001. Based upon the odor of smoke, we concluded that compliance with the law was higher within restaurant-bars than stand-alone bars, although smoking continued in some restaurant-bars.

In year 1 (with a follow-up in year 3), a telephone survey of a cross-sectional sample of Long Beach residents was conducted with over 1500 respondents. A key result was that approval for the SFB Law increased from 66% (in year 1) to 73% in year 3. Other results demonstrated that 68% approved a ban on smoking on a nearby, wooden ocean pier; 75% approved of a cigarette tax to fund early childhood development programs, and 83% approved of smokefree zones in parks frequented by children. In conclusion, this case study demonstrated how epidemiologic methods (e.g., cross-sectional surveys and other analyses of population-based data) could be used in public health policy evaluation. ∎

Supported by Grant 7RT-0185, University of California Tobacco-Related Disease Research Program

Working of Health Services: Operations Research and Program Evaluation

Epidemiology applied to operations research involves the study of the placement of health services in a community and the optimum utilization of such services. "The usual epidemiologic approaches—descriptive, analytic, and experimental—are all used in health services research and, in addition, methods of evaluation have been expanded through their application to problems in health services."[14(p140)] A major contribution of epidemiology to operations research is in the development of research designs, analytic techniques, and measurement procedures. Operations research strives to answer the following kinds of questions, among others:

Using Epidemiology for Operations Research: Examples of Questions Asked

- *What health services are not being supplied by an agency in the community?*
- *Is a particular health service excessively duplicated in the community?*
- *What segments of the community are the primary utilizers of a service, and which segments are being underserved?*
- *What is the most efficient organizational and staffpower configuration?*
- *What characteristics of the community, providers, and patients affect service delivery and outcome?*
- *What procedures could be used to assess, match, and refer patients to service facilities?*

From the community perspective, there may be a wide variety of uncoordinated programs operated by providers who are not in adequate communication with one another. The results may be low efficiency, duplication, service gaps, delays in securing services, fragmented services, and a lack of service continuity. It is often impossible for one agency or program to provide all the needed services to individuals who are afflicted with severe health problems, such as multiple sclerosis or mental illnesses. One agency may specialize in diagnosis, evaluation, and treatment of the client's medical problems, whereas another may emphasize mental health issues. Because the mental and physical dimensions of the person may be intertwined, the holistic medical concept argues that there should be greater coordination among various health care agencies that specialize in a subaspect of health. Furthermore, coordination and integration of services probably would yield the fringe benefit of better utilization of available funds or services.

During the 1970s, Robert Friis directed a project to improve the coordination of health services to severely developmentally disabled children in the Bronx, New York. Some of the goals of the project were to identify unmet needs for services, to identify overlapping services, and to assist the referral of clients from one agency to another. In brief, for every severely developmentally disabled youngster in the Bronx (individuals with an IQ lower than 50) who was under the age of 21, the following representative items of information were collected:

- the facility from which medical treatment or follow-up was received
- drugs or medications that the person received
- diagnostic tests received in the past
- enrollment in educational, recreational, and other specified programs
- specific conditions and disabilities presented

Through statistical analyses, the project aimed to provide information about characteristics of service utilization. For example, it would be possible to tabulate the number of separate agencies that each client visited, to develop a profile of the types of services provided by each agency by cross-tabulating the medical conditions and functional disabilities prevalent in the population with services being received, and to determine quantitatively how many kinds of services would be needed in the community to make projections for sufficient funding of health services. Although this description is a simplification of the goals of the project, it provides an illustration of how the epidemiologic approach may be utilized for operations research purposes.

Another example of the use of epidemiologic methods for operations research comes from the National Ambulatory Medical Care Survey, which is a "survey of the private office-based, non-Federal physicians practicing in the United States."[15(p1)] Figure 2-6 presents data from this source for the percent distribution of office visits by primary expected source of payment according to patient's age. Figure 2-6 shows the relative importance of various methods of payment, such as Medicare, Medicaid, private medical insurance, and self-pay. Such information contributes to improvement of access to health care in the United States.

The foregoing examples illustrate the role of epidemiology in evaluation of health care utilization and needs assessment. A related application is for program evaluation. Specifically, how well does a health program meet certain stated goals? To illustrate, if the goal of a national health insurance program is to provide equal access to health services, an evaluation of the program should include utilization by socioeconomic status variables. The program would be on target if the analysis revealed little discrepancy in service utilization by social class. Epidemiologic methods may be employed to answer this question by providing the following methodologic input:

- methods for selecting target populations to be included in the evaluation
- design of instruments for data collection
- delimitation of types of health-related data to collect
- methods for assessment of health care needs

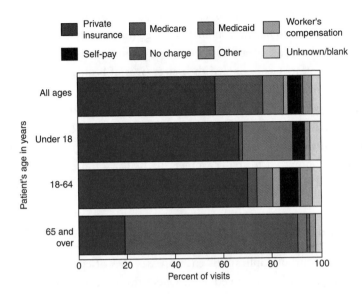

FIGURE 2-6 Percent distribution of office visits by primary expected source of payment according to patient's age: United States, 2000. *Source: Data are from DK Cherry and DA Woodwell, National Ambulatory Medical Care Survey: 2000 Summary. Advance data from vital and health statistics: No 328. Hyattsville, Maryland: National Center for Health Statistics, 2002.*

Evaluation of a clinic program or other health service can make use of epidemiologic tools. An example of an issue to include in the evaluation is the extent to which a program reaches minority individuals or socially and economically disadvantaged persons, the aged, or other targeted groups. An evaluation also might address the issue of changes or improvements in the overall health status of a target population. Other epidemiologic evaluations have studied patient satisfaction with medical care.

Socioeconomic indices may be employed in the epidemiologic evaluation of utilization of surgical operations. Data from the National Health Interview Survey suggest that differentials in surgical utilization between advantaged and disadvantaged socioeconomic groups decreased between 1963 and 1970, although some difference in utilization by race and place of residence remained in 1970.[16] Surgical utilization increased among the aged, lower educated, and nonwhites in urban areas. Income was positively associated with surgical utilization, standardizing for age and sex, although the relationship was weaker in 1970 than in 1963.

Another example of this use of epidemiology is in the evaluation of minority populations' access to health insurance coverage. In an analysis of epidemiologic data from the Hispanic Health and Nutrition Examination Survey (HHANES), 1982–1984, researchers examined the percentages of health insurance coverage among three major subpopulations (Mexican, Puerto Rican, and Cuban) of adult Latino women. The findings demonstrated that Mexican-origin women had the lowest level of any health insurance coverage, about 64% in comparison to the two other groups (about 74% and 81%, respectively). The disparity was even more pronounced for older women, particularly those between 50 to 64 years of age.[17]

Applications Relevant to Disease Etiology

The second group of applications encompasses uses of epidemiology that are closely connected with disease etiology. Under this general area, Morris[1] noted the search for causes, individual risks, and specific clinical concerns.

Causality in Epidemiologic Research

As an observational science, epidemiology is frequently subject to criticism. The prestigious journal *Science* ran a special news report entitled, "Epidemiology Faces Its Limits."[18] The subtitle read: "The Search for Subtle Links between Diet, Life Style, or Environmental Factors and Disease Is an Unending Source of Fear—but Often Yields Little Certainty." A portion of the report follows:

> The news about health risks comes thick and fast these days, and it seems almost constitutionally contradictory. In January of last year, for instance, a Swedish study found a significant association between residential radon exposure and lung cancer. A Canadian study did not. Three months later, it was pesticide residues. *The Journal of the National Cancer Institute* published a study in April reporting—contrary to previous, less powerful studies—that the presence of DDT metabolites in the bloodstream seemed to have no effect on the risk of breast cancer. In October, it was abortions and breast cancer. Maybe yes. Maybe no. In January of this year it was electromagnetic fields (EMF) from power lines. . . .

> These are not isolated examples of the conflicting nature of epidemiologic studies; they're just the latest to hit the newspapers. Over the years, such studies have come up with a mind-numbing array of potential disease-causing agents, from hair dyes (lymphomas, myelomas, and leukemia) to coffee (pancreatic cancer and heart disease), to oral contraceptives and other hormone treatments (virtually every disorder known to woman). The pendulum swings back and forth, subjecting the pub-

lic to an "epidemic of anxiety," as Lewis Thomas put it over a decade ago. Indeed, last July, the *New England Journal of Medicine (NEJM)* published an editorial by editors Marcia Angell and Jerome Kassirer asking the pithy question, "What Should the Public Believe?" Health-conscious Americans, wrote Angell and Kassirer, "increasingly find themselves beset by contradictory advice. No sooner do they learn the results of one research study than they hear of one with the opposite message."[18]

Part of the reason for the skepticism about epidemiologic research is the inability of the discipline to "prove" anything. Recall from Chapter 1 the contributions of Koch. His postulates, first developed by Henle, adapted in 1877, and further elaborated in 1882, also are referred to as the Henle-Koch postulates. They were instrumental in efforts to prove (or disprove) the causative involvement of a microorganism in the pathogenesis of an infectious disease. The postulates specified that the agent must be present in every case of the disease, must be isolated and grown in pure culture, must reproduce the disease when reintroduced into a healthy susceptible animal, and must be recovered and grown again in a pure culture. In addition, the agent should occur in no other disease—the one agent-one disease criterion. This classical Henle-Koch concept of causality, sometimes referred to as *pure determinism,* becomes problematic when one attempts to apply it to the chronic diseases prevalent in modern eras. Let us examine separately three of the four criteria that form part of Koch's concept of causality:

1. *Agent present in every case of the disease.* How would this criterion apply to cardiovascular heart disease (CVD)? Decades of research have established that individuals who develop CVD tend to be overweight, physically inactive, male, cigarette smokers, and have high blood pressure and high total cholesterol. If we were to apply Koch's postulates strictly, then every case of CVD would have all these characteristics—clearly not true.

2. *One agent-one disease.* How would this criterion hold up against cigarette smoking? We just pointed out that smokers are more likely to develop CVD than nonsmokers. Is CVD the only disease associated with smoking? No. In fact, smoking is associated with lung cancer, pancreatic cancer, oral cancer, nasopharyngeal cancer, cervical cancer, emphysema, chronic obstructive pulmonary disease, and stroke, to name just a few. Therefore, the one agent-one disease criterion is not particularly helpful, especially for diseases of noninfectious origin.

3. *Exposure of healthy subjects to suspected agents.* The ethical conduct of research on humans forbids exposure of subjects to risks that exceed potential benefits. Would it be reasonable to suspect the smoking-lung

cancer association even if such an experiment was never conducted? As pointed out in the introduction to this chapter, there are simply some exposures that cannot be evaluated in the context of controlled experimental studies. Epidemiology must be relied upon to provide such information.

In addition to the three issues just discussed that are direct tests of Koch's postulates, there are others that must be considered. It is relatively straightforward to categorize individuals with respect to the presence or absence of an exposure when the exposure is an infectious agent; one is either exposed or not exposed. However, even this simplification ignores the complicating issue of biologically effective dose. What about something such as blood pressure? Individuals with "elevated" blood pressure are more likely to develop a stroke than individuals with "low" blood pressure. Where does one draw the line between elevated and normal (or low)? At what level should an individual be considered obese?

A more subtle concept to consider is the fact that, for diseases of unknown etiology, we are dealing with imperfect knowledge. For example, although we may know that smokers are 20 times more likely to develop lung cancer than nonsmokers, why is it that not all smokers develop the disease? There must be other factors (diet, alcohol intake, host susceptibility, etc) that are part of the total picture of causality. When not all the contributing factors are known, it is problematic indeed to know truly and accurately the complete cause of a given disease. The issue of causality and epidemiology has been the focus of debate for decades. Some of the early writings are still fascinating and relevant today. An excellent text in this regard is the collection of readings assembled by Greenland[19] as well as *Causal Thinking in the Health Sciences,* by Susser.[20]

To summarize, it is now widely accepted that there is no single causal agent but rather multiple factors that produce chronic diseases such as CVD. Cassel, in the fourth Wade Hampton Frost Lecture, noted that early theories stated "disease occurred as a result of new exposure to a pathogenic agent." The single agent causal model was extended to "the well-known triad of host, agent and environment in epidemiologic thinking."[21(pp107-108)] (covered in Chapt. 12). The formulation was satisfactory to explain diseases of importance during the late 19th century and early 20th century, when agents of overwhelming pathogenicity and virulence produced conditions such as typhoid and smallpox. Cassel suggested that the triad of agent, host, and environment is no longer satisfactory because "In a modern society the majority of citizens are protected from these overwhelming agents and most of the agents associated with current diseases are ubiquitous in our environment. . . . [There may be] categories or classes of environmental factors that are capable of changing human resistance in important ways." Cassel argued that the social environment ("presence of other members of the same species") might be capable of profoundly influencing host susceptibility to environmental disease agents, whether they are microbiologic or physiochemical.[21]

Risk Factors Defined

Because of the uncertainty of "causal" factors in epidemiologic research, it is customary to refer to an exposure that is associated with a disease as a risk factor. There are three requisite criteria for risk factors:

1. *The frequency of the disease varies by category or value of the factor.* Consider cigarette smoking and lung cancer. Light smokers are more likely to develop lung cancer than nonsmokers, and heavy smokers are more likely still to develop the disease.
2. *The risk factor must precede the onset of disease.* Continuing with the smoking-lung cancer example, if individuals with lung cancer began to smoke after the onset of disease, it would be incorrect to assign smoking as the cause of the disease. This issue is particularly relevant to chronic diseases of long duration.
3. *The observed association must not be due to any source of error.* There are several points during the conduct of an epidemiologic investigation where error may be introduced: in the selection of the study groups, in the measurement of exposure and disease, and in the analysis. These topics are covered in Chapter 10.

Modern Concepts of Causality

Causal inferences derived from epidemiologic research (especially in the realm of noninfectious diseases) gained increasing popularity as a topic of formal discussion as a result of findings in the early 1950s of the association between smoking and lung cancer.[22] The publication of *Smoking and Health, Report of the Advisory Committee to the Surgeon General of the Public Health Service* listed five criteria for the judgment of the causal significance of an association[23] (Exhibit 2-4). These criteria were addressed subsequently in other writings by Susser,[24] Rothman, and Hill.[25] One of the seminal articles that elaborated on the five criteria for causality in epidemiologic research was published in 1965 by Sir Austin Bradford Hill, then Professor Emeritus of Medical Statistics at the University of London.[25] The

EXHIBIT 2-4

Case Study: Does Smoking Cause Lung Cancer?

The first Surgeon General's report on smoking and health was published in 1964.[23] The report generated global reaction by stating that cigarette smoking is a cause of lung cancer in men and is linked to other disabling or fatal diseases. This document identified five criteria necessary for the establishment of a causal relationship between smoking and lung cancer. The authors concluded that, to judge the causal significance of the association between cigarette smoking and lung cancer, several of these criteria would have to be taken into account in combination and no single criterion would, in itself, be "pathognomonic" (*pathognomonic* means characteristic or diagnostic). The criteria of judgment were strength of association, time sequence, consistency of relationship upon repetition, specificity of association, and coherence of explanation.

- *Strength of association:* The report stated that the relative risk ratio* is the most direct measure of the strength of association between smoking and lung cancer; several retrospective* and prospective* studies completed up to the time of the report demonstrated high relative risks for lung cancer among smokers and nonsmokers. Thus, it was concluded that the criterion of strength of association was supported.
- *Time sequence:* The report argued that early exposure to tobacco smoke and late manifestation seem to meet the criterion of time sequence, at least superficially.
- *Consistency upon repetition:* With regard to the causal relationship between smoking and health, the report asserted that this criterion was strongly confirmed for the relationship between smoking and lung cancer. Numerous retrospective and prospective studies demonstrated highly significant associations between smoking and lung cancer; it is unlikely that these findings would be obtained unless the association were causal or else due to unknown factors.
- *Specificity:* The hypothesis that smoking causes lung cancer has been attacked because of the lack of specificity of the relationship; smoking

continues

EXHIBIT 2-4 *continued*

> has been linked to a wide range of conditions, including cardiovascular disease (CVD), low birth weight, and bladder cancer. The report claimed, however, that rarely in the biologic realm does an agent always predict the occurrence of a disease; in addition, accumulating evidence about chronic diseases suggests that a given disease may have multiple causes.
>
> - *Coherence of explanation:* The report contended that the association between cigarette smoking and lung cancer was supported for this criterion. Evidence noted included the rise in lung cancer mortality with increases in per capita consumption of cigarettes and increases in lung cancer mortality as a function of age cohort* patterns of smoking among men and women; the sex differential in mortality was consistent with sex differences in tobacco use. General smoking rates were higher among men than among women; the report noted that young women were increasing their rates of smoking, however. ■
>
> *The terms *cohort, relative risk ratio, retrospective,* and *prospective* are defined in Chapters 6 and 7.

article, which was his President's Address to the Section of Occupational Medicine of the Royal Society of Medicine, lists nine aspects of an empirical association to consider when one is trying to decide whether the association is consistent with cause and effect. These were not intended to be interpreted as criteria of causality, but nonetheless they have been presented as such in several textbooks. The following is a quotation from his article:

> I have no wish, nor the skill, to embark upon a philosophical discussion of the meaning of "causation." The "cause" of illness may be immediate and direct, it may be remote and indirect, underlying the observed association. But with the aims of occupational, and almost synonymously preventive, medicine in mind the decisive question is whether the frequency of the undesirable event B will be influenced by a change in the environmental feature A. How such a change exerts that influence may call for a great deal of research. However, before deducing "causation" and taking action we shall not invariably have to sit around awaiting the results of that research. The whole chain may have to be unraveled or a few links may suffice. It will depend upon circumstances.[25(p295)]

This landmark article identified nine issues that are relevant to causality and epidemiologic research.

1. *Strength of association.* One example cited by Hill was the observation of Percival Pott that chimney sweeps in comparison to other workers had an enormous increase in scrotal cancer; the mortality was more than 200 times that of workers not exposed to tar and mineral oils. A strong association is less likely to be the result of errors.

2. *Consistency upon repetition.* This term refers to whether the association between agent and putative health effects has been observed by different persons in different places, circumstances, and times. The Surgeon General's report of 1964 cited a total of 36 different studies that found an association between smoking and lung cancer.[23] Hill felt that consistency was especially important when the exposure was rare.

3. *Specificity.* With respect to occupational exposures, Hill noted that if "the association is limited to specific workers and to particular sites and types of disease and there is no association between the work and other modes of dying, then clearly that is a strong argument in favor of causation."[25(p297)] He later went on to acknowledge that specificity should be used as evidence in favor of causality, not as refutation against it.

4. *Time sequence.* In Hill's words, "Which is the cart and which is the horse?" For example, if one is trying to identify the role of diet in the pathogenesis of colon cancer, one has to be careful to sort out dietary preferences that lead to colon cancer versus dietary changes that result from early stages of the disease. There is some evidence that low intakes of calcium are associated with increased risk of colon cancer. If early stages of disease create problems with digestion of milk products (which are good sources of calcium), individuals may lower their intake of milk (and calcium) as a consequence of the disease. The shorter the duration between exposure to an agent and development of the disease (i.e., the latency period), the more certain one is regarding the hypothesized cause of the disease. For this reason, many of the acute infectious diseases or chemical poisonings are relatively easy to pinpoint as to cause. Diseases having longer latency periods—many forms of cancer, for example—are more difficult to relate to a causal agent; it is said that the onset of chronic diseases is insidious and that one is ignorant of the precise induction periods for chronic diseases. Many different causal factors could intervene during the latency period. This is why a great deal of detective work was needed to link early exposure to asbestos in shipyards to subsequent development of mesothelioma, a form of cancer of the lining of the abdominal cavity.

5. *Biologic gradient.* Evidence of a dose-response curve is another important criterion. Hill notes "the fact that the death rate from lung cancer increases linearly with the number of cigarettes smoked daily adds a great deal to the simpler evidence that cigarette smokers have a higher death rate than non-smokers."[25(p298)] MacMahon and Pugh state "the existence of a dose-response relationship—that is, an increase in disease risk with increase in the amount of exposure—supports the view that an association is a causal one."[3(p235)] Figure 2-7 illustrates a dose-response relationship between number of cigarettes smoked per day and lung cancer mortality among male British physicians.

6. *Plausibility.* If an association is biologically plausible, it will be helpful. The weakness of this line of evidence is that it is necessarily dependent upon the biologic knowledge of the day.

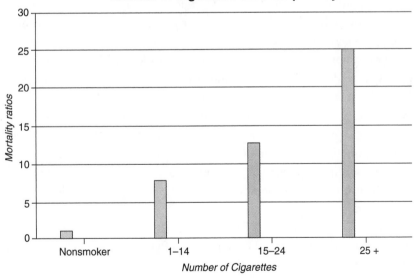

FIGURE 2-7 Dose-response relationships between smoking and lung cancer mortality among British physicians. *Source:* Data are from R Doll, R Peto. Mortality in Relation to Smoking: 20 Years' Observations on Male British Doctors. *British Medical Journal,* vol 2 (6051), pp 1525–1536, BMJ Publishing Group, © 1976.

7. *Coherence of explanation.* The association must not seriously conflict with what is already known about the natural history and biology of the disease. Data from laboratory experiments on animals may be most helpful. For example, the ability of tobacco extracts to cause skin cancer in mice is coherent with the theory that consumption of tobacco products in humans causes lung cancer.

8. *Experiment.* In some instances there may be "natural experiments" that shed important light on a topic. The observation that communities with naturally fluoridated water had fewer dental caries among their citizens than communities without fluoridated water is one example.

9. *Analogy.* The examples Hill cites are thalidomide and rubella. Given that such associations have already been demonstrated, "we would surely be ready to accept slighter but similar evidence with another drug or another viral disease in pregnancy."[25(p299)]

Although it is not critical that all these lines of evidence be presented to support the concept of causality, the more that are supported, the more the case of causality is strengthened. More important, careful consideration of these concepts is helpful in trying to decide at what point one needs to take action. One of Hill's concluding remarks was particularly poignant: "All scientific work is incomplete—whether it be observational or experimental. All scientific work is liable to be upset or modified by advancing knowledge. That does not confer upon us a freedom to ignore the knowledge we already have, or to postpone the action that it appears to demand at a given time."[25(p300)] It also should be noted that the processes of causal inference and statistical inference (refer to Chapt. 9) frequently overlap yet represent different principles. According to Susser, "Formal statistical tests are framed to give mathematical answers to structured questions leading to judgments, whereas in any field practitioners must give answers to unstructured questions leading from judgment to decision and implementation."[24(p1)]

Evans,[26] in a compelling discussion of causality, drew an analogy between ascertainment of causality and establishment of guilt in a criminal trial. Evans' detailed arguments are found in Exhibit 2-5.

Study of Risks to Individuals

Epidemiologic research on disease etiology typically involves collection of data on a number of individual members of different study groups or study populations. Two main types of observational studies are employed. These are discussed

EXHIBIT 2-5

Rules of Evidence:
Criminality and Causality

Mayhem or murder and criminal law	Morbidity, mortality, and causality
1. Criminal present at scene of crime.	Agent present in lesion of the disease.
2. Premeditation.	Causal events precede onset of disease.
3. Accessories involved in the crime.	Cofactors and/or multiple causality involved.
4. Severity or death related to state of victim.	Susceptibility and host response determine severity.
5. Motivation—The crime must make sense in terms of gain to the criminal.	The role of the agent in the disease must make biologic and common sense.
6. No other suspect could have committed the crime.	No other agent could have caused the disease under the circumstances given.
7. The proof of the guilt must be established beyond a reasonable doubt.	The proof of causation must be established beyond reasonable doubt or role of chance.

"In criminal law, the presence of the criminal at the scene of the crime would be equivalent to the presence of the agent in a lesion of the disease. Premeditation would be similar to the requirement that the causal exposure should precede the onset of the disease. The presence of accessories at the scene of the crime might be compared to the presence of cofactors and/or multiple causes for human diseases. The severity of the crime or the consequence of death might be loosely equivalent to susceptibility and the host responses which determine the severity of the illness. The motivation involved in a crime should make sense in terms of reward to the criminal, just as the role of the causal agent should make biologic sense. The absence of other suspects and their elimination in a criminal trial would be similar to that of the exclusion of other putative causes in human illness. Finally, need

continues

EXHIBIT 2-5 *continued*

that the proof of guilt must be established beyond a reasonable doubt would be true for both criminal justice and for disease causation." ■

Source: Adapted from AS Evans, Causation and Disease: A Chronological Journey, *American Journal of Epidemiology,* vol 108, No 4, pp 254-255, with permission of the Johns Hopkins University, School of Hygiene and Public Health. © 1978.

in greater detail in Chapters 6 and 7, but at this time suffice it to say that the case-control design compares a group of well individuals with a group of individuals who have the disease of interest. The two groups are compared with respect to a variety of exposures (e.g., diet, exercise habits, or use of sunscreens). Differences that are observed between the two groups may be the reason why one group is healthy and the other is not. Another research method is the cohort study. In this approach, a study group free of disease is assembled and measured with respect to a variety of exposures that are hypothesized to increase (or decrease) the chance of getting the disease. One then follows the group over time for the development of disease, comparing the frequency with which disease develops in the group exposed to the factor and the group not exposed to the factor. Either type of study may demonstrate that a disease or other outcome is more likely to occur in those with a particular exposure.

The issue of whether the results of an epidemiologic study influence clinical decision-making is in part determined by the criteria of causality covered in the previous section. How large is the effect? How consistent is the finding with previous research? Is there biologic plausibility? All these issues are important, but a major issue for the clinician is the relevance to each particular patient. Epidemiologic studies are studies of groups of individuals; the studies provide evidence that groups that have particular exposures or lifestyle characteristics are more or less likely to develop disease than groups of individuals without the exposures. Extrapolation to the individual from findings based on observations of groups should be made with caution. The observation that cigarette smokers are 20 times more likely to develop lung cancer than nonsmokers does not necessarily entitle someone to tell a smoker "You are 20 times more likely to get lung cancer than a nonsmoker." The problem is that there are a number of other factors that may be important contributors to the cause of lung cancer. A more accurate statement would be "Collectively, groups of individuals who smoke are 20 times more likely to develop lung cancer than nonsmokers." The difference is subtle, yet important.

Another issue for the clinician is the size of the risk; an example is the slight risk of mortality from CVD associated with a high serum cholesterol level. If the risk is small, a person may reasonably not wish to change his or her lifestyle.[27] The 1990 editorial in the *New England Journal of Medicine* is particularly illustrative.[2] Suppose that the 10-year risk of death is 1.7% in middle-aged men with cholesterol levels below 200 mg/dL but 4.9% if the cholesterol level is above 240 mg/dL.[28] This difference in risk of approximately 3.0% may be insufficient to induce an otherwise healthy man to try to lower his cholesterol level. Conversely, even if the risk factor is strong, it may still be unimportant to individual patients if the disease is rare.

The extrapolation of epidemiologic research to individuals thus is complicated. Another aspect of risk concerns public health implications. A risk factor that may be relatively unimportant for individuals may indeed be important when the effect is multiplied over the population as a whole, especially if the disease is common. Refer to Chapter 9 for more detail.

This application of epidemiology also makes possible the prediction of the individual's prognosis and likelihood of survival if afflicted by a serious disease. Such information can be used to inform the patient about his or her chances for survival and ultimate recovery. It also demonstrates the efficacy of medical intervention by showing whether the practice yields an increase in long-term survival for a population of cases. Some illustrations of the use of epidemiology to study risks to the individual are predictions of mortality from cancer and other serious chronic diseases and studies of the relationship between longevity and coronary bypass surgery.

Epidemiologic research indicates that there is a low, but nevertheless important, contribution to mortality from frequently occurring infectious diseases, such as influenza and the common cold. Mortality results from complications that occur in the neonatal and elderly groups or in debilitated individuals. Without population-based data, mortality from these "minor" diseases might not be obvious. In 1978, influenza was responsible for slightly less than 1 death per 100,000 individuals in the United States.

Epidemiologic data may be used to predict cancer prognosis and mortality. Both vary by site of the tumor, type, and a number of social variables, such as socioeconomic status, race, and sex. Figure 2-8 presents the five-year relative survival rate for selected forms of cancer by race from 1975 to 1984. Differences in survival are evident by both cancer type and race. Among African Americans in comparison to whites, the five-year survival rates for all cancer sites were 39.6 and 51.9, respectively.

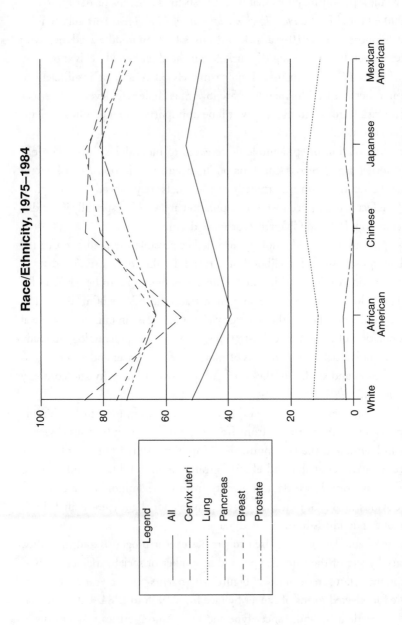

FIGURE 2-8 Five-year relative survival rates by race/ethnic group, 1975 to 1984. *Source:* Data are from *Cancer Facts and Figures for Minority Americans* by the American Cancer Society, Inc, p 7. © 1991.

Another illustration of the study of risks to the individual draws upon studies of prognosis of survival from coronary bypass surgery. The Veterans Administration Cooperative Study[29] traced the survival of 596 patients treated by medication or by surgery for chronic stable angina in a large-scale prospective, randomized study. Findings indicated no differences in survival at 21 and 36 months between surgery patients and medically treated patients. Thus, the factors of mortality from surgery itself and expense of the operation need to be weighed against increases in life expectancy and improvement in the quality of life due to improved arterial circulation. This is an epidemiologic question that may be raised about risks associated with other types of surgical procedures as well.

Enlargement of the Clinical Picture of Disease

When a new disease first gains the attention of health authorities, it is usually the most dramatic cases that are the ones observed. It may be concluded incorrectly that the new disease is an extremely acute or fatal condition; later epidemiologic studies may reveal that the most common form of the new disease is a mild, subclinical illness and that it occurs widely in the population. To develop a complete clinical picture of the disease, careful studies are necessary to find out about the subacute cases; an adequate study requires a survey of a population.

An instance in which epidemiology has added to clinical knowledge about a disease that appeared to be new and highly virulent was the Legionnaires' disease situation. During July of 1976, public attention and concern were evoked by the outbreak of a mysterious illness that ravaged participants at a convention of the American Legion in Philadelphia. Local and federal epidemiologists were called in to investigate the outbreak. It was found subsequently that Legionnaires' disease is associated with a previously unidentified bacterium, that about 15% of the people who developed the disease died of it, and that the disease had probably occurred sporadically in other areas of the country before 1976.

Prevention of Disease

One of the potential applications of research on disease etiology is to identify where, in the disease's natural history, effective intervention might be implemented. The natural history of disease refers to the course of disease from its beginning to its final clinical end points. The period of *prepathogenesis* occurs before the precursors of disease (e.g., the bacterium that causes Legionnaires' disease) have interacted with the host (the person who gets the disease). The period of *pathogenesis* occurs after the precursors have interacted with the host, an event that is marked by initial appearance of disease (the presymptomatic stage) and is characterized by tissue and physiologic changes. Later stages of the natural history include development of active signs and symptoms and eventually recovery, disability, or death (all examples of clinical end points). It is possible to consider three strategies for disease prevention: primary, secondary, and tertiary.

Primary Prevention

Primary prevention activities, designed to reduce the occurrence of disease, occur during the period of prepathogenesis. Education about the hazards of starting smoking is an example of primary prevention. Interventions to reduce the number of alcohol-related traffic accidents similarly may focus on education, media campaigns, and warning labels on alcohol-containing beverages. Other examples of primary prevention are wearing protective devices to prevent occupational injuries, utilization of dietary supplements to prevent nutritional deficiency diseases, and immunizations against infectious diseases.

Primary prevention activities may be either active or passive. Active prevention requires some sort of behavior change on the part of the subject. Wearing protective devices and obtaining vaccinations require involvement of the individual to receive the benefit. Passive interventions, on the other hand, do not require any behavior change. Fluoridation of public water supplies and vitamin fortification of milk and bread products achieve their desired effects without any voluntary effort of the recipients.

Secondary Prevention

Secondary prevention occurs when the intent is to reduce the progress of disease and takes place during the pathogenesis phase of the natural history of disease. Cancer screening programs, which are efforts to detect cancer in early stages (when it is more successfully treated) among apparently healthy individuals, provide one example of secondary prevention. One should note that in this situation cancer is already present; however, detection of the tumor before the onset of clinical symptoms reduces the likelihood of progress to death. Most cancer screening programs are secondary prevention. However, screening for colorectal cancer also can be considered primary prevention. This is because most colorectal cancers arise through a precancerous lesion (adenomatous polyp). Screening that detects and removes polyps therefore prevents cancer, rather than merely detecting cancer early.

Tertiary Prevention

Tertiary prevention includes activities designed to limit disability from disease. Thus, disease already has occurred and has been treated clinically, but rehabilitation is needed to limit the sequelae and restore the patient to an optimal functional level. Tertiary prevention also includes efforts to minimize the side effects of clinical treatment (such as drug side effects). Examples include physical therapy for stroke victims, halfway houses for persons recovering from alcohol abuse, sheltered homes for the developmentally disabled, and fitness programs for heart attack patients.

Conclusion

This chapter identified seven uses of epidemiology. The historical use of epidemiology traced changes in rates of disease from early in this century to the present. Dramatic changes in morbidity and mortality rates were noted. Predictions of future trends in health status employ population dynamics, or shifts in the demographic composition of populations. Operations research and program evaluation are examples of using epidemiologic methods to improve health care services. Epidemiology also is used to describe the health of the community, to identify causes of disease, and to study risks to individuals. One of the most important applications is the study of the causality of disease; a detailed discussion of causality was provided. The chapter concluded with a review of primary, secondary, and tertiary prevention of diseases.

Study Questions and Exercises

1. Define in your own words the following terms:
   a. secular changes
   b. operations research
   c. risk factor
   d. the natural history of disease
   e. demographic transition
   f. disorders: disappearing, residual, persisting, epidemic
   g. population pyramid
2. Name three approaches for primary, secondary, and tertiary prevention of the following health problems/conditions:
   a. motor vehicle accidents
   b. obesity

    c. hepatitis A

    d. hepatitis B and C

    e. foodborne illness on cruise ships

    f. mortality due to gang violence

3. State the seven uses of epidemiology according to Morris.[1] Are the uses of epidemiology defined in the chapter distinct or overlapping? Can you think of other uses of epidemiology not identified in the chapter? Do all the uses belong exclusively to the domain of epidemiology?

4. Describe a role for epidemiology in the field of policy evaluation. Consider how the field of epidemiology might inform policy evaluation of laws that regulate tobacco consumption in public places.

5. How are the rules of evidence for criminality similar or different from the rules of evidence for disease causality? (Refer to Exhibit 2-5 to help with your answer.)

6. Clinicians and epidemiologists differ in their assessment of the importance of risks. State how the clinical and epidemiologic approaches differ. Give an example by using a disease or condition that is important for society.

7. Describe how it is possible for an infectious disease, when it first comes to the attention of public health authorities, to be considered an extremely acute or fatal condition—and then later found to be mild or benign in its most common form. Give an example of such a disease.

8. This chapter stated how epidemiology may be applied to the study of the causality of disease. Suggest other examples of how epidemiology might be applied to study the causality of disease.

9. The following questions refer to Table 1 in Appendix 2 at the end of this chapter.

    a. Calculate the percentage decline in the death rate. What generalizations can be made about changes in disease rates that have occurred between 1900 and the present?

    b. Contrast the changes in death rates due to cancer, heart disease, and stroke. What additional information would be useful to specify better the changes in these conditions?

    c. Note the decline in mortality for the four communicable diseases (1, 2, 3, and 10). With the exception of pneumonia and influenza, these are no longer among the 10 leading causes of death. Can you speculate regarding how much of each is due to environmental improvements and how much to specific preventive and curative practices?

d. Among the 10 leading causes of death in 1996 are pulmonary disease (40.0, rank 4), diabetes (23.2, rank 7), human immunodeficiency virus (HIV) infection (12.3, rank 8), and chronic liver disease and cirrhosis (9.5, rank 10). In 1900, these were not among the 10 leading causes of death. How do you account for these changes?

10. The following questions refer to Figure 2-2.

a. List and describe the trends in death rates by the five leading causes of death.

b. Describe the trend for influenza and pneumonia. Can you suggest an explanation for the peaks in influenza and pneumonia deaths?

c. Does the curve for accidental deaths correspond to our expectations from various publicity reports?

d. What is the trend for HIV infection? Can you offer an explanation?

References

1. Morris JN. *Uses of Epidemiology, 3rd ed.* Edinburgh, UK: Churchill Livingstone; 1975.
2. Angell M. The interpretation of epidemiologic studies. Editorial, *N Engl J Med.* 1990;323:823–825.
3. MacMahon B, Pugh TF. *Epidemiology Principles and Methods.* Boston, MA: Little, Brown; 1970.
4. Susser MW, Watson W, Hopper K. *Sociology in Medicine,* 3rd ed. New York, NY: Oxford University Press; 1985.
5. Mausner JS, Kramer S. *Epidemiology: An Introductory Text,* 2nd ed. Philadelphia: Saunders; 1985.
6. Rothman KJ. *Modern Epidemiology.* Boston, MA: Little, Brown; 1986.
7. U.S. Department of Health and Human Services. *Healthy People 2010: Understanding and Improving Health,* 2nd ed. Washington, DC: U.S. Government Printing Office, November 2000.
8. National Institutes of Health. *Addressing Health Disparities: The NIH Program of Action.* Available at: http://healthdisparities.nih.gov/welcome.html. Accessed February 8, 2003.
9. Ibrahim MA. *Epidemiology and Health Policy.* Gaithersburg, MD: Aspen Publications; 1985.
10. Samet JM, Lee NL. Bridging the gap: Perspectives on translating epidemiologic evidence into policy. *Am J Epidemiol.* 2001;154(12 Suppl):S1–S3.
11. Weed DL, Mink PJ. Roles and responsibilities of epidemiologists. *Ann Epidemiol.* 2002;12:67–72.
12. Matanoski GM. Conflicts between two cultures: Implications for epidemiologic researchers in communicating with policy-makers. *Am J Epidemiol.* 2001;154(12 Suppl):S36–S42.

13. Spasoff RA. *Epidemiologic Methods for Health Policy.* New York, NY: Oxford University Press; 1999.

14. Hulka BS. Epidemiological applications to health services research. *J Community Health.* 1978;4:140–149.

15. Woodwell DA. *Office Visits to General Surgeons 1989–90, National Ambulatory Medical Care Survey.* Advance Data from Vital and Health Statistics. Report 228. Hyattsville, MD: National Center for Health Statistics; December 22, 1993.

16. Bombardier C, Fuchs VR, Lillard LA, et al. Social economic factors affecting the utilization of surgical operations. *N Engl J Med.* 1977;297:699–705.

17. de la Torre A, Friis R, Hunter HR, Garcia L. The health insurance of U.S. Latino women: a profile from the 1982-1984 HHANES. *Am J Public Health.* 1996;86:533–537.

18. Epidemiology faces its limits. *Science.* 1995;269:164–169.

19. Greenland S. *Evolution of Epidemiologic Ideas: Annotated Readings on Concepts and Methods.* Chestnut Hill, MA: Epidemiology Resources; 1987.

20. Susser M. *Causal Thinking in the Health Sciences.* New York, NY: Oxford University Press; 1973.

21. Cassel J. The contribution of the social environment to host resistance. *Am J Epidemiol.* 1976;104:107–123.

22. Winkelstein W Jr. Invited commentary on "Judgment and causal inference: criteria in epidemiologic studies." *Am J Epidemiol.* 1995;141:699–700.

23. U.S. Department of Health, Education and Welfare, Public Health Service. *Smoking and Health, Report of the Advisory Committee to the Surgeon General of the Public Health Service.* Public Health Service publication 1103. Washington, DC: Government Printing Office; 1964.

24. Susser M. Judgment and causal inference: criteria in epidemiologic studies. *Am J Epidemiol.* 1977;105:1–15.

25. Hill AB. The environment and disease: association or causation? *Proc R Acad Med.* 1965;58:295–300.

26. Evans AS. Causation and disease: a chronological journey. *Am J Epidemiol.* 1978;108:254–255.

27. Brett AS. Treating hypercholesterolemia: how should practicing physicians interpret the published data for patients? *N Engl J Med.* 1989;321:676–680.

28. Pekkanen J, Linn S, Heiss G, et al. Ten-year mortality from cardiovascular disease in relation to cholesterol level among men with and without preexisting cardiovascular disease. *N Engl J Med.* 1990;322:1700–1707.

29. Murphy M, Hultgren HN, Detre K, et al. Treatment of chronic stable angina: a preliminary report of survival data of the randomized Veterans Administration Cooperative Study. *N Engl J Med.* 1977;297:621–627.

APPENDIX
2

Data for Study Question 9

Table 2A Leading Causes of Death and Rates for Those Causes in 1900 and 1996, United States

Rank, 1900	Cause of Death*	Rate per 100,000 Population	
		1900	1996
	All cases	1,719.1	875.4
1	Influenza and pneumonia, except pneumonia of newborn	202.2	31.1
2	Tuberculosis, all forms	194.4	NA†
3	Gastroenteritis	142.7	NA
4	Disease of heart	137.4	276.6
5	Cerebrovascular diseases	106.9	60.5
6	Chronic nephritis	81.0	NA
7	Accidents and adverse effects	72.3	35.4
8	Malignant neoplasms	64.0	205.2
9	Certain diseases of early infancy	62.6	NA
10	Diphtheria	40.3	NA

*Some categories may not be strictly comparable because of change in classification.

†NA: These are no longer listed among the top 10 causes of death for 1996.

Source: Data are from SJ Ventura, et al, US Bureau of the Census, *Statistical Abstract of the United States: 1957,* p 69: and National Center for Health Statistics, Births and Deaths: United States, 1996; *Monthly Vital Statistics Report,* Vol 46, No 1, p 5, 1997.

Measures of Morbidity and Mortality Used in Epidemiology

LEARNING OBJECTIVES

By the end of this chapter the reader will be able to:

- define and distinguish among proportions, rates, and ratios
- explain the term *population at risk*
- identify and calculate commonly used rates for morbidity, mortality, and natality
- state the meanings and applications of incidence rates and prevalence
- discuss limitations of crude rates and alternative measures for crude rates
- apply direct and indirect methods to adjust rates
- list situations where direct and indirect adjustment should be used

CHAPTER OUTLINE

Introduction

Chapter 1 stated that, because the work of the epidemiologist involves the enumeration of cases of diseases and health-related phenomena, epidemiology tends to be a quantitative discipline. This chapter defines several of the more common measures of disease frequency that are employed in epidemiology. The ability to measure carefully and accurately the occurrence of morbidity and mortality forms the foundation of studies designed to identify etiology, monitor trends, and evaluate public health interventions designed to decrease disease frequency.

Definitions of Count, Proportion, Ratio, and Rate

Count

The simplest and most frequently performed quantitative measure in epidemiology is a count. As the term implies, a count merely refers to the number of cases of a disease or other health phenomenon being studied. Several examples of counts include the number of:

- cases of influenza reported in Westchester County, New York, during January of a particular year
- traffic fatalities in the borough of Manhattan during a 24-hour period
- participants screened positive in a hypertension screening program organized by an industrial plant in northern California
- college dorm residents who had hepatitis
- stomach cancer patients who were foreign born

Proportion

For a count to be descriptive of a group, however, it must usually be seen relative to the size of the group. Referring to the foregoing examples, suppose there were 10 college dorm residents who had hepatitis. How large a problem did these 10 cases represent? To answer this question, one would need to know whether the dormitory housed 20 students or 500 students. If there were only 20 students, then 50% (or 0.50) were ill. Conversely, if there were 500 students in the dormitory, then only 2% (or 0.02) were ill. Clearly, these two scenarios paint a completely different picture of the magnitude of the problem. In this situation, expressing the count as a proportion is indeed helpful.

In most situations it will be informative to have some idea about the size of the denominator. Although the construction of a proportion is straightforward, one of the central concerns of epidemiology is to find and enumerate appropriate denominators to describe and compare groups in a meaningful and useful way.

The previous discussion may leave the reader with the impression that counts, in and of themselves, are of little value in epidemiology; this is not true, however. In fact, case reports of patients with particularly unusual presentations or combinations of symptoms often spur epidemiologic investigations. In addition, for some diseases even a single case is sufficient to be of public health importance. For example, if a case of smallpox or Ebola virus were reported, the size of the denominator would be irrelevant. That is, in these instances a single case, regardless of the size of the population at risk, would stimulate an investigation.

Ratio

A ratio, like a proportion, is a fraction and therefore consists of a numerator and a denominator. The difference is that in a ratio there is not necessarily any specified relationship between the numerator and denominator. In a proportion, however, the numerator is always part of the denominator. A ratio may be expressed as follows: ratio = X/Y. For example, of 1,000 motorcycle fatalities, 950 victims are men and 50 are women. The sex ratio for motorcycle fatalities is:

$$\frac{\text{Number of male cases}}{\text{Number of female cases}} = \frac{950}{50} = 19:1 \text{ male to female}$$

A proportion is a type of ratio in which the numerator is a part of the denominator; proportions may be expressed as percentages. The following example illustrates the calculation of the proportion of African-American male deaths among African-American and white boys aged 5 to 14 years:

A	B	Total (A + B)
Number of deaths among African-American boys	Number of deaths among white boys	Total
1,150	3,810	4,960

Proportion = A/(A + B) × 100 = (1,150/4,960) × 100 = 23.2%

Rate

A rate differs from a proportion because the denominator involves a measure of time. The numerator consists of the frequency of a disease over a specified period of time, and the denominator is a unit size of population (Exhibit 3-1). It is critical to remember that, to calculate a rate, two periods of time are involved: the beginning of the period and the end of the period.

EXHIBIT 3-1

Rate Calculation

Rate: A ratio that consists of a numerator and a denominator and in which time forms part of the denominator.

Epidemiologic rates contain the following elements:
- disease frequency
- unit size of population
- time period during which an event occurs

Example:

$$\text{Crude death rate} = \frac{\text{Number of deaths in a given year}}{\substack{\text{Reference population} \\ \text{(during midpoint of the year)}}} \times 100,000$$

(Either rate per 1,000 or 100,000 is used as the multiplier)

Calculation problem (crude death rate in the United States):

Number of deaths in the United States during 1990 = 2,148,463
Population of the United States as of June 30, 1990 = 248,709,873

$$\text{Crude death rate} = \frac{2,148,463}{248,709,873} = 863.8 \text{ per } 100,000$$

Medical publications may use the terms *ratio, proportion,* and *rate* without strict adherence to the mathematical definitions for these terms. Hence one must be alert to how a measure is defined and calculated.[1] In the formula shown in Exhibit 3-1, the denominator also is termed the reference population and by definition is the population from which cases of a disease have been taken. For example, in calculating the annual death rate (crude mortality rate) in the United States, one would count all the deaths that occurred in the country during a certain year and assign this value to the numerator. The value for the denominator would be the size of the population of the country during a particular year. The best estimate of the population would probably be the population around the midpoint of the year, if such information could be obtained. Referring to Exhibit 3-1, one calculates the U.S. crude mortality rate as 863.8 per 100,000 persons for 1990.

Rates improve one's ability to make comparisons. This is because rates of mortality or morbidity for a specific disease (see the section on cause-specific mortality rates later in this chapter) reduce that standard of comparison to a common denominator, the unit size of population. To illustrate, the U.S. crude death rate for diseases of the heart in 1991 was 285.9 per 100,000. One also might calculate the heart disease death rate for geographic subdivisions of the country (also expressed as frequency per 100,000 individuals). These rates could then be compared with one another and with the rate for the United States to judge whether the rates found in each geographic area are higher or lower. For example, the crude death rates for diseases of the heart in New York and Texas were 353.1 and 226.7 per 100,000, respectively. It would appear that the death rate is higher in New York than in Texas based on the crude death rates. This may be a specious conclusion, however, because there may be important differences in population composition, for example age differences between populations, that would affect mortality experience. Later in this chapter, the procedure to adjust for age differences or other factors is discussed.

Rates can be expressed in any form that is convenient (e.g., per 1,000, per 100,000, or per 1,000,000). Many of the rates that are published and routinely used as an indicator of public health are expressed in a particular convention. For example, cancer rates are typically expressed per 100,000 population, and infant mortality is expressed per 1,000 live births. One of the determinants of the size of the denominator is whether the numerator is large enough to permit the rate to be expressed as an integer or an integer plus a trailing decimal (e.g., 4 or 4.2). For example, it would be preferable to describe the occurrence of disease as 4 per 100,000 rather than 0.04 per 1,000, even though both are perfectly correct. Throughout this chapter, the multiplier for a given morbidity or mortality statistic is provided.

Exhibit 3-2 describes the Iowa Women's Health Study (IWHS). The data collected illustrate the various measures of disease frequency defined in this chapter.

EXHIBIT 3-2

The Iowa Women's Health Study

The IWHS is a longitudinal study of mortality and cancer occurrence in older women.[2,3] The state of Iowa was chosen as the site of this study because of the availability of cancer incidence and mortality data from the State Health Registry of Iowa. This registry is a participant in the National Cancer Institute's Surveillance, Epidemiology, and End Results Program. The sample was selected from a January 1985 current drivers list obtained from the Iowa Department of Transportation. The list contained the names of 195,294 women aged 55 to 69 and represented approximately 94% of the women in the state of Iowa in this age range.

In December 1985, a 50% random sample of the eligible women was selected, yielding 99,826 women with an Iowa mailing address. A 16-page health history questionnaire was mailed on January 16, 1986, followed by a reminder postcard one week later and a follow-up letter four weeks later; a total of 41,837 women responded. Information was collected about basic demographics, medical history, reproductive history, personal and family history of cancer, usual dietary intake, smoking and exercise habits, and medication use. A paper tape measure also was provided along with detailed instructions for the subject to record selected body measurements: height, weight, and circumferences of the waist and hips.

The primary focus of the study was to determine whether distribution of body fat centrally (i.e., around the waist) rather than peripherally (i.e., on the hips) is associated with increased risk of cancer. The occurrence of cancer was determined by record linkage with the State Health Registry. A computer program was used to match new cancer cases in the registry with study participants on name, ZIP code, birth date, and Social Security number. ■

Prevalence

The term *prevalence* refers to the number of existing cases of a disease or health condition in a population at some designated time.[4] Prevalence data provide an indication of the extent of a health problem and thus may have implications for the scope of health services needed in the community. Consider three examples: The prevalence of diarrhea in a children's camp on July 13 was 33%, the prevalence of phenylketonuria-associated mental retardation in institutions for the developmentally disabled was 15%, and the prevalence of obesity among women aged 55 to 69 years was 367 per 1,000. These examples illustrate that the designated time can be specified, (e.g., one day) or unspecified; when the time period is unspecified, prevalence usually implies a particular point in time. More specifically, these examples refer to *point prevalence*.

$$\text{Point prevalence} = \frac{\text{Number of persons ill}}{\text{Total number in the group}} \text{ at a time point}$$

Example: In the IWHS, respondents were asked "Do you smoke cigarettes now?" The total number in the group was 41,837. The total number who responded yes to the smoking question was 6,234. Therefore, the prevalence of current smokers in the IWHS on January 16, 1985, was 6,234/41,837. This result could be expressed as a percentage (14.9%) or as a frequency per 1,000 (149.0).

A second type of prevalence measure is *period prevalence*, which denotes the total number of cases of a disease that exist during a specified period of time, for instance a week, month, or longer time interval. To determine the period prevalence, one must combine the number of cases at the beginning of the time interval (the point prevalence) with the new cases that occur during the interval. Because the denominator may have changed somewhat (the result of people entering or leaving during the period of observation), one typically refers to the average population. Note that for period prevalence, cases are counted even if they die, migrate, or recur as episodes during the period.

$$\text{Period prevalence} = \frac{\text{Number of persons ill}}{\text{Average population}} \text{ during a time period}$$

Example: In the IWHS, women were asked: "Have you ever been diagnosed by a physician as having any form of cancer, other than skin cancer?" Note that the question did not ask about current disease but rather about the lifetime history. Thus it refers to period prevalence, the period being the entire life span. To calculate the period prevalence, one needs to know the average population (still 41,837) and the number who responded yes to the question (2,293). Therefore, the period prevalence of cancer in the study population was 2,293/41,837, or 5.5%.

Technically speaking, both measures of prevalence are proportions. As such, they are dimensionless and should not be described as rates—a mistake that is commonly made.

To illustrate the distinction between point and period prevalence, consider as an example the issue of homelessness in the United States. The conditions surrounding homelessness present a serious public health problem, particularly in the control of infectious diseases and the effect on homeless persons' physical and mental health. Consequently, there is a legitimate need to estimate the magnitude of the problem, an issue that has produced intense debate. Surveys of currently homeless people pose extremely challenging methodologic difficulties that have led some authorities to believe that point prevalence may lead to serious underreporting. According to Link and colleagues, "The first problem is finding people who are currently homeless. Surveys may miss the so-called hidden homeless, who sleep in box cars, on the roofs of tenements, in campgrounds, or in other places that researchers cannot effectively search. [Even if located] . . . respondents may refuse to be interviewed or deliberately hide the fact that they are homeless."[5(p1907)] People who experience relatively short or intermittent episodes of literal homelessness are likely to be missed in brief surveys. To address these problems, Link et al. conducted a national household telephone survey to provide lifetime and five-year period prevalence estimates. They found that 14.0% of the sample had ever been homeless, 4.6% in the last five years. Compared with previous estimates based on point prevalence, the investigators concluded that the magnitude of the problem was much greater than previous estimates had indicated.

Prevalence data are useful in describing the health burden of a population, to estimate the frequency of an exposure, and in allocation of health resources, such as facilities and personnel. Typically, prevalence data are not as helpful for studies of etiology. There are several reasons for this, but the main concern has to do with the possible influences of differential survival. That is, for a case to be included in a prevalence study, he or she would have had to survive the disease long enough to participate. Cases who died before participation would obviously be missed, resulting in a truncated sample of eligible cases. Risk factors for rapidly fatal cases may be quite different from risk factors for less severe manifestations. One situation in which the use of prevalent cases may be justified for studies of disease etiology arises when a condition has an indefinite time of onset, such as occurs in mental illness.[1]

Incidence Rate (Cumulative Incidence)

The term *incidence* describes the rate of development of a disease in a group over a certain time period; this period of time is included in the denominator. An incidence rate (Exhibit 3-3) includes three important elements:

1. a numerator—the number of new cases
2. a denominator—the population at risk
3. time—the period during which the cases accrue

EXHIBIT 3-3

Incidence Rate

$$\text{Incidence rate} = \frac{\text{Number of new cases}}{\text{Total population at risk}} \quad \begin{array}{c}\text{over a time period} \times \\ \text{multiplier (e.g., 100,000)}\end{array}$$

The denominator consists of the population at risk (i.e., those who are at risk for contracting the disease).

Example: Calculate the incidence rate of postmenopausal breast cancer in the IWHS. The population at risk in this example would not include women who were still premenopausal ($n = 569$), women who had had their breasts surgically removed ($n = 1,870$), and women with a previous diagnosis of cancer ($n = 2,293$). Thus, the denominator is 37,105 women. After eight years of follow-up, 1,085 cases were identified through the State Health Registry. The incidence rate is therefore 1,085/37,105 per eight years. To express this rate per 100,000 population: divide 1,085 by 37,105 (answer: 0.02924). This is the rate over an eight-year period. Therefore, divide this number by eight years (answer: 0.003655) and multiply by 100,000. ■

Answer: 365.5 cases of postmenopausal breast cancer per 100,000 women per year.

Number of New Cases

The incidence rate uses the frequency of new cases in the numerator. This means that individuals who have a history of the disease are not included.

Population at Risk

The denominator for incidence rates is the population at risk. One therefore should exclude individuals who have already developed the disease of interest (e.g., those who have had heart attacks) or are not capable of developing the disease. For example, if one wanted to calculate the rate of ovarian cancer in the IWHS, women who had had their ovaries removed (oophorectomized women) should be excluded from the cohort at risk. It is not uncommon, however, to see some incidence rates based on the average population as the denominator rather than the population at risk. This distinction really must be made for those infectious diseases that confer lifetime immunity against recurrence. Regarding chronic diseases to which most people appear to be susceptible, the distinction is less critical. The population at risk may include those exposed to a disease agent or unimmunized or debilitated people, or it may consist of an entire population (e.g., a county, a city, or a nation). The population at risk may represent special risk categories; occupational injury and illness incidence rates are calculated for full-time workers in various occupations, for example, because these are the populations at risk.

Specification of a Time Period

The definition of incidence entails the designation of a time period, such as a week, a month, a year, or a multiyear time period. To determine an incidence rate, one must be able to specify the date of onset for the condition during the time period. Some acute conditions (e.g., a severe stroke or an acute myocardial infarction) may have a readily identifiable time of onset. Other conditions (e.g., cancer) may have an indefinite time of onset, which is defined by the initial definitive diagnosis date for the disease.[6]

Attack Rate

The attack rate (AR) is an alternative form of the incidence rate that is used when the nature of the disease or condition is such that a population is observed for a short time period, often as a result of specific exposure.[1] In reporting outbreaks of *Salmonella* infection or other foodborne types of gastroenteritis, epidemiologists employ the AR. The formula for the AR is:

$$AR = Ill/(Ill + well) \times 100 \text{ (during a time period)}$$

As shown in the formula, the numerator consists of people who are ill as a result of exposure to the suspected agent, and the denominator consists of all people, whether well or ill, who were exposed to the agent during a time period.

Although the AR often is used to measure the incidence of disease during acute infectious disease epidemics, it may also be used for the incidence of other conditions where the risk is limited to a short time period or the etiologic factors operate only within certain age groups. An example is hypertrophic pyloric stenosis, which occurs predominantly in the first three months of life and is practically unknown after the age of six months. Illustrations of the methods to calculate an AR and secondary AR are given in Chapter 12.

Risk Versus Rate

Epidemiologists have been known to use the terms risk and rate interchangeably. If pressed to explain the difference, however, they would be able (one hopes) to identify several key distinctions. First, risk is a statement of the probability or chance that an individual will develop a disease over a specified period, conditioned on that individual's not dying from any other disease during the period.[7] As such, risk ranges from 0 to 1 and is dimensionless. Statements of risk also require a specific reference period, for example, the five-year risk of developing asthma. Risk can be estimated as the cumulative incidence of a particular disease. The cumulative incidence is the proportion of a fixed population that becomes diseased during a stated period of time. The illustration regarding the incidence of postmenopausal breast cancer in the IWHS is an example of a cumulative incidence.

Because the population is fixed, no individuals are allowed to enter the denominator after the start of the observation period, and the numerator can include only individuals who were members of that fixed population. Calculation of cumulative incidence also requires that disease status be determined for everyone in the denominator. That is, once a group of individuals is selected for follow-up for disease occurrence, subsequent information about the occurrence of disease is obtained for everyone selected, which is difficult to achieve even in the best of circumstances. Most of the regions where we live and work contain dynamic populations; people move into and out of the area. Some individuals who were not in the study population at the baseline period may move into the region and become ill. Thus, the numerator has increased but the denominator has not. Conversely, if an individual moves away and then develops the disease, he or she would be counted in the denominator but not in the numerator. One solution to the problem of geographic mobility and loss to follow-up is to use rates as an indicator of risk. A simple perspective is that groups with high rates of disease are at greater risk than are groups with low rates of disease. The issue is a bit more complicated than that perspective (and beyond the scope of this book). The main caveat is that rates can be used to estimate risk only when the period of follow-up is short and the rate of disease over that interval is relatively constant. Thus, to estimate small risks, one simply multiplies the average rate times the duration of follow-up.[8]

A special problem occurs when a population or study group is under observation for different lengths of time. This may occur for a variety of reasons, including attrition or dropout, mortality, or development of the disease under study.

Consider the calculation of the incidence of postmenopausal breast cancer in the IWHS. Although the study was able to identify all cancers diagnosed within the state, some women may have moved out of state after the initial questionnaire administration. Any cancers diagnosed among these women would be unknown to the investigators. Other women died before the end of the follow-up period. In the previous calculation, we merely counted the number of cases over the eight-year period of follow-up ($n = 1,042$) and divided by the number of women at risk ($n = 37,105$). The implicit assumption of this calculation is that each of the 37,105 women was "observed" for the full eight-year period. Clearly, this could not be the case. To allow for varying periods of observation of the subjects, one uses a modification of the formula for the incidence in which the denominator becomes person-time of observation. Incidence density is defined in Exhibit 3-4.[1] An example of how to calculate person-years is shown in Table 3-1.

EXHIBIT 3-4

Incidence Density

$$\text{Incidence density} = \frac{\text{Number of new cases during the time period}}{\text{Total person-time of observation}}$$

When the period of observation is measured in years, the formula becomes:

$$\text{Incidence density} = \frac{\text{Number of new cases during the time period}}{\text{Total person-years of observation}}$$

Example: In the IWHS, the 37,105 women at risk for postmenopausal breast cancer contributed 276,453 person-years of follow-up. Because there were 1,085 incident cases, the rate of breast cancer using the incidence density method is 1,085/276,453 = 392.5 per 100,000 per year. Note that, had each woman been followed for the entire eight-year period of follow-up, the total person-years would have been 296,840. Because the actual amount of follow-up was 20,000 person-years less than this, the estimated rate of breast cancer was higher (and more accurate) using the incidence density method. ∎

In Table 3-1, person-years were derived simply by summing the product of each category of length of observation and the number of subjects in the category. A more difficult issue is how one actually determines the length of observation for each individual. Visiting again the IWHS example, a computer program was used to tabulate,

Table 3-1 Person-Years of Observation for Hypothetical Study Subjects in a 10-Year Heart Disease Research Project

A Number of Subjects	B Length of Observation (Years)	A × B Person-Years
30	10	300
10	9	90
7	8	56
2	7	14
1	1	1
Totals 50		461

Number of health events (heart attacks) observed during the 10-year period: 5

Incidence density = (5/461) × 100 = 1.08 per 100 person-years of observation

for each individual, the amount of time that elapsed from receipt of the mailed questionnaire until the occurrence of one of the following events (listed in order of priority): breast cancer diagnosis, death (if in Iowa), a move out of Iowa (if known through the National Change of Address Service), midpoint of interval between date of last contact and December 30, 1993, or midpoint of interval between date of last contact and date of death (for deaths that occurred out of Iowa, identified through the National Death Index). Women who did not experience any of these events were assumed to be alive in Iowa and contributed follow-up until December 30, 1993. This real-life example illustrates that actual computation of person-years, although conceptually straightforward, can be a fairly complicated procedure.

Interrelationship Between Prevalence and Incidence

Interrelationship: $P \cong ID$

The prevalence (P) of a disease is proportional to the incidence rate (I) times the duration (D) of a disease.

For conditions of short duration and high incidence, one may infer from this formula that, when the duration of a disease becomes short and the incidence is high, the prevalence becomes similar to incidence. For diseases of short duration, cases recover rapidly or are fatal, eliminating the build-up of prevalent cases. Some of the infectious diseases of short duration, such as the common cold, are examples. Many chronic diseases generally have a low incidence and long duration; as the duration of the disease increases, even though incidence is low the prevalence of the disease increases relative to incidence.

Figure 3-1 illustrates the relationship between incidence and prevalence. Suppose that there is an outbreak of meningococcal disease in a summer school class of 10 students. The frequency of the disease is recorded for two weeks. Individual cases plotted by the duration of each case for the period July 1 through July 14 are shown in Figure 3-1. For the 10-day period (July 5 through July 14), the period prevalence of meningococcal disease was 8/10; the point prevalence of disease on July 5 was 5/10. Because the disease in this example is one that can affect individuals more than once (no lifetime immunity after initial infection) the incidence rate of disease was 3/10. Note that on July 5 cases A, B, C, D, and F were existing cases of disease and were not included in the count for incidence; subsequently, case A was a recurrent case and should be counted once for incidence and twice for period prevalence. The measure of incidence would be more accurate if the cumulative duration of observation (person-days) were used in the denominator. If one was interested only in the first occurrence of meningococcal disease, then students A, B, C, D, and F would not have been included in the estimation of incidence, since they were prevalent cases on July 5. In that situation, the incidence would have been 2/5.

Applications of Incidence Data

It was noted earlier that prevalence data are useful for determining the extent of a disease (particularly chronic diseases) or health problem in the community. Prevalence data are not as helpful as incidence data for studies of etiology because of the possible influence of differential survival. Incidence data (e.g., cumulative incidence rates) help in research on the etiology of disease because they provide estimates of risk of developing the disease. Thus, incidence rates are considered to be fundamental tools in research that pursues the causality of diseases. Note how the incidence rate of postmenopausal breast cancer was calculated in the IWHS. As we shall see in Chapter 7, comparison of incidence rates in population groups that differ in exposures permits one to estimate the effects of exposure to a hypothesized factor of interest. This topic is discussed also in Chapter 9.

Crude Rates

The basic concept of a rate can be broken down into three general categories: crude rates, specific rates, and adjusted rates. Crude rates are summary rates based on the actual number of events in a population over a given time period.

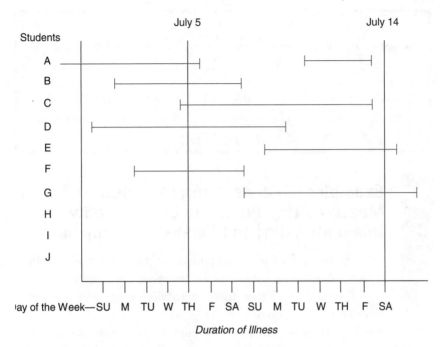

FIGURE 3-1 Outbreak of meningococcal infections in a summer school class of 10 students. *Note:* Students H, I, and J were not ill.

An example is the crude death rate, which approximates the proportion of a population that dies during a time period of interest.[4] Refer to the study questions and exercises at the end of this chapter for calculation problems. Some of the more commonly used crude rates are presented in Exhibit 3-5. The definitions for measures of natality (statistics associated with births) come from *Health United States 1990.*[9]

Birth Rate

The crude birth rate refers to the number of live births during a specified period of time (e.g., one calendar year) per the resident population during the midpoint of the time period (expressed as rate per 1,000). The crude birth rate is a useful measure of population growth and is an index for comparison of developed and developing countries; as noted in Chapter 2, the crude birth rate is generally higher in less developed areas than in more developed areas of the world. As an illustration of this measure, Figure 3-2 presents birth rates categorized by age of mother for the United States for 1960 to 1995.

$$\text{Crude birth rate} = \frac{\substack{\text{Number of live births} \\ \text{within a given period}}}{\substack{\text{Population size at the} \\ \text{middle of that period}}} \times 1{,}000 \text{ population}$$

Sample calculation: 4,111,000 babies were born in the United States during 1991, when the US population was 252,688,000. The birth rate was 4,111,000/252,688,000 = 16.3 per 1,000.

EXHIBIT 3-5

Examples of Crude Rates: Overview of Measures That Pertain to Birth, Fertility, Infant Mortality, and Related Phenomena

- *Crude birth rate:* used to project population changes; it is affected by the number and age composition of women of childbearing age.
- *Fertility rate:* used for comparisons of fertility among age, racial, and socioeconomic groups.
- *Infant mortality rate:* used for international comparisons; a high rate indicates unmet health needs and poor environmental conditions.
- *Fetal death rate (and late fetal death rate):* used to estimate the risk of death of the fetus associated with the stages of gestation.
- *Fetal death ratio:* provides a measure of fetal wastage (loss) relative to the number of live births.
- *Neonatal mortality rate:* reflects events happening after birth, primarily:
  1. Congenital malformations
  2. Prematurity (birth before gestation week 28)
  3. Low birth weight (birth weight less than 2,500 g)
- *Postneonatal mortality rate:* reflects environmental events, control of infectious diseases and improvement in nutrition. Since 1950, neonatal mortality in the United States has declined; postneonatal mortality has not declined greatly.
- *Perinatal mortality rate:* reflects events that occur during pregnancy and after birth; it combines mortality during the prenatal and postnatal periods.
- *Maternal mortality rate:* reflects health care access and socioeconomic factors; it includes maternal deaths resulting from causes associated with pregnancy and puerperium (during and after childbirth). ■

NOTE: Rates are plotted on a log scale.

FIGURE 3-2 Birth rates by age of mother: United States, 1960–1995. Source: Reprinted from SJ Ventura et al., *Monthly Vital Statistics Report*, vol 45, No 11, Suppl 2, 1997, National Center for Health Statistics.

Fertility Rate

There are several types of fertility rates; one of the most noteworthy is the general fertility rate. This rate consists of the number of live births reported in an area during a given time interval (for example, during 1 year), divided by the number of women aged 15 to 44 years in that area. The population size for the number of women aged 15 to 44 years is assessed at the midpoint of the year. Sometimes the age range of 15 to 49 years is used. Figure 3-3 illustrates fertility rates for the United States from 1950 to 1992. (The general fertility rate is often referred to more generically as the fertility rate.)

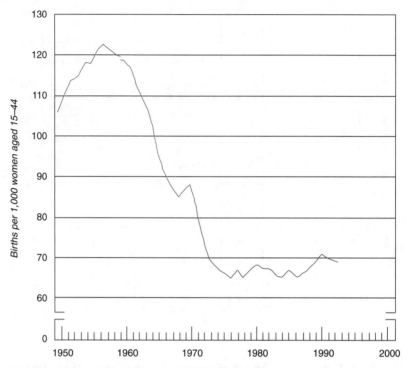

NOTE: Beginning with 1959, trend line is based on registered live births; trend line for 1950–1959 is based on live births adjusted for underregistration.

FIGURE 3-3 Fertility rates: United States, 1950–1992. *Source:* Reprinted from National Center for Health Statistics, Annual Summary of Births, Marriages, Divorces and Deaths, United States, 1992, *Monthly Vital Statistics Report,* vol 41, No 13, p 3, 1993.

$$\text{General fertility rate} = \frac{\text{Number of live births within a year}}{\text{Number of women aged 15–44 years during the midpoint of the year}} \times 1{,}000 \text{ women aged 15–44}$$

Sample calculation: During 1991, there were 59,139,000 women aged 15 to 44 in the United States. There were 4,111,000 live births. The general fertility rate was 4,111,000/59,139,000 = 69.5 per 1,000 women aged 15 to 44.

Infant Mortality Rate

The infant mortality rate measures the risk of dying during the first year of life among infants born alive. Note that not all infants who die in a calendar year are born in that year, which represents a source of error. Typically, however, the number of infant deaths from previous years' births is balanced by an equal number of deaths during the following year among the current year's births. The following is the definition of the infant mortality rate:

$$\text{Infant mortality} = \frac{\substack{\text{Number of infant deaths} \\ \text{among infants aged 0-365 days} \\ \text{during the year}}}{\substack{\text{Number of live births} \\ \text{during the year}}} \times 1{,}000 \text{ live births}$$

Sample calculation: In the United States during 1991, there were 36,766 deaths among infants under 1 year of age and 4,111,000 live births. The infant mortality rate was (36,766/4,111,000) × 1,000 = 8.9 per 1,000 live births.

Infant mortality rates are highest among the least developed countries of the world (approximately 120 per 1,000 births in 1991) in comparison with developing countries (70 per 1,000), Eastern Europe (20 per 1,000), and developed market economies (10 per 1,000).[10] Figure 3-4 shows trends in U.S. infant mortality by race from 1950 to 1995. Note how infant mortality rates have steadily declined, although the disparity between whites and African Americans is maintained.

Fetal Mortality

Fetal mortality indices depend on estimation of fetal death after a certain number of weeks of gestation. In the following three definitions, the gestation time is stated or presumed. The fetal death rate is defined as the number of fetal deaths after 20 weeks or more gestation divided by the number of live births plus fetal deaths (after 20 weeks or more gestation). It is expressed as rate per 1,000 live births and fetal deaths. The late fetal death rate refers to fetal deaths after 28 weeks or more gestation. Both measures pertain to a calendar year.

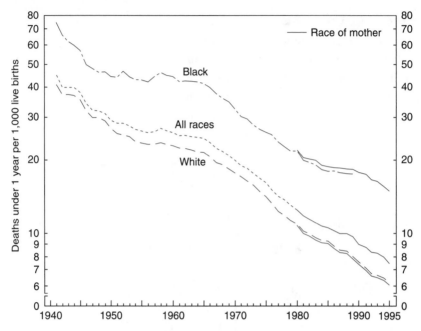

NOTE: Infant deaths are classified by race of descedent. 1940–90, live births are classified by race of child and for 1980–94, by race of mother.

FIGURE 3-4 Infant mortality rates by race: United States, 1950–1995. *Source:* Reprinted from RN Anderson, KD Kochanek, and SL Murphy, Report of Final Monthly Statistics, 1995, *Monthly Vital Statistics Report,* vol 45, No 11, Suppl 2, 1997, National Center for Health Statistics.

Fetal death rate (per 1,000 live births plus fetal deaths) =

$$\frac{\text{Number of fetal deaths after 20 weeks or more gestation}}{\text{Number of live births + number of fetal deaths after 20 weeks or more gestation}} \times 1{,}000$$

Late fetal death rate (per 1,000 live births plus late fetal deaths) =

$$\frac{\text{Number of fetal deaths after 28 weeks or more gestation}}{\text{Number of live births + number of fetal deaths after 28 weeks or more gestation}} \times 1{,}000$$

The fetal death ratio refers to the number of fetal deaths after gestation of 20 weeks or more divided by the number of live births during a year. It is expressed as rate per 1,000 live births.

Fetal death ratio =

$$\frac{\text{Number of fetal deaths after 20 weeks or more gestation}}{\text{Number of live births}} \times 1,000 \text{ (during a year)}$$

Sample calculation: During 1 year there were 134 fetal deaths with 20 weeks or more gestation and 10,000 live births. The fetal death ratio is (134/10,000) = 13.4 per 1,000. Note that the fetal death rate is (134/10,134) = 13.2 per 1,000, which is slightly lower than the fetal death ratio.

Neonatal Mortality Rate

The neonatal mortality rate measures risk of dying among newborn infants who are under the age of 28 days for a given year. The formula is as follows:

Neonatal mortality rate =

$$\frac{\text{Number of infant deaths under 28 days of age}}{\text{Number of live births}} \times 1,000 \text{ live births (during a year)}$$

Postneonatal Mortality Rate

A statistic that is related to the neonatal mortality rate is the postneonatal mortality rate. The postneonatal mortality rate measures risk of dying among older infants during a given year.

Postneonatal mortality rate =

$$\frac{\text{Number of infant deaths from 28 days to 365 days after birth}}{\text{Number of live births} - \text{neonatal deaths}} \times 1,000 \text{ live births}$$

Figure 3-5 illustrates trends in infant mortality rates, neonatal mortality rates, and postneonatal mortality rates in the United States. Note that infant and neonatal mortality rates showed a downward trend between 1960 and 1988; the

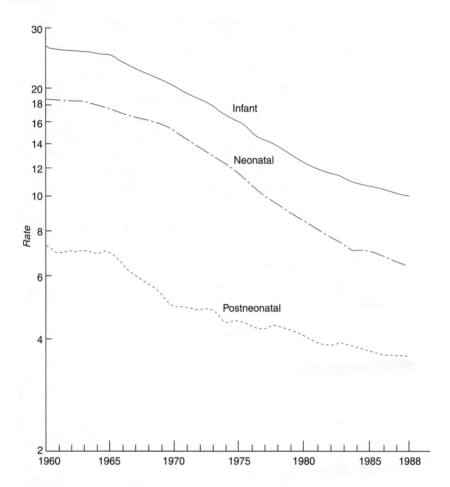

FIGURE 3-5 Infant, neonatal, and postneonatal mortality rates: United States, 1960–1988. Source: Reprinted from MF MacDorman and HM Rosenberg, Trends in Infant Mortality by Cause of Death and Other Characteristics, 1960–88, *Vital Health Statistics,* vol 20, No 20, p 5, 1993.

postneonatal mortality rate also declined during this time period, but not as steeply. The infant mortality rate is higher than neonatal and postneonatal mortality rates; in addition, both infant and neonatal mortality rates are higher than the postneonatal mortality rate.

Perinatal Mortality

Two measures of perinatal mortality are the perinatal mortality rate and the perinatal mortality ratio. The perinatal period used in these measures captures late fetal deaths plus infant deaths within seven days of birth.

Perinatal mortality rate =

$$\frac{\text{Number of late fetal deaths after}}{\text{28 weeks or more gestation +}} \times 1{,}000 \text{ live births and fetal deaths}$$

$$\frac{\text{infant deaths within 7 days of birth}}{\text{Number of live births +}} \times 1{,}000 \text{ live births and fetal deaths}$$
number of late fetal deaths

Perinatal mortality ratio =

$$\frac{\text{Number of late fetal deaths after}}{\text{28 weeks or more gestation +}} \\ \frac{\text{infant deaths within 7 days of birth}}{\text{Number of live births}} \times 1{,}000 \text{ live births}$$

Maternal Mortality Rate

The maternal mortality rate is the number of maternal deaths ascribed to childbirth (i.e., pregnancy and puerperal causes) per 10,000 or 100,000 live births. Factors that affect maternal mortality include maternal age, socioeconomic status, nutritional status, and health care access.

Maternal mortality rate
(per 100,000 live births, including multiple births) =

$$\frac{\text{Number of deaths assigned to}}{\text{causes related to childbirth}} \times 100{,}000 \text{ live births (during a year)}$$

Specific Rates

Although the crude rates described so far are important and useful summary measures of the occurrence of disease, they are not without limitations. A crude rate should be used with caution in making comparative statements about disease frequencies in populations. Observed differences between populations in crude rates of disease may be the result of systematic factors within the populations rather than true variations in rates. Systematic differences in sex or age distributions would affect observed rates. To correct for factors that may influence the make-up of populations and in turn influence crude rates, one may construct specific and adjusted rates. Specific rates refer to a particular subgroup of the population defined, for example, in terms of race, age, or sex, or they may refer to the entire population but be specific for some single cause of death or illness. Two other measures that have been defined previously also can be considered specific rates: incidence and prevalence. That is, both are typically specific to a particular end point.

Cause-Specific Rate

Cause-specific rate =

$$\frac{\text{Mortality (or frequency of a given disease)}}{\text{Population size at midpoint of time period}} \times 100,000$$

An example of a cause-specific rate is the cause-specific mortality rate. As the name implies, it is the rate associated with a specific cause of death. A sample calculation is shown in Table 3-2. The number of deaths among the 25- to 44-year age group (population 83,761,000) due to human immunodeficiency virus (HIV) infection was 22,795 during 1996. The cause-specific mortality rate due to HIV was (22,795/83,761,000), or 27.2 per 100,000.

Table 3-2 The 10 Leading Causes of Death, 25–44 Years, All Races, Both Sexes, United States, 1996 (Population 83,761,000)

Rank Order	Cause of Death	Number	Proportional Mortality Ratio (%)	Cause-Specific Death Rate per 100,000
1	Accidents and adverse effects	26,554	17.8	31.7
2	HIV infection	22,795	15.3	27.2
3	Malignant neoplasms	22,147	14.9	26.4
4	Diseases of heart	16,261	10.9	19.4
5	Suicide	12,536	8.4	15.0
6	Homicide and legal intervention	9,261	6.2	11.1
7	Chronic liver disease and cirrhosis	4,230	2.8	5.1
8	Cerebrovascular diseases	3,418	2.3	4.1
9	Diabetes mellitus	2,520	1.7	3.0
10	Pneumonia and influenza	1,972	1.3	2.4
	All causes	148,904		

Source: Data are from Births and Deaths: United States, 1996, *Monthly Vital Statistics Report,* vol 46, No 1, Suppl 2, p 33, 1997, National Center for Health Statistics; and *Statistical Abstract of the United States, 1997,* p 15, U.S. Bureau of the Census.

Proportional Mortality Ratio

The proportional mortality ratio (PMR) is the number of deaths within a population due to a specific disease or cause divided by the total number of deaths in the population.

PMR (%) =

$$\frac{\text{Mortality due to a specific cause during a time period}}{\text{Mortality due to all causes during the same time period}} \times 100$$

Sample calculation: In a certain community there were 66 deaths due to coronary heart disease during a year. There were 200 deaths due to all causes in that year. The PMR is (66/200) × 100 = 33%.

Refer to Table 3-2 for a more detailed example of a PMR. In Table 3-2, the PMR is calculated according to the formula given above. For example, the proportional mortality ratio for HIV among the 25- to 44-year group was 15.3% (22,795/148,904). This PMR should be used with caution when comparisons are made across populations, especially those that have different rates of total mortality. To illustrate, consider that two countries have identical death rates from cardiovascular disease (perhaps 5 per 100,000 per year) and that each country has exactly 1 million inhabitants. Therefore, one would expect 50 deaths from cardiovascular disease to occur in each country (5 per 100,000 per year × 1,000,000). Suppose further, however, that in country A the total death rate per 100,000 per year is 30 and that it is only 10 in country B. Therefore, the expected total number of deaths would be 300 in country A and only 100 in country B. When these data are used to construct a PMR, one sees that the proportion of deaths from cardiovascular disease is higher in country B (0.50) than in country A (0.17). The PMR is not a measure of the risk of dying of a particular cause. It merely indicates, within a population, the relative importance of a specific cause of death. For a health administrator, such information may be useful to determine priorities and planning. To an epidemiologist, such differences may indicate an area for further study. For example, why does country A have such higher total mortality rates than country B? Is it merely because of differences in age structure? Is the difference a result of access to health care or certain behavioral or lifestyle patterns associated with elevated mortality? The PMR is not to be confused with a case fatality rate (see Chapt. 12). The case fatality rate expresses the proportion of fatal cases among all cases of disease during a specific time period.

Age-Specific Rates

To calculate age-specific rates, one subdivides (or stratifies) a population into age groups, such as those defined by 5- or 10-year intervals. Then, one divides the frequency of a disease in a particular age stratum by the total number of persons within that age stratum to find the age-specific rate. A similar procedure may be employed to calculate sex-specific rates. An example of an age-specific cancer mortality rate is shown in Exhibit 3-6. A second example of the calculation of age-specific mortality rates for the U.S. population is shown in Table 3-3 (some age-specific death rates shown in Table 3-3 differ from published rates because of differences in estimation of population size and use of different intervals for age groups).

Table 3-4 presents a summary of unadjusted measures of morbidity and mortality discussed in Chapter 3. We provide this table to assist you with future review and reference to these measures.

Adjusted Rates

Specific rates are a much better indicator of risk than crude rates, especially if it is possible to construct rates specific to refined subsets of the population (e.g., age, race, and sex specific). However, in some instances, the stratum-specific data to derive such rates may not be available. In situations where this occurs, the use of

---

EXHIBIT 3-6

Age-Specific Rate

Age-specific rate: The number of cases per age group of population (during a specified time period).

Example:

$$\frac{\text{Number of deaths among those aged 5–14 years}}{\substack{\text{Number of persons who are aged 5–14 years} \\ \text{(during time period)}}} \times 100,000$$

Sample calculation: In the United States during 1991, there were 1,106 deaths due to malignant neoplasms among the age group 5 to 14 years, and there were 35,904,000 persons in the same age group. The age-specific malignant neoplasm death rate in this age group is (1,106/35,904,000) = 3.1 per 100,000. ∎

Table 3-3 Method of Calculation of Age-Specific Death Rates

Age Group (Years)	Number of Deaths in 1990	Number In Population as of April 1, 1990	Age-Specific Rate per100,000
Under 1	38,351	3,217,312	1,192.0
1–4	6,931	15,137,131	45.8
5–9	3,995	18,099,179	22.1
10–14	4,441	17,114,249	25.9
15–19	15,711	17,754,015	88.5
20–24	21,022	19,020,312	110.5
25–29	26,579	21,313,045	124.7
30–34	33,512	21,862,887	153.3
35–39	39,093	19,963,117	195.8
40–44	44,469	17,615,786	252.4
45–49	51,856	13,872,573	373.8
50–54	66,752	11,350,513	588.1
55–59	97,865	10,531,756	929.2
60–64	154,831	10,616,167	1,458.4
65–69	217,333	10,111,735	2,149.3
70–74	260,616	7,994,823	3,259.8
75–79	301,114	6,121,369	4,919.1
80–84	300,325	3,933,739	7,634.6
85+	463,105	3,080,165	15,035.1
Not stated	562	NA	NA
Totals	2,148,463	248,709,874	863.8*

*The crude mortality rate for the United States.

Source: Data are from US Department of Commerce, *1990 Census of the Population: General Population Characteristics,* p 425, November 1992, and from National Center for Health Statistics, Advance Report of Final Mortality Statistics, 1990, *Monthly Vital Statistics Report,* vol 41, No 7, p 15, 1993.

adjusted rates can be an extremely valuable alternative for evaluation of the magnitude of a health problem. In addition, specific rates can make it difficult to see the "big picture" in those situations where data are stratified on several factors. For example, Table 3-5 shows the age-specific cancer incidence rates by sex, age group, and year of diagnosis. Most people would find it difficult to synthesize the data from a 30 × 15 array and see any specific trends. Some readers may find it helpful to consider summary-adjusted rates for each individual year as a function of time (i.e., a 1 × 15 array of rates adjusted for age and sex). Adjusted rates are summary measures of the rate of morbidity or mortality in a population in which statistical procedures have been applied to remove the effect of differences in composition of the various populations. Note that each rate in Table 3-5 is age adjusted.

A common factor for rate adjustment is age, which is probably the most important variable in risk of morbidity and mortality, although rates can be adjusted for other variables. There are two methods for the adjustment of rates: the direct method and the indirect method. An easy way to remember how they differ is that

Table 3-4 Summary of Unadjusted Measures of Morbidity and Mortality Discussed in This Chapter*

Measure	Numerator (x)	Denominator (y)	Expressed per Number at Risk (10^n)
Age-specific rate (e.g., mortality rate)	Number of deaths among a specific age group of the population during a specified time period	Number of persons who comprise that age group during the same time period	100,000
Attack rate	Number ill during a time period	Number ill + well during the same time period	100 (or percent)
Case fatality rate (discussed in Chapt. 12)	Number of deaths due to disease "X" during a given time interval	Number of new cases of that disease reported during the same time interval	100 (or percent)
Cause-specific rate, e.g., cause-specific death or mortality rate	Number of deaths (mortality) assigned to a specific cause during a year	Estimated population size during the midpoint of that same year	100,000
Crude birth rate	Number of live births within a given period	Population size at the midpoint of that time period	1,000
Crude death rate	Number of deaths during a given year	Reference population during the midpoint of the year	100,000
Fetal death rate	Number of fetal deaths after 20 weeks or more gestation during a year	Number of live births + number of fetal deaths after 20 weeks or more gestation during the same year	1,000
Fetal death ratio	Number of fetal deaths after 20 weeks or more gestation during a year	Number of live births during the same year	1,000
General fertility rate	Number of live births within a year	Number of women aged 15–44 years during the midpoint of the year	1,000
Incidence density	Number of new cases during a time period	Total person-years of observation during the same time period	Varies, e.g., 100,000
Incidence rate	Number of new cases during a time period	Total population at risk during the same time period	Varies, e.g., 100,000

continues

Table 3-4 *continued*

Measure	Numerator (x)	Denominator (y)	Expressed per Number at Risk (10^n)
Infant mortality rate	Number of infant deaths under 1 year of age (0–365 days) during a year	Number of live births reported during that same year	1,000
Late fetal death rate	Number of fetal deaths after 20 weeks or more gestation during a year	Number of live births + number of fetal deaths after 28 weeks or more gestation during the same year	1,000
Maternal mortality rate	Number of deaths assigned to causes related to childbirth during a year	Number of live births during the same year	100,000
Neonatal mortality rate	Number of infant deaths under 28 days of age during a year	Number of live births during the same year	1,000
Perinatal mortality rate	Number of late fetal deaths after 28 weeks or more gestation + infant deaths within 7 days of birth during a year	Number of live births + number of late fetal deaths during the same year	1,000
Perinatal mortality ratio	Number of late fetal deaths after 28 weeks or more gestation + infant deaths within 7 days of birth during a year	Number of live births during the same year	1,000
Postneonatal mortality rate	Number of infant deaths from 28 days to 365 days after birth during a year	Number of live births - neonatal deaths during the same year	1,000
Proportional mortality ratio	Mortality due to a specific cause during a year	Mortality due to all causes during that same year	100 or 1,000

Note: The foregoing measures are expressed in the general form $\frac{x}{y} \times 10^n$.

direct and indirect refer to the source of the rates. The direct method may be used if age-specific death rates in a population to be standardized are known and a suitable standard population is available. The direct method is presented in Table 3-6. Note that each age-specific rate found in Table 3-3 is multiplied by the number of persons in the age group in the standard population. The U.S. population in 1940 is used as

Table 3–5 15-Year Trends: Age-Specific Cancer Incidence Rates* (By Sex, Age Group, and Year of Diagnosis, SEER Program, 1973–1987; All Sites Combined, All Races)

Sex/Age	Year of Diagnosis														
	1973	1974	1975	1976	1977	1978	1979	1980	1981	1982	1983	1984	1985	1986	1987
Males & Females	319.9	332.3	331.8	337.2	336.6	336.7	340.2	344.0	349.7	350.2	355.4	362.4	368.9	369.9	377.2
0-54	97.2	101.7	98.7	100.7	99.9	98.9	98.0	97.5	98.3	97.3	97.8	100.9	103.7	105.4	106.6
0-14	12.6	13.0	11.3	12.7	12.7	13.0	12.9	12.7	12.1	12.8	12.7	13.6	14.0	13.7	13.4
15-34	35.8	37.8	38.1	37.5	39.0	38.2	37.9	37.9	38.2	38.5	39.1	39.4	40.7	41.7	40.0
35-44	160.3	159.4	159.2	151.8	156.5	159.3	152.1	154.3	155.5	156.6	160.8	169.3	172.2	176.1	178.0
45-54	405.0	431.8	413.9	433.3	419.3	410.9	412.7	407.6	412.5	402.1	399.9	410.5	422.7	429.6	441.2
55-64	844.4	896.7	900.6	899.6	887.9	896.9	893.4	897.5	925.3	929.7	943.0	955.1	982.5	953.4	961.7
65+:	1660	1700	1717	1756	1767	1768	1814	1853	1878	1887	1924	1958	1976	1998	2055
65-74	1457	1483	1496	1520	1532	1529	1583	1614	1632	1650	1686	1720	1741	1773	1806
75+	1992	2054	2076	2139	2151	2158	2192	2242	2280	2274	2312	2345	2359	2364	2461
Males	365.2	372.1	377.8	388.9	392.7	394.8	400.5	407.5	411.5	411.7	419.2	423.0	426.8	430.7	441.9
0-54	77.5	79.4	77.9	80.4	83.0	81.6	81.4	83.2	82.0	81.5	83.3	84.9	87.7	90.9	91.1
0-14	14.1	14.3	12.3	13.6	12.7	13.9	13.3	12.7	12.9	13.6	13.8	13.9	14.9	15.0	14.1
15-34	30.8	31.4	32.3	30.9	32.7	31.9	33.0	33.8	33.8	33.4	36.1	36.3	38.0	40.0	38.0
35-44	106.0	99.8	104.7	102.2	115.5	107.9	104.4	107.6	106.4	111.6	117.0	121.1	128.9	132.3	136.4
45-54	328.5	346.3	333.3	353.9	356.4	353.7	354.0	363.3	355.2	346.2	345.9	352.1	356.9	371.4	375.6
55-64	882.6	910.0	924.4	948.2	936.6	960.2	963.2	979.1	1010	1007	1024	1032	1059	1019	1025
65+:	2245	2274	2331	2401	2429	2439	2496	2538	2560	2568	2613	2632	2623	2672	2779
65-74	1854	1884	1914	1948	1991	1997	2040	2071	2102	2100	2142	2164	2165	2213	2283
75+	2883	2911	3012	3139	3143	3160	3239	3298	3305	3331	3381	3394	3370	3419	3588

continues

Table 3-5 *continued*

Sex/Age	1973	1974	1975	1976	1977	1978	1979	1980	1981	1982	1983	1984	1985	1986	1987
Females	293.2	311.0	306.7	307.7	303.5	302.3	304.3	305.4	312.3	313.4	316.5	326.3	334.5	333.4	338.4
0-54:	116.1	123.1	118.6	120.2	116.2	115.5	114.0	111.4	114.0	112.6	111.8	116.6	119.1	119.5	121.7
0-14	11.0	11.6	10.3	11.9	12.6	12.0	12.5	12.7	11.3	12.0	11.5	13.4	13.0	12.3	12.7
15-34	40.8	44.1	43.8	44.1	45.3	44.4	42.6	41.9	42.5	43.5	42.1	42.6	43.4	43.3	42.0
35-44	212.7	217.2	212.2	200.1	196.3	209.4	198.8	200.1	203.7	200.8	203.7	216.7	214.8	219.1	218.9
45-54	477.4	513.1	490.4	508.8	479.2	465.3	468.5	449.7	467.1	455.6	451.5	466.4	485.7	485.5	504.3
55-64	809.5	885.1	879.3	856.0	844.1	839.8	830.6	824.2	849.6	860.4	870.4	885.8	914.3	894.6	905.0
65+:	1268	1320	1318	1337	1339	1336	1377	1416	1441	1453	1483	1528	1563	1568	1591
65-74	1148	1173	1176	1192	1181	1170	1231	1262	1267	1300	1330	1375	1410	1429	1432
75+	1463	1559	1550	1574	1597	1607	1617	1668	1724	1702	1732	1777	1813	1793	1849

*Rates are per 100,000 and are age adjusted to the 1970 US standard population. Each rate has been age-adjusted by 5-year age group.

Source: Reprinted from CL Kosary et al, *SEER Cancer Statistics Review, 1973–1992: Tables and Graphs,* p II.23, 1995, NIH Pub No 96-2789, National Cancer Institute.

Table 3–6 Direct Method for Adjustment of Death Rates

Age Group (Years)	1990 Age-Specific Death Rate per 100,000	Number in Population, 1940	Expected Number of Deaths
Under 5	246.7	10,541,524	26,007.0
5–9	22.1	10,684,622	2,358.1
10–14	25.9	11,745,935	3,042.2
15–19	88.5	12,333,523	10,913.9
20–24	110.5	11,587,835	12,806.9
25–29	124.7	11,096,638	13,838.6
30–34	153.3	10,242,388	15,699.5
35–39	195.8	9,545,377	18,692.7
40–44	252.4	8,787,843	22,184.0
45–49	373.8	8,255,225	30,858.0
50–54	588.1	7,256,846	42,677.5
55–59	929.2	5,843,865	54,303.5
60–64	1,458.4	4,728,340	68,958.1
65–69	2,149.3	3,806,657	81,816.9
70–74	3,259.8	2,569,532	83,761.9
75+	8,104.5	2,643,125	214,211.3
Totals		131,671,215	702,130.2

Age-adjusted rate per 100,000 =
(total expected number of deaths/1940 population) x 100,000 .... 533.2

Source: Age-specific death rates are from Table 3–3. Data are from U.S. Bureau of the Census, *Statistical Abstract of the United States,* 1957, p 28.

the standard in Table 3-6 (see Exhibit 3-7 for information on the development of the year 2000 standard for age adjustment). The result is the expected number of deaths in each age group, which is then summed across all age groups to determine the total number of expected deaths. The age-adjusted rate is the total expected number of deaths divided by the total 1940 population times 100,000: $[(702{,}130.2/131{,}671{,}215) \times 100{,}000] = 533.2$ per 100,000. To summarize, direct adjustment requires the application of the observed rates of disease in a population to some standard population to derive an expected number (rate) of mortality. The same procedure would be followed for other populations that one might wish to compare. By standardizing the observed rates of disease in the populations being compared to the same reference population, one is thereby assured that any observed differences that remain are not simply a reflection of differences in population structure with respect to factors such as age, race, and sex.

A second method of age adjustment is the indirect method, which may be used if age-specific death rates of the population for standardization are unknown or unstable (e.g., because the rates to be standardized are based on a small population). The stratum-specific rates of a larger population, such as that of the United

EXHIBIT 3-7

The National Center for Health Statistics Adopts a New Standard Population for Age Standardization of Death Rates

The crude death rate is a widely used measure of mortality. However, crude rates are influenced by the age composition of the population. As such, comparisons of crude death rates over time or between groups may be misleading if the populations being compared differ in age composition. This is relevant, for example, in trend comparisons of U.S. mortality, given the aging of the U.S. population. . . . The crude death for the United States rose from 852.2 per 100,000 population to 880.0 during 1979–1995. This increase in the crude death rate was due to the increasing proportion of the U.S. population in older age groups that have higher death rates. Age standardization, often called *age adjustment*, is one of the key tools used to control for the changing age distribution of the population, and thereby to make meaningful death comparisons of vital rates over time and between groups. In contrast to the rising crude rate, the age-adjusted death rate for the United States dropped from 577.0 per 100,000 U.S. standard population to 503.9 during 1979-1995. This age-adjusted comparison is free from the confounding effect of changing age distribution and therefore better reflects the trend in U.S. mortality. To use age adjustment requires a standard population, which is a set of arbitrary population weights.

The new standard is based on the year 2000 population, and beginning with data year 1999 will replace the existing standard based on the 1940 population. . . . Currently, at least three different standards are used among Department of Health and Human Services agencies. Implementation of the year 2000 standard will reduce confusion among data users and the burden on state and local agencies. Use of the year 2000 standard also will result in age-adjusted death rates that are substantially larger than those based on the 1940 standard. Further, the new standard will affect trends in age-adjusted rates for certain causes of death and will narrow race differentials in age-adjusted death rates. ■

Source: Adapted from RN Anderson and HM Rosenberg, Age Standardization of Death Rates: Implementation of the Year 2000 Standard, *National Vital Statistics Reports,* Vol 47, No 3, p 1, 1998, National Center for Health Statistics.

States, are applied to the number of persons within each stratum of the population of interest to obtain the expected numbers of deaths. Thus, the indirect method of standardization does not require a knowledge of the actual age-specific incidence or mortality rates among each age group for the population to be standardized. By applying the rates of disease from a standard population to the observed structure of the population of interest, one is left with an expected number of cases (or deaths) in the study population if the rates of disease were the same as in the standard population. One way to evaluate the result is to construct a standardized morbidity ratio or a standardized mortality ratio (SMR).

> SMR =
>
> $\dfrac{\text{Observed deaths}}{\text{Expected deaths}} \times 100$
>
> *Sample calculation:* The number of observed deaths due to heart disease is 600 in a certain county during year 2003. The expected number of deaths is 1,000. The SMR = (600/1,000) × 100 = 60% (0.6).

If the observed and expected numbers are the same, the SMR would be 1.0, indicating that the observed morbidity or mortality in the study population is not unusual. An SMR of 2.0 is interpreted to mean that the death (or disease) rate in the study population is two times greater than expected.

A second example of the indirect method of adjustment is shown in Table 3-7. Note that the standard age-specific death rates from Table 3-3 (the standard population) were multiplied by the number in each age group of the population of interest to obtain the expected number of deaths. To calculate the SMR, the observed number of deaths was divided by the expected number. The crude mortality rate is 502/230,109 = 218.2 per 100,000. The SMR is (502/423)×100 = 118.7%. From the SMR, one may conclude that the observed mortality in this population exceeds expectations, because the SMR is greater than 1.0 or 100%. Note that construction of an SMR is not the only way to interpret the net effect of the indirect adjustment procedure. An alternative is to use, rather than the observed number of events in the study population as the numerator, the expected number of deaths (or morbid events) based on the rates observed in your standard population. Referring to the example in Table 3-7, the total population size was 230,109 and the total expected number of deaths was 423. The adjusted death

Table 3-7 Illustration of Indirect Age Adjustment: Mortality Rate Calculation for a Fictitious Population of 230,109 Persons

Age (Years)	Number in Population of Interest	Death Rates (per 100,000) in Standard Population	Expected Number of Deaths in Population of Interest
20–24	7,989	110.5	8.8
25–29	37,030	124.7	46.2
30–34	60,838	153.3	93.3
35–39	68,687	195.8	134.5
40–44	55,565	252.4	140.3
Total expected number of deaths			423
Observed number of deaths in this population			502

Source: Standard death rates are from Table 3-3.

rate would be $423/230,109 \times 100,000 = 183.8$ per 100,000 per year. In comparison, the unadjusted death rate was $502/230,109$ or 218.2 per 100,000 per year.

It is important to be aware that the numeric magnitude of an SMR in this situation is a reflection of the standard population. That is, if one were to use the age distribution of the 1970 U.S. population instead of the 1940 U.S. population for age adjustment, the adjusted rates that one would find would be quite different. Accordingly, SMRs for different populations typically cannot be compared with one another unless the same standard population has been applied to them. In addition, SMRs sometimes can be misleading: As a summary index, the overall SMR can be equal to 1.0 across different populations being compared, yet there might still be important differences in mortality in various subgroups. Finally, the longer a population is followed, the less information the SMR provides. Because it is expected that everyone in the population will die eventually, the SMR will tend to be equal to 1.0 over time.

Conclusion

This chapter defined several measures of disease frequency that are commonly employed in epidemiology. Counts or frequency data refer to the number of cases of a disease or other health phenomenon being studied. A ratio consists of a numerator and a denominator that express one number relative to another (e.g., the sex ratio). Prevalence is a measure of the existing number of cases of disease in a population at a point in time or over a specified period of time. A rate is defined as a proportion in which the numerator consists of the frequency of a disease during a period of time and the denominator is a unit size of population. Rates improve one's ability to make comparisons of health indices across contrasting populations. Examples of rates include the crude mortality rate, incidence rates, and infant mortality rates. Other examples of rates discussed were the birth rate, fertility rate, and perinatal mortality rate. Specific rates are more precise indicators of risk than crude rates. It was noted that, to make comparisons across populations, adjusted rates also may be used. Two techniques were presented on how to adjust rates. Finally, the chapter gave illustrations of how the standardized mortality ratio (an example of indirect adjustment) is used.

Study Questions and Exercises

1. Define the following terms:
   a. crude death rate
   b. age-specific rate
   c. cause-specific rate
   d. proportional mortality ratio (PMR)
   e. maternal mortality rate
   f. infant mortality rate
   g. neonatal mortality rate
   h. fetal death rate and late fetal death rate
   i. fetal death ratio
   j. perinatal mortality rate
   k. postneonatal mortality rate
   l. crude birth rate
   m. general fertility rate
   n. age-adjusted (standardized) rate
   o. direct method of adjustment
   p. indirect method of adjustment
   q. standardized mortality ratio (SMR)
2. Using Table 3A-1 in the Appendix at the end of this chapter, calculate age-specific lung cancer death rates. What inferences can be made from the age-specific death rates for lung cancer?
3. Using Table 3A-2 in the Appendix at the end of this chapter, calculate the following for the United States: The age-specific death rates and age- and sex-specific death rates per 100,000 (for age groups 15 to 24, 25 to 34, and 35 to 44 years). Note that there are nine calculations and answers.

One answer is as follows: The age- and sex-specific death rate for females aged 15 to 24 years is 48.1 per 100,000 [(8,467/17,594,565)×100,000].

4. Refer to Table 3A-3 in the Appendix at the end of this chapter. The total population in 1995 was 262,755,720 (males = 128,313,798; females = 134,441,472).

   a. Calculate the crude death rate (per 100,000) and the cause-specific death rates (per 100,000) for accidents, neoplasms, and viral hepatitis. Repeat these calculations for males and females separately.

   b. What is the PMR (percent) for accidents, neoplasms, and viral hepatitis? Repeat these calculations for males and females separately.

5. Refer to both Table 3A-2 and Table 3A-3 in the Appendix at the end of this chapter. For 1995, the total number of live births was 3,899,598. Calculate the:

   a. maternal mortality rate (per 100,000 live births)
   b. infant mortality rate (per 1,000 live births)
   c. crude birth rate (per 1,000 population)
   d. general fertility rate (per 1,000 women aged 15 to 44 years)

6. Give definitions of the terms prevalence and incidence. What are appropriate uses of prevalence and incidence data? State the relationships among prevalence, incidence, and duration of a disease.

7. Suppose that "X" represents the name of a disease. An epidemiologist conducts a survey of disease "X" in a population. The prevalence of disease "X" among women is 40/1,000 and among men is 20/1,000. Assuming that the data have been age adjusted, is it correct to conclude that women have twice the risk of disease "X" as men? Explain.

References

1. Hennekens CH, Buring JE. *Epidemiology in Medicine.* Boston, MA: Little, Brown; 1987.
2. Folsom AR, Kaye SA, Sellers TA, et al. Body fat distribution and 5-year risk of death in older women. *JAMA.* 1993;269:331–339.
3. Sellers TA, Kushi LH, Potter JD, et al. Effect of family history, body-fat distribution, and reproductive factors on the risk of postmenopausal breast cancer. *N Engl J Med.* 1992;326:1323–1329.
4. Last JM, ed. *A Dictionary of Epidemiology,* 3rd ed. New York, NY: Oxford University Press; 1995.
5. Link BG, Susser E, Stueve A, Phelan J, Moore RE, Struening E. Lifetime and five-year prevalence of homelessness in the United States. *Am J Public Health.* 1994;84:1907–1912.

6. Mausner JS, Kramer S. *Epidemiology: An Introductory Text.* 2nd ed. Philadelphia, PA: Saunders; 1985.

7. Kleinbaum DG, Kupper LL, Morgenstern H. *Epidemiologic Research: Principles and Quantitative Methods.* Belmont, CA: Lifetime Learning; 1982.

8. Rothman KJ. *Modern Epidemiology.* Boston, MA: Little, Brown; 1986.

9. National Center for Health Statistics. *Health United States 1990.* Hyattsville, MD: Public Health Service; 1991.

10. World Health Organization (WHO). *World Health Statistics Annual 1992.* Geneva, Switzerland: WHO; 1993.

APPENDIX
3

Data for Study Questions 2 Through 5

Table 3A-1 Lung Cancer Deaths by Age Group, United States, 1995

Age (Years)	Population	Lung Cancer* Deaths
5–14	38,134,488	11
15–24	35,946,635	41
25–34	40,873,139	303
35–44	42,467,719	2,709
45–54	31,078,760	12,356

*Includes ICD-9, 1975 codes 160–165.

Source: Data are from Report of Final Mortality Statistics, 1995, *Monthly Vital Statistics Report,* vol 45, No 11, Suppl 2, pp 34 and 76, 1997, National Center for Health Statistics.

Table 3A-2 Mortality by Selected Age Groups, Males and Females, United States, 1995

Age (Years)	Males Population	Males Number of Deaths	Females Population	Females Number of Deaths	Total Population	Total Number of Deaths
15–24	18,352,070	25,777	17,594,565	8,467	35,946,635	34,244
25–34	20,431,915	41,826	20,441,224	15,919	40,873,139	57,745
35–44	21,061,683	70,131	21,406,036	32,139	42,467,719	102,270

Source: Data from Report of Final Mortality Statistics, 1995, *Monthly Vital Statistics Report,* vol 45, No 11, Suppl 2, pp 60 and 76, 1997, National Center for Health Statistics.

Table 3A-3 Total Mortality from Selected Causes, Males and Females, United States, 1995

	Males	Females	Total
All causes	1,172,959	1,139,173	2,312,132
Accidents [a]	61,401	31,919	93,320
Malignant neoplasms [a]	281,611	256,844	538,455
Viral hepatitis	2,076	1,324	3,400
Infant deaths	16,622	12,961	29,583
Maternal deaths	NA	277	277

Source: Data are from Report of Final Mortality Statistics, 1995, *Monthly Vital Statistics Report,* vol 45, No 11, Suppl 2, pp 40, 42, and 71, 1997, National Center for Health Statistics..

Descriptive Epidemiology: Person, Place, Time

Introduction

The basic premise of epidemiology is that disease does not occur randomly, but rather in patterns that reflect the operation of underlying factors. Therefore, it is critical to the ultimate elucidation of etiology that these patterns be carefully and accurately described. The purpose of this chapter is to provide a brief survey of some of the ways that one can describe the pattern of disease. Each of the characteristics falls into one of three categories: person, place, or time. By using the tools in Chapter 3 regarding how to measure the frequency of disease, one can now extend the process to consider more intimately the details of the occurrence of disease. Person characteristics speak to the question of who is being affected: young versus old? males versus females? rich versus poor? overnourished versus undernourished? more educated versus less educated? Throughout the remainder of the chapter, a variety of personal characteristics are identified that may help describe the pattern of disease and help generate hypotheses regarding the underlying causes. Place speaks to the question of where the problem is occurring: urban versus rural? some states more than others? only in particular cities? national versus international variation? in regions of high altitude or low altitude? where there is plentiful rainfall or little rainfall? in polluted areas more than unpolluted areas? Time refers to the issue of when the problem is occurring: Was there a sudden increase over a short period of time? Is the problem greater in winter than in summer? Is the problem gradually increasing over long periods of time or increasing greatly over just a few years? The occurrence of disease with respect to the characteristics of person, place, and time is central to the field of epidemiology.

Person, place, and time may directly or indirectly relate to the occurrence of illness because they affect a wide range of exposures associated with lifestyle, behavior patterns, access to medical care, and exposure to environmental hazards, to name a few. Being male, for example, is more likely to be associated with accidental death or injury than being female; behavior patterns characteristic of a particular ethnic group may affect subcultural levels of stress and methods for coping with social stresses. Suchman[1] referred to these variables as social group membership factors that affect perceptions, interpretations, and reactions to the social and physical environment. Membership in specific groups influences "exposure to and patterns of perceiving, interpreting, and reacting to health hazards."[1(p109)] We shall observe also that combinations of variables, for example, age and sex, are noteworthy.

Descriptive Versus Analytic Epidemiology

It is important at this point to make a distinction between two broad categories of epidemiologic studies. Descriptive studies are concerned with characterizing the amount and distribution of disease within a population. Analytic studies, on the other hand, are concerned with the determinants of disease, the reasons for relatively high or low frequency of disease in specific population subgroups. Descriptive studies generally precede analytic studies: The former are used to identify any health problems that may exist, and the latter proceed to identify the cause(s) of the problem.

Objectives of Descriptive Epidemiology

It is possible to identify three broad objectives that characterize the utility of descriptive epidemiology:

1. to permit evaluation of trends in health and disease and comparisons among countries and subgroups within countries; this objective includes monitoring of known diseases as well as the identification of emerging problems
2. to provide a basis for planning, provision, and evaluation of health services; data needed for efficient allocation of resources often come from descriptive epidemiologic studies
3. to identify problems to be studied by analytic methods and to suggest areas that may be fruitful for investigation

The acquired immune deficiency syndrome (AIDS) epidemic illustrates how these objectives are implemented. Descriptive data on the epidemiology of AIDS provided an indication of the emergence of the epidemic (objective 1), were useful for allocation of hospital beds and treatment centers (objective 2), and spurred etiologic studies into why intravenous drug users and gay and bisexual men were more likely than other groups to develop the disease (objective 3).

Descriptive Studies and Epidemiologic Hypotheses

The third objective relates to the use of descriptive epidemiology to aid in the creation of hypotheses. "For any public health problem, the first step in the search for possible solutions is to formulate a reasonable and testable hypothesis."[2(p112)] "*Hypotheses* are suppositions that are tested by collecting facts that lead to their acceptance or rejection. They are not assumptions to be taken for granted, neither are they beliefs that the investigator sets out to prove. They are 'refutable predictions.'"[3(p40)] Three common ways of stating hypotheses are as follows[3]:

1. Positive declaration (research hypothesis): The infant mortality rate is higher in one region than another.
2. Negative declaration (null hypothesis): There is no difference between the infant mortality rates of two regions.
3. Implicit question: To study the association between infant mortality and geographic region of residence.

Hypotheses should be made as explicit as possible and not left as implicit.

Mill's Canons

What is the source of hypotheses that guide epidemiologic research? The logical processes for deriving hypotheses are patterned after John Stuart Mill's canons of inductive reasoning.[4] The following are four of his canons:

1. the method of difference
2. the method of agreement
3. the method of concomitant variation
4. the method of residues

The Method of Difference

All of the factors in two or more places are the same except for a single factor. The frequency of a disease that varies across the two settings is hypothesized to result from variation in the single causative factor. The method of difference has been employed widely in epidemiologic research. It is similar to classic experimental design. A hypothetical example of its use would be the study of the role of physical activity in reducing morbidity from coronary heart disease (CHD). Suppose groups of workers in the same factory were compared when the factors of age, diet, socioeconomic status, and other variables were constant. The hypothesis would be that differences in morbidity from CHD are due to level of physical activity, that is, sedentary workers are at greater risk of developing heart attacks than physically active workers.

The Method of Agreement

A single factor is common to a variety of different settings. It is hypothesized that the common factor is a cause of the disease. Wherever air pollution is present, for example, there is an increased prevalence of chronic respiratory diseases, such as emphysema. This finding leads to the hypothesis that air pollution, if present, is a contributing factor to lung diseases.

The Method of Concomitant Variation

The frequency of a disease varies according to the potency of a factor, and this linked association suggests that the factor is the causative agent for the disease. An example confirmed by a large body of research is that the incidence of bronchitis, emphysema, and lung cancer is directly related to the number of cigarettes smoked by an individual. That is, the greater the number of cigarettes smoked, the greater the risk of incurring these conditions.

The Method of Residues

The method of residues involves subtracting potential causal factors to determine which individual factor or set of factors makes the greatest impact upon a dependent variable. In research on heart disease, statistical methods similar to the method of residues (e.g., multiple regression analysis) have been used to determine which of a number of risk factors may be associated with coronary attack or death from CHD. The individual contribution to CHD of one's heredity, diet, stress level, amount of exercise, and blood lipid level can be quantified. One then can determine which has the greatest impact.

The Method of Analogy

The fifth method for developing hypotheses is taken from MacMahon and Pugh.[5] The mode of transmission and symptoms of a disease of unknown etiology bear a pattern similar to that of a known disease. It is suggested by this information that the unknown disease is caused by an agent similar to that of the known disease. There are many examples of this method in the field of infectious diseases. The symptoms of Legionnaires' disease are similar to those produced by an infectious respiratory disease agent of either viral or bacterial origin.

Categories of Descriptive Epidemiology

In Chapter 3 we covered the role of counts in epidemiology. It was argued that, although counts are sometimes useful, they are usually more informative when expressed relative to a denominator (as a proportion). One could view case reports (counts) as the simplest category of descriptive epidemiology. Astute clinical observations on unusual cases may spur additional investigation to determine whether there is a large number of cases with similar presentations and to explore underlying mechanisms. Because it can be difficult to draw firm conclusions from a single case report, one may wish to extend the observations to include a case series. Typically this series involves a summary of the characteristics of a consecutive listing of patients from one or more major clinical settings. Having a large number of observations permits the generation of summary measures to help derive typical features. The third major category of descriptive epidemiology comprises cross-sectional studies. These are surveys of the population to estimate the prevalence of a disease or exposures. One can sometimes use data from repeated cross-sectional surveys at different points in time to examine time trends in prevalence of disease or risk factors. Cross-sectional studies are covered in greater detail in Chapter 6.

Characteristics of Persons

Age

Age is perhaps the most important factor to consider when one is describing the occurrence of virtually any disease or illness. This is because there is greater variation in age-specific disease rates than in rates defined by almost any other personal attribute. That is why public health professionals use age-specific rates when comparing the disease burden between populations. Otitis media (ear infections), measles, mumps, and chickenpox tend to occur most commonly in childhood. Acne is generally a problem among teenagers. Chronic diseases become the dominant sources of morbidity and mortality in later life (Fig. 4-1). For example, cancer incidence tends to increase with age, as demonstrated by the generally log-linear increase in age-specific incidence rates that decelerate later in life. Note in Figure 4-1 how the cancer incidence rates by sex and race increase with increasing age groups. The apparent decline around age 70 is somewhat deceptive because the rates are presented on a log scale and because the size of the numerators and denominators for the very elderly categories are smaller than for other age groups, resulting in unstable estimates.

Some health conditions may show multimodal age-specific curves, meaning that there are several peaks and declines in the frequency of the diseases at various ages. One example is tuberculosis, which has two peaks, one between age 0 and 4 years and another around age 20 to 29 years. Another example is Hodgkin's disease, which shows a peak in the mid-20s and another in the early 70s.[5] Bimodal (two-peak) distributions for these conditions may suggest two different causal mechanisms. For example, in the case of tuberculosis the increase in prevalence of the disease in the early years of life may be due to the increased susceptibility of

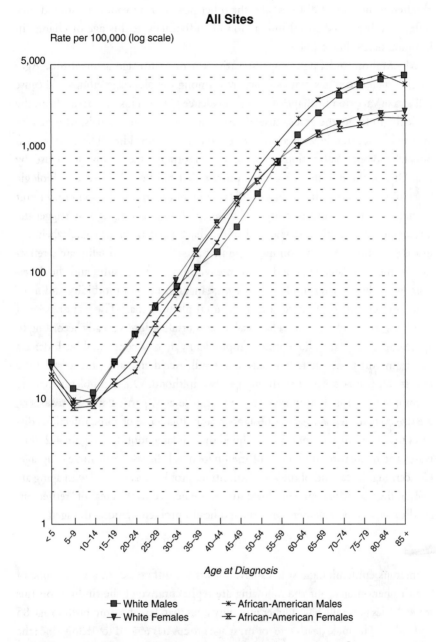

FIGURE 4-1 Age-specific incidence rates for all cancer sites by race and sex, 1986-1990, United States. *Source:* Reprinted from *SEER Cancer Statistics Review: 1973–1990* by BA Miller et al., p II.33, National Cancer Institute, National Institutes of Health, Publication No 93-2789, 1993.

children to infectious diseases, and the other peak during young adulthood may reflect the increased social interaction of individuals at this age or change in immune status due to puberty.

MacMahon and Pugh[5] suggest various reasons for age associations. Age-specific incidence rates may be inaccurate among the older age groups and cause artifactual variation in shape of an age-incidence graph. This may result from the difficulty in fixing the exact cause of death among older individuals, who may be afflicted concurrently with a number of sources of morbidity. There are several possible biologic explanations for increases in mortality due to chronic diseases by age. One of these is an endogenous process that has been likened to a biologic clock phenomenon. After a certain age, waning of the immune system may result in increasing tissue susceptibility to disease, or chronologic aging may trigger the appearance of conditions that are believed to have a genetic basis (e.g., Alzheimer's disease). Another explanation might be that age effects on mortality are a reflection of the long latency period between environmental exposures and the development of disease later in life. Many age changes in rates of morbidity and mortality are related to life cycle and behavioral phenomena.[6] The importance of accidents, homicide, and suicide as causes of mortality differs greatly according to age group. For infants, developmental problems, such as congenital birth defects and immaturity are the major causes of death. Accidents and violence take the largest toll from adolescence through early adulthood. Other problems that are becoming increasingly important to American society, particularly for teenagers, are unplanned pregnancy and substance abuse. Incidence of some infectious diseases may be more common in childhood than in later adult life. Figure 4-2 illustrates the decreasing incidence of meningococcal disease with increasing age. Concerning the far end of the age distribution, problems associated with aging are also on the rise. More epidemiologic studies are needed in the areas of "retirement syndrome," the bereavement process, and health problems among the aged.

Sex

Numerous epidemiologic studies have shown sex differences in a wide scope of health phenomena, but the following are representative of the findings on this topic. Males generally have higher mortality rates than females from birth to age 85 and older.[7] The male death rate for most age groups has tended to decline since the late 1960s; an exception is the death rate among the 34- to 44-year age group, which declined until 1983 and 1984, when it began to rise and continued to rise as of the early 1990s. With some exceptions, the female age-specific death rates have generally shown decreases since 1950. In the early 1990s the age-adjusted death

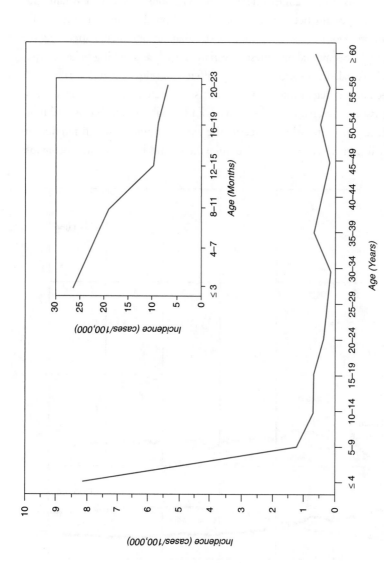

FIGURE 4-2 Incidence of meningococcal disease, by age group, selected U.S. areas, 1989–1991. *Source:* Reprinted from Centers for Disease Control and Prevention, Laboratory-Based Surveillance for Meningococcal Disease in Selected Areas—United States, 1989–1991, *MMWR*, vol 42, No SS-2, p 25, June 4, 1993.

rate for males was 1.7 times that for females, which compares to a ratio of 1.5:1 in 1950.[6] Male versus female morbidity differences are the reverse of this, however, because females have higher age-standardized morbidity rates for acute conditions, chronic conditions, and disability due to acute conditions.[8] Data for mortality due to lung cancer, especially between 1975 and 1990, show that the mortality rate for this cause among women increased much faster than among men, supporting the view that certain behavioral and lifestyle variables, such as smoking behavior may relate to male/female lung cancer mortality differences (Figs. 4-3 and 4-4).

The speculations regarding the sources of sex differences in mortality are as fascinating as the discrepancy between males and females in morbidity and mortality. An interesting question concerns the extent to which sex differences in mortality will narrow as the lifestyle, employment, and health-related behaviors

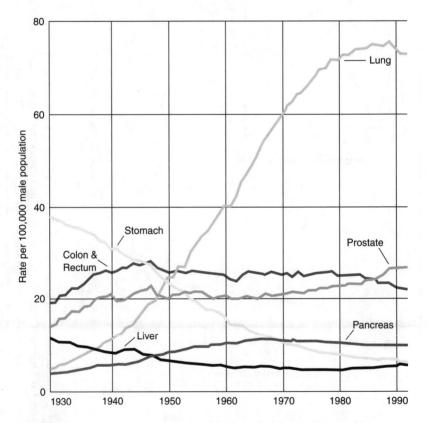

FIGURE 4-3 Age-adjusted cancer death rates, males, by site, United States, 1930–1993. *Source:* Reprinted by permission of the American Cancer Society, Inc.

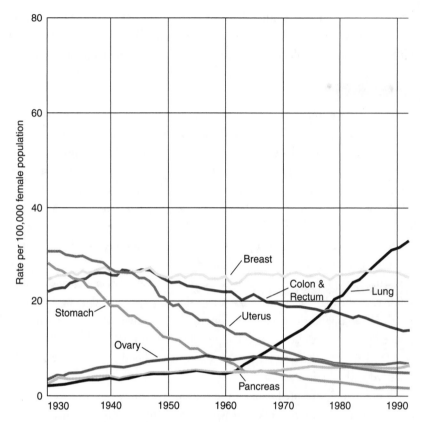

FIGURE 4-4 Age-adjusted cancer death rates, females, by site, United States, 1930–1993. *Source:* Reprinted by permission of the American Cancer Society, Inc.

of women become equalized to those of men. Specific research studies have investigated genetic and environmental factors, differentials in exposure to stress, reporting of illness, and the effects of women's changing role in society upon mortality. Waldron[9] attributed higher male mortality to greater frequency of smoking, a greater prevalence of the coronary-prone behavior pattern, higher suicide and motor vehicle accident rates, and other behavioral patterns that are expected of and condoned among men. Sex differences in mortality may result from social factors that have not yet been delineated.[10]

Coronary heart disease (CHD) is the leading cause of death for both men and women. However, sex differences in mortality from CHD persist between men and women, even when both have high-risk factor status for serum cholesterol, blood pressure, and smoking. This finding implicates important biologic parameters as the basis for the observed differences (e.g., differences in hormonal profiles). Production of estrogen changes during menopause; the result is that heart disease typically does not leave its mark on women until after age 60.

Marital Status

In general, epidemiologic research has shown that married individuals have lower rates of morbidity and mortality than those who are single, divorced, or widowed (especially men). An analysis of nationwide trends showed lower rates of mortality from chronic diseases among married individuals for coronary diseases, ulcer, and many forms of cancer as well as for many of the infectious diseases, suicide, and motor vehicle accidents.[11] Divorced persons, especially divorced men, have the highest death rates among the unmarried groups.[12] Over the past several decades, divorced and widowed persons in their 20s and 30s have had a higher risk of dying than married persons of the same age.

Marital status is related to suicide rates. In a northern urban area with a high suicide rate, the highest suicide rates occurred among widows, the lowest among married persons, and the next lowest among single individuals. The rate among divorced persons was also high and approached about 60% of the rate for widows.[13] Other research, however, suggests that widowhood may not be adversely associated with physical health.[14]

Schottenfeld[15] presented data on the risk of developing breast cancer among single compared with ever-married women and for ever-married nulliparous women compared with parous married women. Married women had reduced risk of cancer mortality in comparison with single women, and among all married women childbirth slightly reduced the risk of breast cancer. A prospective study of survival of melanoma and breast cancer patients found that marital status was unrelated to cancer survival once the disease process was established.[16]

Marriage may operate as either a protective or a selective factor in health.[17] The marital state somehow may provide a beneficial environment that makes a positive contribution to health, perhaps through its influence on lifestyle factors or because of social support. According to the marital selection model, married people may be less likely than nonmarried people to possess physical characteristics, such as obesity, that are perceived by some as unattractive. This model did not appear to be supported in research that found the marital role to be associated with obesity among men, but not women.[18] Married men were *more* likely to be obese or overweight than never-married or previously married men. Among women, in comparison, marital status was not associated with being overweight. Another aspect of the selection model is that people who become married are healthier in the first place, resulting in lower mortality rates among married persons. In summary, the marital environment or factors associated with marriage apparently reduces risk of death and, therefore, should be considered a possible source of differences in disease rates.[17]

Race and Ethnicity

Race and ethnicity are, to some extent, ambiguous characteristics that tend to overlap with nativity and religion. In Census 2000, the U.S. Bureau of the Census classified race into five major categories: white; black or African American; American Indian and Alaska Native; Asian; Native Hawaiian and other Pacific Islander. To a degree, race tends to be synonymous with ethnicity because people who come from a particular racial stock also may have a common ethnic and cultural identification. Also, assignment of some individuals to a particular racial classification on the basis of observed characteristics may be difficult. Often, one must ask the respondent to elect the racial group with which he or she identifies. The response one elicits from such a question may not be consistent: Individuals may change ethnic or racial self-identity or respond differently on different occasions, depending on their perception of the intent of the race question. Classification of persons of mixed racial parentage also may be problematic.[19] The 2000 census allowed respondents to check a multiracial category, which was used for the first time. Changes in the definitions of racial categories affect the denominators (i.e., the numbers in a particular racial subgroup) of rates used to track various health outcomes and the consequent assessments of unmet needs and social inequalities in health.[20] Assuming that race can be measured with some degree of truth, it does have implications for differences in incidence and prevalence of disease, as numerous epidemiologic studies have determined. Noteworthy variations in the rates of disease and risk factors for disease have been identified by using race as a variable in epidemiologic and public health research.[21] For more definitions and explanations of the race questions used in Census 2000, refer to Exhibit 4-1.

An illustration of variation by race from the National Center for Health Statistics for U.S. infants born in 1983 shows that infant mortality rates due to birth defects were highest among American Indians (2.9 deaths per 1,000 live births), followed by Asians and Hispanics (2.6) and African Americans (2.5).[22] Other illustrations follow.

African Americans

According to a study of differential mortality in the United States, African Americans had the highest mortality of any of several racial groups examined.[11] The age-standardized mortality rates for African Americans were 47% and 28%

EXHIBIT 4-1

Overview of Race and Hispanic Origin, Census 2000

Understanding Race and Hispanic Origin Data From Census 2000

The 1990 census questions on race and Hispanic origin were changed for Census 2000

The federal government considers race and Hispanic origin to be two separate and distinct concepts. For Census 2000, the questions on race and Hispanic origin were asked of every individual living in the United States. The question on Hispanic origin asked respondents if they were Spanish, Hispanic, or Latino. The question on race asked respondents to report the race or races they considered themselves to be. Both questions are based on self-identification. The question on Hispanic origin for Census 2000 was similar to the 1990 census question, except for its placement on the questionnaire. For Census 2000, the question on Hispanic origin was asked directly before the question on race. For the 1990 census, the order was reversed—the question on race preceded questions on age and marital status, which were followed by the question on Hispanic origin. The question on race for Census 2000 was different from the one for the 1990 census in several ways. Most significantly, respondents were given the option of selecting one or more race categories to indicate their racial identities. Because of these changes, the Census 2000 data on race are not directly comparable with data from the 1990 census or earlier censuses. Caution must be used when interpreting changes in the racial composition of the U.S. population over time.

[Refer to Figure 1 for the questions on race and Hispanic origin used in Census 2000.]

How are the race categories used in Census 2000 defined?

"White" refers to people having origins in any of the original peoples of Europe, the Middle East, or North Africa. It includes people who

continues

EXHIBIT 4-1 *continued*

indicated their race or races as "White" or wrote in entries such as Irish, German, Italian, Lebanese, Near Easterner, Arab, or Polish.

"Black or African American" refers to people having origins in any of the black racial groups of Africa. It includes people who indicated their race or races as "Black, African Am., or Negro," or wrote in entries such as African American, Afro American, Nigerian, or Haitian.

"American Indian and Alaska Native" refers to people having origins in any of the original peoples of North and South America (including Central America), and who maintain tribal affiliation or community

Continues on next page.

NOTE: Please answer BOTH Questions 5 and 6.

5. **Is this person Spanish/Hispanic/Latino?** *Mark* ☒ *the "No" box if not Spanish/Hispanic/Latino.*
   - ❏ **No**, not Spanish/Hispanic/Latino
   - ❏ Yes, Mexican, Mexican Am., Chicano
   - ❏ Yes, Puerto Rican
   - ❏ Yes, Cuban
   - ❏ Yes, other Spanish/Hispanic/Latino—*Print group.*

6. **What is this person's race?** Mark ☒ **one or more races** to indicate what this person considers himself/herself to be.
   - ❏ White
   - ❏ Black, African Am., or Negro
   - ❏ American Indian or Alaska Native—Print name of enrolled or principal tribe.

❏ Asian Indian	❏ Japanese	❏ Native Hawaiian
❏ Chinese	❏ Korean	❏ Guamanian or Chamorro
❏ Filipino	❏ Vietnamese	❏ Samoan
❏ Other Asian—*Print race.*		❏ Other Pacific Islander—*Print race.*

   - ❏ Some other race—*Print race.*

EXHIBIT 4-1, FIGURE 1 Reproduction of questions on race and Hispanic origin from Census 2000. *Source:* U.S. Census Bureau, Census 2000 questionnaire.

continues

EXHIBIT 4-1 *continued*

attachment. It includes people who indicated their race or races by marking this category or writing in their principal or enrolled tribe, such as Rosebud Sioux, Chippewa, or Navajo.

"Asian" refers to people having origins in any of the original peoples of the Far East, Southeast Asia, or the Indian subcontinent. It includes people who indicated their race or races as "Asian Indian," "Chinese," "Filipino," "Korean," "Japanese," "Vietnamese," or "Other Asian," or wrote in entries such as Burmese, Hmong, Pakistani, or Thai.

"Native Hawaiian and Other Pacific Islander" refers to people having origins in any of the original peoples of Hawaii, Guam, Samoa, or other Pacific Islands. It includes people who indicated their race or races as "Native Hawaiian," "Guamanian or Chamorro," "Samoan," or "Other Pacific Islander," or wrote in entries such as Tahitian, Mariana Islander, or Chuukese.

[Refer to Table 1 for a distribution of the U.S. population according to race.]

Exhibit 4-1, Table 1: Population by race and Hispanic origin for the United States, 2000

Race and Hispanic or Latino	Number	Percent of Total Population
RACE		
Total population	281,421,906	100.0
One race	274,595,678	97.6
White	211,460,626	75.1
Black or African American	34,658,190	12.3
American Indian and Alaska Native	2,475,956	0.9
Asian	10,242,998	3.6
Native Hawaiian and Other Pacific Islander	398,835	0.1
Some other race	15,359,073	5.5
Two or more races	6,826,228	2.4
HISPANIC OR LATINO		
Total population	281,421,906	100.0
Hispanic or Latino	35,305,818	12.5
Not Hispanic or Latino	246,116,088	87.5

Source: U.S. Census Bureau, Census 2000 Redistricting (Public Law 94-171) Summary File, Tables PL1 and PL2.

Source for Exhibit 4-1: Adapted and reprinted from EM Grieco and RC Cassidy. *Overview of race and Hispanic origin: Census 2000 brief.* Available at: http://www.census.gov/ prod/2001pubs /c2kbr01-1.pdf. Accessed July 16, 2003.

above the rates for white males and females, respectively. Figure 4-5 presents life expectancy by race and sex in the United States between 1970 and 1995. African-American males have the lowest life expectancy rates of the four groups shown.

The Hypertension Detection and Follow-Up Program found that, among both sexes, 37.4% of African Americans and 18.0% of whites age 30 years and older were hypertensive.[23] Apparently, higher blood pressure levels among African Americans result in higher rates of hypertensive heart disease and higher mortality from hypertension and stroke than are found among whites.[24] A number of factors could account for increased rates of hypertension among African Americans, including dietary factors and exposure to stress. Among psychologic and physical correlates of elevated blood pressure in a sample of urban African American adolescents, obesity was the single strongest predictor of elevated blood pressure.[25]

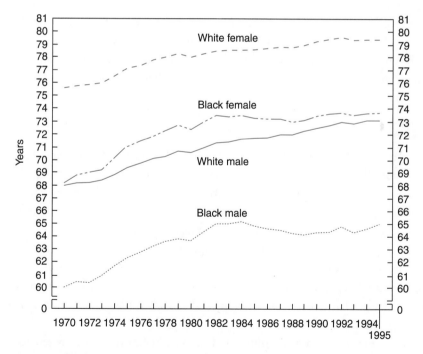

FIGURE 4-5 Life expectancy by sex, United States, 1970-1995. *Source:* Reprinted from RN Anderson, KD Kochanek, and SL Murphy, *Monthly Vital Statistics Report*, Vol 45, No 11, Supp 2, p 6, 1997, National Center for Health Statistics.

Among adolescent boys, impaired psychologic well-being (i.e., having an emotional or personal problem) was associated with elevated blood pressure.

American Indians

Knowler et al.[26] studied the incidence and prevalence of diabetes mellitus in nearly 4,000 Pima Indians aged 5 years and older over a 10-year period. This is a group of North American Indians who are native to Arizona. The investigators reported a diabetes prevalence of about 21%, adjusting for age and sex; the incidence rate was about 26 cases per 1,000. Diabetes incidence was about 19 times greater than that of a predominantly white comparison population in Rochester, Minnesota.

During 1975 through 1984, the Pima Indians who resided in the Gila River Indian community had a death rate of 1.9 times that for all races in the United States. Among men aged 25 to 34 years, the Pima death rate was 6.6 times that for all races in the United States. Diseases of the heart and malignant neoplasms accounted for 59% of the U.S. deaths in 1980, but only 19% for the American Indian community. The age- and sex-adjusted mortality rate was 5.9 times the rate for all races in the United States for accidents, 6.5 times for cirrhosis of the liver, 7.4 times for homicide, 4.3 times for suicide, and 11.9 times for diabetes. Tuberculosis and coccidioidomycosis also were important causes of death in the Pima, for whom infectious disease was the 10th leading cause of death among all causes of death.[27]

Asians

The Japanese, in comparison with other racial groups in the United States, have low mortality rates: one-third the rates for whites of both genders.[11] The Japanese culture seems to afford a protective influence that results in lower mortality, especially from chronic diseases, such as CHD and cancer. The orientation of the Japanese culture even in this age of industrialization is toward conformity and group consensus rather than toward the "rugged individualism" and competitiveness that pervade the American culture.[28] Degree of acculturation to Japan was related to low rates of CHD mortality.[28] Acculturation is defined as modifications that individuals or groups undergo when they come into contact with another culture.[29]

According to Marmot,[30] "Among industrialised countries, Japan is remarkable for its low rate of ischaemic heart disease. It is unlikely to be the result of some genetically-determined protection, as Japanese migrants to the USA lose this apparent protection."[30(p378)] The Honolulu Heart Study prospectively followed a large population of men of Japanese ancestry who resided on the island of Oahu at the beginning of the study.[31,32] Various measures of the degree of early exposure to Japanese culture were collected, including: birthplace in Japan; total number of years of residence in that country; ability to read, write, and speak Japanese; and a preference for the Japanese diet. After adjusting for the influence of well-established risk factors for CHD (age, serum cholesterol, systolic blood pressure, and cigarette smoking), there was a gradient in incidence of CHD across variables related to identification with the Japanese culture. For example, men who could read and write Japanese well had an incidence rate about half that reported for those who could neither read nor write Japanese. Other studies of Japanese men living in Japan, Hawaii, and California have shown an increasing gradient in mortality, prevalence, and incidence of CHD from Japan to Hawaii to California. Observed lower rates of CHD in Japan in comparison with the United States have been attributed to a low-fat diet among the Japanese and to institutionalized stress-reducing strategies (e.g., community bonds and group cohesion) within Japanese society.[33]

Studies of acculturation among the Japanese provide evidence that environmental and behavioral factors influence chronic disease rates and provide a rationale for intervention and prevention of chronic disease.[34] The Japanese who migrated shared a common ethnic background. After migrating to diverse geographic and cultural locales, they experienced a shift in rates of chronic disease to rates more similar to those found in the host countries.

Hispanics/Latinos

In the United States, Hispanic/Latino populations include the major groups— Mexican Americans, Puerto Ricans, and Cubans—as well as other groups that have migrated to the United States from Latin America. In comparison with other whites, Latinos have unique morbidity and mortality profiles. Mexican Americans represent one of the dominant ethnic minorities in the southwestern United States. However, this group has been relatively under-researched for prevalence of hypertension, CHD, diabetes, and other chronic diseases. The first special population survey of Hispanics in the United States was the Hispanic Health and Nutrition Examination Survey (HHANES). Conducted by the National Center for Health Statistics, HHANES assessed the health and nutritional status of Mexican Americans, mainland Puerto Ricans, and Cuban Americans.[35] An entire supplement of the *American Journal of Public Health* covered findings from HHANES.[36] As more research is conducted among Latinos, it is becoming apparent that they are highly diverse and should be studied as distinct subpopulations (e.g., Cuban Americans or Salvadoran Americans). Low rates of CHD among Mexican

Americans may be due to cultural factors, such as dietary preferences and the availability of social support mechanisms found in large and extended family systems. A study of CHD among Puerto Ricans reported a low prevalence of this condition.[37]

A major epidemiologic investigation of diabetes and other cardiovascular risk factors in Mexican Americans and non-Hispanic whites is the San Antonio Heart Study.[38] Among the findings were the high prevalence of obesity and non–insulin-dependent diabetes mellitus among the Mexican-American population.

Nativity and Migration

Nativity refers to the place of origin of the individual or his or her relatives. A common subdivision used in epidemiology is foreign born or native born. Thus, nativity is inextricably tied to migration because foreign-born persons have immigrated to their host country. As a result, nativity and migration frequently overlap the epidemiologic categories of race, ethnicity, and religion, because streams of immigrants may bring their cultural and religious practices to the new land, or may comprise a common racial background.

The phenomenon of migration meets the criteria for a natural experiment in which the effects of change from one environment can be studied. For example, migration research has examined various health dimensions, including stress, acculturation, chronic disease, and infectious disease. Classic epidemiologic research conducted in the late 1930s examined rates of admission to mental hospitals in New York State. Admission rates were higher among foreign-born than native-born persons, suggesting that foreign-born individuals may experience stresses associated with migration to a new environment.[5]

Another impact of migration has been to modify the profile of infectious diseases seen in public health departments throughout the developed world. Some immigrants from Southeast Asia and Mexico may import "Third World" diseases to the United States. For example, local health departments in Southern California have found that intestinal parasites, malaria, and certain other tropical diseases may occur among newly arrived immigrants from endemic areas in developing countries; the same conditions are rare in the resident U.S. population. One of the implications of migration from developing countries has been the need to establish specialized tuberculosis and nutritional screening programs for refugees and the need to reeducate physicians with respect to formerly uncommon (in the United States) tropical diseases. The inadequate immunization status of some migrants and refugees with respect to measles and other vaccine-preventable diseases has hampered the efforts of health officials to eradicate these conditions in the United States.

Researchers who strive to examine the health of migrants are confronted with significant methodologic challenges. One of them is the difficulty in separating environmental influences in the host country from selective factors operative among those who choose to migrate. The term *healthy migrant effect* acknowledges the observation that healthier, younger persons usually form the majority of migrants. Nevertheless, despite methodologic difficulties, such as the healthy migrant effect, migration research is a fascinating area that has already yielded many intriguing findings. For a review, refer to Friis, Yngve, and Persson.[39]

Religion

One's religious beliefs also may exert important influences on the rates of morbidity and mortality to the extent that certain religions stipulate prescribed lifestyles or that religiosity has health impacts. A thoughtful review of the subject of religion and health pointed out that the epidemiologic literature on this topic is extensive, with several hundred epidemiologic studies reporting statistically significant associations between religious indicators and morbidity and mortality.[40] While there is definitive evidence of an association between these two dimensions, the question remains unanswered as to whether the association is causal. We provide several examples of work in this area that examine the occurrence of morbidity and mortality among population subgroups classified by religious membership.

The Seventh-Day Adventist church endorses a lacto-ovovegetarian diet (meat, poultry, or fish less than once per week with no restriction on egg or dairy consumption). Members are required to abstain from alcohol, tobacco, and pork products.[41] The low rates of CHD observed among this religious group suggest that the corresponding lifestyle has health benefits. The Seventh-Day Adventists also have been reported to have low mortality rates from other chronic diseases. Armstrong et al.[42] studied Seventh-Day Adventists in western Australia and found that mean systolic and diastolic blood pressures were significantly lower than those of the comparison population. Phillips[43] also reported findings of reduced risk of cancer and other chronic diseases among the Seventh-Day Adventist population.

Jarvis[44] summarized findings on Mormons and other groups and presented data on Mormon mortality rates in Canada. He noted that, compared with the general U.S. population, Mormons have lower incidence and mortality rates due to cancer and other diseases. The study of mortality rates among Mormons in Alberta, Canada, generally confirmed mortality findings for the United States. Jarvis speculated that mortality differences may be due to restrictions on the intake of coffee, tea, and meats and lifestyle variables related to physical fitness, social support, and a stress-reducing religious ideology. Data on Mormons in Alameda County, California, corroborate findings from previous descriptive studies of an unusually low risk for cancer.[45]

Socioeconomic Status (SES)

Social class variations in health have been observed, formally and informally, since the beginning of organized society. The relationship between social class and health is remarkably consistent, having been demonstrated for a wide range of health outcomes and confirmed by a massive body of evidence.[46] Particularly noteworthy are social class differences in mortality, with persons lower in the social hierarchy having higher mortality rates than do persons in upper levels.[47] Link, et al. wrote, "This dynamic connection between SES and risk factors has led to the observation of a persistent association between SES and mortality. We refer to social conditions whose association with mortality persists in this manner as 'fundamental social causes' of inequalities in health."[48(p377)] Enduring low income is especially consequential for mortality.[49] Berkman and Syme[50] concluded that low social class standing is related to excess mortality, morbidity, and disability rates. Some of the more obvious explanations for the negative health effects of low social class membership are poor housing, crowding, racial disadvantages, low income, poor education, and unemployment. A complex web of factors includes exposure to environmental and work-related hazards, both material and social deprivation, lack of access to health care, and negative lifestyle. Socioeconomic factors also may play a role in the association of race and ethnicity with health.[51]

> There is a striking consistency in the distribution of mortality and morbidity between social groups. The more advantaged groups, whether expressed in terms of income, education, social class or ethnicity, tend to have better health than the other members of their societies. The distribution is not bipolar (advantaged vs. the rest) but graded, so that each change in the level of advantage or disadvantage is in general associated with a change in health.[52(p903)]

Measurement

Much of the terminology of social class that is used in epidemiologic research has been derived from sociology, in particular the branch of sociology dealing with social class and social stratification. Social class also is related to ethnicity, race, religion, and nativity. This is because some ethnic and other minority groups often occupy the lowest social class rankings in the United States. There are several different measures of social class that draw upon the individual's economic position in society. Such measures include the prestige of the individual's occupational or social position, educational attainment, income, or combined indices of two or more of these variables. Occupational prestige is often employed as a measure of social class. For example, learned professionals (e.g., physicians, college professors, lawyers, and similar occupational groups) are accorded the highest occupational prestige, and other occupations are ranked below them. A measure of occupational prestige derived by the British Registrar General has five levels of occupational prestige. The U.S. Bureau of the Census has derived a ranked measure of occupational status that has more levels with finer categories within each one of the major levels. Some measures of social class represent a composite of variables, including occupation, education, and income.[53] Two approaches are illustrative of the work in this field. Hollingshead and Redlich[54] derived a two-factor measure of social class that combines level of education with occupational prestige. Duncan[55] also developed a three-factor socioeconomic status index that has been used in epidemiologic research.

Problems arise in the assignment of social class to unemployed or retired persons and to students, who may ultimately occupy a high social class position in society upon graduation but who temporarily have low income and occupational prestige. It is difficult to assign social class ranking to a family when both mother and father work and have occupations that are disparate in occupational prestige. People who occupy the same category of occupational prestige may be quite diverse in income and other characteristics.

Measurement of income also is fraught with difficulty. The individual may not want to reveal income information or may not actually know the precise income of the family, as in the case of children, when it is necessary for the researcher to measure their social class. Also, two workers who have low-status occupations may have a combined family income that is higher than the total family income of one professional worker. The correct method for assigning social class in these situations may not be readily discernible.

Education (measured by number of years of formal schooling completed) is another component of socioeconomic status. Higher levels of education, in contrast to income or occupation, appear to be the strongest and most important predictor of positive health status.[53]

Findings

In spite of the unreliability of measures of social class, studies of the association between social class and health have yielded noteworthy findings, and thus social class usually should be considered when one is evaluating the occurrence of disease. Among the major illustrations of the association between social class and health are the findings on the frequency of mental illness. Exhibit 4-2 is one of the most noteworthy studies in this field, carried out by Hollingshead and Redlich,[54] who surveyed New Haven, Connecticut, and reported that as socioeconomic status increased, the severity of mental illness decreased.

Dunham[56] and others proposed two alternative hypotheses for the finding of highest incidence of severe mental illness among the lowest social classes. One, the social causation explanation (known as the breeder hypothesis), suggested that conditions arising from membership in the low social class groups produced schizophrenia and other mental illnesses.[57] However, an equally plausible explanation was the downward drift hypothesis, which stated that the clustering of psychosis was an artifact of drift of schizophrenics to impoverished areas of a city. Murphy et al.[58] indicated that during the 1950s and the 1960s the prevalence of depression

---

EXHIBIT 4-2

Socioeconomic Status and Mental Illness Survey of New Haven, Connecticut

Hollingshead and Redlich[54] classified New Haven, Connecticut, into five social class levels according to prestige of occupation, education, and address. These were some of the findings of the study:

- There was a strong inverse association between social class and the likelihood of being a mental patient under treatment.
- With respect to severity of mental illness, upper socioeconomic individuals were more likely to be neurotics, whereas lower socioeconomic individuals were more likely to be psychotics (i.e., less severe forms of mental illness occurred in the upper social class strata, and the highest incidence of schizophrenia was found in the lowest social classes).
- The type of treatment varied by socioeconomic status ranking. It was more common for upper socioeconomic individuals to receive treatment from a psychiatrist, whereas lower socioeconomic status individuals were treated in state and public hospitals, where they received organic modes of treatment, such as shock therapy.

was significantly and persistently higher in the low socioeconomic status population than at other socioeconomic levels. Stresses associated with poverty may be linked to depression, which in turn may be associated with subsequent downward social mobility. This hypothesis is consonant with the view that the concentration of depressed people at the lower end of the social hierarchy may result from handicapping aspects of the illness. Although epidemiologic research that shows variation in mental disorders by position in social structures has generated great excitement, additional work is needed to develop adequate theories to explain these findings.[56]

Low social class standing correlates with increased rates of infectious disease, including tuberculosis, rheumatic fever, influenza, and pneumonia, and other respiratory diseases.[50] It is reasonable to attribute increased rates of these conditions to overcrowding, increased exposure to infection, lack of medical care, nutritional deficiencies, and poor sanitary conditions.

In comparison with upper socioeconomic groups, lower socioeconomic groups have higher infant mortality rates and overall mortality rates and lower life expectancy.[59] The influence of psychosocial and behavioral factors on differential health outcomes associated with varying socioeconomic status levels is not fully understood.[60] Social class differences in mortality and morbidity have persisted over time, even with overall reductions in infant mortality and infectious diseases.[50] Life expectancies, based on data from the National Longitudinal Mortality Study for 1979 to 1985, were estimated for white men and white women by education, family income, and employment status. Life expectancy varied directly with amount of schooling and family income.[61] Although inadequate medical care and exposure to environmental hazards may account for some of the social differences in morbidity and mortality, other factors also may be relevant, such as exposure to stressful life events, stresses associated with social and cultural mobility, and poverty. For example, mortality among African-American infants in the United States is approximately twice that among white infants. The disparity has been attributed in large part to the higher incidence of poverty and limited access to health care among African Americans. Infant mortality rates among the dependents of African-American military personnel, who were guaranteed access to health care and who had levels of family income and education that were higher than those of the U.S. African-American population, were somewhat lower than the infant mortality rates for the general U.S. population.[62] For persons who are younger than 65 years of age, mortality rates are lower among those with higher family income for both African Americans and whites and for both men and women. However, at each level of income, African Americans have higher mortality rates than whites. Higher levels of family income also are associated with lower death rates from cardiovascular diseases and cancer.[63]

Wide differentials in cancer survival were observed among socioeconomic groups in England and Wales.[64] Lower socioeconomic groups tended to have a larger proportion of cancers with poor prognoses in comparison with upper socioeconomic groups. Poor survival rates among the lower socioeconomic groups might have been due to delay in seeking health care. Health system barriers, such as lack of access to care and the financial burden of diabetes care in the United States, may affect the health of insulin-dependent diabetes mellitus patients, which increases mortality rates among people 25 to 37 years of age.[65]

Among the other conditions that vary by social class is a specific form of mental retardation: mild mental retardation (IQ 60 through 75). Research reported a gradation of the frequency of mild mental retardation by social class; low social class groups had the highest prevalence of mild retardation. More severe forms of mental retardation tended to be more uniformly distributed across social classes.[66]

Characteristics of Place

Types of Place Comparisons

International
Geographic (within-country) variations
Urban/rural differences
Localized occurrence of disease

International Comparisons of Disease Frequency

The World Health Organization (WHO), which sponsors and conducts ongoing surveillance research, is a major source of information about international variations in rates of disease. WHO statistical studies portray international variations in infectious and communicable diseases, malnutrition, infant mortality, suicide, and other conditions. As might be expected, both infectious and chronic diseases show great variation from one country to another. Some of these differences may be attributed to climate, cultural factors, and national dietary habits.

Coronary heart disease, hypertension, stroke, and diabetes are among the "diseases of affluence," conditions formerly confined primarily to the developed world, but now occurring more frequently in developing regions as living standards improve. Nevertheless, mortality due to CHD is the leading cause of death in the United States and tends to be increasingly common in other areas as well. Countries that have high economic standards tend to foster behavioral and lifestyle factors implicated in CHD and other chronic diseases: lack of exercise, rich diets, and use of tobacco products. Fortunately, CHD mortality in the United States is on the decline due to preventive efforts that aim to modify these behavioral and lifestyle factors.

Cancer rates are increasing worldwide, especially as the population ages.[67] Lung cancer is the most common form of cancer in the world, showing declines in nations where it was formerly on the rise: Britain and the United States. The eastern European countries have the highest rates of lung cancer in the world. High rates occur in parts of the developing world where smoking is common, although exposure to environmental pollution may play a small role.

According to WHO statistics reported in 1977, stomach cancer was the second most common form of cancer worldwide.[67] Japan, as well as parts of Central and South Asia, formed a high-risk area. Risk factors for stomach cancer include consumption of preserved, cured, or salted foods. Decline in stomach cancer rates in some areas is related to improved diet (e.g., greater consumption of fresh vegetables). Stomach cancer death rates in Japan declined from 70.3 per 100,000 and 37.0 per 100,000 in 1958–1962 to 34.5 per 100,000 and 15.2 per 100,000 in 1988–1992 for males and females, respectively.[68] Nevertheless, despite a declining trend, stomach cancer death rates remained higher in Japan than rates observed in many other countries.

There are numerous examples of international variations in infectious diseases and related conditions. Schistosomiasis (see Chapt. 12) is endemic to the Nile River area of Africa and to sections of Latin America, but it rarely occurs in the United States unless it is imported into the country from an endemic area. Yaws tends to be localized in tropical climates and does not ordinarily occur in the temperate climate of the United States. Countries in tropical Africa account for more than 80% of all clinical cases of parasitic infections and more than 90% of all parasite carriers.[69] The WHO African Region reported 800,000 children's deaths per year (based on 1991 data). Exacerbations of malaria outbreaks follow major ecologic or social changes, such as agricultural or other economic exploitation of jungle areas or sociopolitical unrest.

Infectious diseases account for only 4.4% of all deaths in developed countries but, alarmingly, 44.1% of deaths in less developed nations. Examples of communicable diseases that show international variation are cutaneous leishmaniasis,

Chagas' disease, dengue fever, malaria, and cholera.[70] Zoonotic diseases (transmitted from animal hosts to humans) vary greatly from one country to another. "Mad cow disease" or BSE (bovine spongiform encephalopathy) has been confined largely to the United Kingdom, although the disease has spread to the Continent and outside of Europe. Refer to case study on BSE that follows. Vampire bat rabies increased during the 1980s as a cause of human death in Peru and Brazil.[71]

Suicide rates for selected countries showed marked differences between the lowest and highest ranked countries (Fig. 4-6). On the basis of the data presented, low rates were found in Mexico, Greece, and Italy; the United States and Canada fell in the middle range; and Belgium, Switzerland, Finland, and Hungary had the highest rates.[72]

There also are widely varying international differences in infant mortality rates, which show that the Central African nations have the highest rates of infant mortality and that the next highest rates are concentrated in North Africa, the Middle East, and India. The lowest rates exist in Japan, the Scandinavian countries, and France. The United States, Great Britain, Canada, and Australia all have higher rates of infant mortality than the foregoing countries. Social factors, education, and availability of medical care may account, in part, for the international variation in infant mortality.

Many countries, especially those in Africa, have had to reduce drastically their budgets for health services in the past decade, creating a wide discrepancy between those countries and the developed world. In developing countries, high population growth also reduces the available resources for health care and prevention programs and at the same time increases the potential for spread of infection through crowding. Korte et al.[73] argue that environmentally related health problems and adverse impacts of industrialization, urbanization, and slum growth will challenge the health care resources of developing countries in the future.

Within-country Geographic Variation in Rates of Disease

Many of the countries of Europe and North America have substantial variations in climate, geology, latitude, environmental pollution, and concentrations of ethnic and racial stock, all of which may be related to differences in frequency of disease. Examples of within-country comparisons made in the United States include case rates by region (e.g., Pacific, Mountain, Central, Atlantic). Sometimes, comparisons in rates are made by states, or, if fine comparisons are to be made across the United States, rates may be calculated by counties. In the United States, infectious diseases (e.g., intestinal parasites, influenza, AIDS, and many others) and chronic diseases (e.g., some forms of cancer and multiple sclerosis) show variation

Case Study: Mad Cow Disease (BSE)

Bovine spongiform encephalopathy (BSE) refers to a group of diseases that are caused by an unconventional agent, for which the name "prion" has been proposed. The mechanism by which the infectious agent replicates is not entirely known. As the name implies, BSE affects cattle (but is also capable of infecting sheep, goats, and some other animals) by causing degenerative diseases of the brain.[1] Strong evidence suggests that there is ". . . a causal relationship between ongoing outbreaks in Europe of . . . [BSE] and a disease in humans originally called new variant Creutzfeldt-Jacob disease or more recently simply variant CJD (vCJD)."[2]

"In 2001, only two countries, the United Kingdom and Portugal, reported a BSE incidence rate of > 100 indigenous cases per million cattle aged over 24 months. Although reported BSE rates must be interpreted with considerable caution because the sensitivity of surveillance may vary over time and by country, for 2001, the reported BSE rates for other countries (in decreasing order) were as follows: Republic of Ireland (62 BSE cases per million), Switzerland (49 cases per million), Belgium (28), Spain (24), Germany (20), France (20), Slovakia (18), Italy (14), and the Netherlands (10). The reported rates for Denmark, Slovenia, Greece, the Czech Republic, Finland, Japan, and Austria were between 1 and 7 BSE cases per million."[2] [In May 2003, a BSE case was reported in Canada.]

"The current risk of acquiring vCJD from eating beef (muscle meat) and beef products produced from cattle in countries with or at possibly increased risk of BSE cannot be precisely determined. . . . To reduce the possible current risk of acquiring vCJD from food, travelers to Europe or other areas with indigenous cases of BSE or at possibly increased risk of BSE may wish to consider either: (1) avoiding beef and beef products altogether or (2) selecting beef or beef products, such as solid pieces of muscle meat (versus calf brains or beef products such as burgers and sausages), which might have a reduced opportunity for contamination with tissues that may harbor the BSE agent."[2] ■

[1] Chin J., ed. *Control of Communicable Diseases in Man*. Washington, DC: American Public Health Association; 2000.

[2] Centers for Disease Control and Prevention. Update 2002: Bovine Spongiform Encephalopathy and Variant Creutzfeldt-Jakob Disease. Available at: http://www.cdc.gov/ncidod/diseases/cjd/bse_cjd.htm. Accessed June 10, 2003.

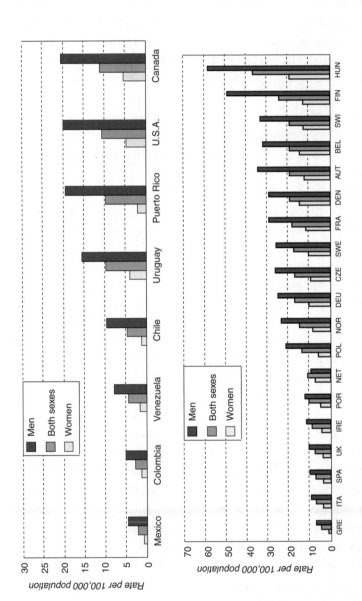

FIGURE 4-6 Suicide rate per 100,000 population by sex for all age groups, selected countries/areas in the Americas and selected countries in Europe, latest available year. *Source:* Reprinted from RFW Diekstra and W Gulbinat, The Epidemiology of Suicidal Behaviour: A Review of Three Continents, *World Health Statistics Quarterly,* vol 46, pp 56–57, World Health Organization, © 1993.

in frequency across the country. For example, high death rates due to leukemia are concentrated in the upper Midwest, whereas malignant melanoma of the skin appears to be related to latitude, the lowest rates occurring in the northern tier of the country and the highest rates being concentrated along the Sunbelt.[74] Multiple sclerosis varies according to latitude in the United States.[75] There is a gradient in rates from 15 per 100,000 in the South (Charleston, New Orleans, and Houston) to intermediate rates in Denver to high rates in Rochester, Minnesota (more than 40 per 100,000).[76]

The frequency of intestinal parasites varies from state to state in the United States, according to the findings of intestinal parasite surveillance programs conducted by the Centers for Disease Control and Prevention. During 1987, the states surrounding the Great Lakes and states in the Northwest had the highest percentage of stool samples positive for *Giardia* species. Stool samples positive for hookworm tended to be found most frequently in nine states (ranging from California to Wisconsin), although no consistency emerged from the distribution of positive specimens. Several factors may account for the variations in the prevalence and geographic distribution of intestinal parasites, including the arrival in the United States of large numbers of immigrants from endemic areas, increases in parasitic infections among patients with AIDS, and the recognition of *Giardia* species as frequently occurring pathogens in day care centers.[77]

Variations in morbidity and mortality rates due to pneumonia and influenza may be seen for different geographic sections of the United States, but the pattern changes from year to year and is also related to the variant of the influenza virus. Influenza epidemics remain an important cause of hospitalization and also are a cause of mortality as well as a factor that exacerbates health problems among the elderly and persons with a chronic disease. During the 2002–2003 influenza season in the United States (for the dates September 29, 2002 through March 8, 2003), the Centers for Disease Control and Prevention reported that influenza activity was mild. Nevertheless, occurrence of influenza varied by region and according to virus strain (i.e., influenza A or influenza B). "For the season, influenza type A viruses have predominated in the New England, East North Central, Mountain, Pacific, and Mid-Atlantic regions, and influenza B viruses have predominated in the West South Central, South Atlantic, West North Central, and East South Central regions."[78] Approximately 14 years earlier, during the 1988-1989 season, influenza appeared with essentially equal frequency regionally, although the predominance of two strains (variants)—influenza A and B—alternated.[79]

Figure 4-7 depicts variations in AIDS cases in the United States. The highest reported rates (greater than 30.0 per 100,000 population, data for 1996 and

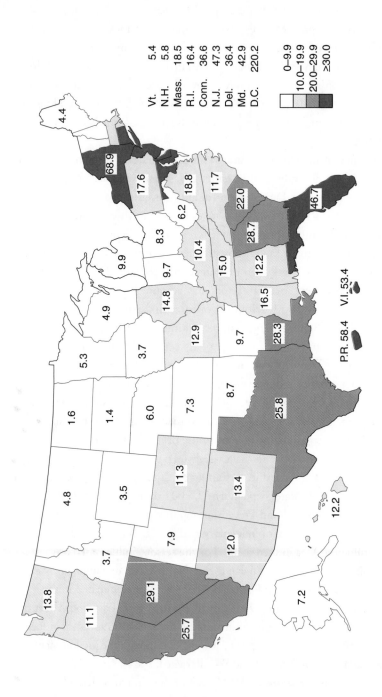

FIGURE 4-7 AIDS annual rates per 100,000 population—United States, July 1996–1997. *Source:* Reprinted from AIDS Rate, *MMWR*, vol 46, No 38, p 903, 1997, Centers for Disease Control and Prevention.

1997) tended to be concentrated in the northeastern, southeastern, and western states. Approximately 4/5 of reported cases could be attributed to the residents of large metropolitan areas (500,000 or more population).[80]

Urban/Rural Differences in Disease Rates

Urban and rural sections of the United States both have characteristic risks for morbidity and mortality. Urban diseases and causes of mortality are those that are more likely to be spread by person-to-person contact, crowding, and poverty or to be associated with urban pollution. Lead poisoning has been associated with inadequate housing and is found in inner city areas, where increased exposure of children occurs through ingestion of lead-based paints. Although such paints are now outlawed for interior residential use, exposure may still be high in poor urban areas. Mortality rates due to atherosclerotic heart disease, tuberculosis, and cirrhosis of the liver are higher in urban areas than in rural areas. Urban areas also show higher rates of bladder, lung, larynx, liver, and oral cancer and cancer of the pharynx and cervix, whereas rural areas show excesses in cancer of the lip in both sexes and cancer of the eye among men.[81] Among African Americans, data for the prevalence, incidence, and mortality of CHD reflect higher rates for urban residents than for rural residents.[82] Such observed differences immediately raise questions as to what might account for them. Taking into consideration what one already knows about differences in urban and rural lifestyles, one might hypothesize that smoking, diet, and physical activity could be associated with the outcomes of interest.

For urban/rural comparisons, data from the standard metropolitan statistical areas (SMSAs) are often employed. SMSAs are standard areas of the United States established by the U.S. Bureau of the Census to make regional comparisons in disease rates and also to make urban/rural comparisons.

Localized Place Comparisons

A local outbreak of a disease, or localized elevated morbidity rate, may be due to the unique environmental or social conditions found in a particular area of interest. Fluorosis, a disease resulting in mottled teeth, is most common in those areas of the world and the United States where there are naturally elevated fluoride levels in the water. Goiter, associated with iodine deficiency in the diet, was historically more common in land-locked areas of the United States, where seafood was not consumed, although this problem has been greatly alleviated by the introduction of iodized salt.

Localized concentrations of ionizing radiation have been studied in relation to cancer incidence. Ohio communities with high risk of exposure to radon had higher rates than the rest of Ohio of all cancers in general and cancer of the respiratory system in particular.[83] Ontario gold miners had excess mortality from carcinoma of the lung. This excess mortality was linked to exposure to radon decay products, arsenic, and high dust concentrations.[84] Local geologic formations may affect water hardness, which, some studies suggest, is a protective factor against heart disease deaths. For 1969 to 1983, one study reported an east-west regional gradient in cardiovascular mortality within seven counties in central Sweden, supporting other reports that have suggested water hardness to be inversely related to cardiovascular mortality.[85] Variation in water hardness accounted for 41% of the variation in the ischemic heart disease mortality rate and 14% of the variation in the stroke mortality rate. A second Swedish study attributed variation in mortality rates for coronary disease to exposure to cold weather, which was positively associated with heart disease and negatively associated with water hardness.[86] However, the evidence for this hypothesis has been both positive and negative.

Geographical Information Systems

Increasingly, public health practitioners are using Geographical Information Systems (GIS) as a method to provide a spatial perspective on the geographic distribution of health conditions. Although GIS has existed for some time, newer software has increased the ease of application of GIS methods by non-experts.[87] As a result, GIS has generated much excitement in the epidemiology community with respect to fresh applications. It is an advance that has enormous possibilities for defining new methods of comprehending data.[88]

A GIS is defined as ". . . computer hardware and software that integrates maps and graphics with a database related to a defined geographical space. . . . The geographical data may be spatial or descriptive in nature. A GIS can be defined as an integrated set of tools within an automated system capable of collecting, storing, handling, analyzing, and displaying geographically referenced information."[89(p2 of 9)] A GIS contains a database, maps, and a method to link these elements.[87] "GIS is, at its heart, a simple extension of statistical analyses that join epidemiological, sociological, clinical, and economic data with references to space. A GIS system does not create data but merely relates data using a system of references that describe spatial relationships."[88(p18.3)]

Although many uses exist, an important application of GIS is to map locations that have higher disease occurrence or mortality risk than do other areas.

Planners then are able to target these high-risk areas with appropriate social and health interventions. Subsequently, GIS facilitates the assessment of the impact of these interventions, which presumably would result in reductions of disease occurrence that could be visualized on a map. Thus, it is apparent that the use of GIS in epidemiology follows from the heritage of John Snow who, as noted in Chapter 1, produced a map of the cholera outbreak in Broad Street, Golden Square, London. At present, epidemiologists use GIS for many purposes, including research and planning in environmental health, infectious disease outbreaks, and policy evaluation.[87] Table 4-1 provides examples of applications of GIS.

To obtain more information about GIS, navigate the CDC web site "Resources for creating public health maps" (http://www.cdc.gov/epiinfo/eihlgeog.htm). The CDC web site lists more than one dozen software packages that are available for purchase or free download. An example is EpiMap 2002, which is freeware developed at CDC. In conclusion, Figure 4-8 presents an example of a GIS map of infant mortality rates in the U.S. state of Idaho. This map is called a *choropleth map,* defined as a map that represents disease rates (or other numerical data) for a group of regions by different degrees of shading.

Reasons for Place Variation in Disease

Concentration or clustering of racial, ethnic, or religious groups within a specific geographic area may result in higher or lower rates of diseases, depending upon the lifestyle and behaviors of the particular religious or ethnic group. The Seventh-Day Adventists, who espouse vegetarianism, are concentrated, among

---

Table 4-1 Representative Applications of
Geographic Information Systems (GIS)

Mapping of environmental health risks
    Pesticide pollution of groundwater
    Drifting of crop pesticides
    Average air pollution concentrations
    Exposure to elevated levels of magnetic fields
    Lead hazards

Portraying the geographic distribution of infectious diseases
    Bovine spongiform encephalopathy (BSE) in Europe
    Surveillance of disease outbreaks, e.g., Lyme disease, hepatitis C
    Mapping of water-borne, vector-borne, and tropical diseases

Health policy/planning
    Risk assessment
    Intervention evaluation
    Health services needs assessment
    Hospital accessibility

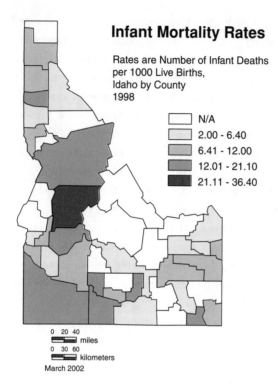

Infant Mortality Rates

Rates are Number of Infant Deaths
per 1000 Live Births,
Idaho by County
1998

- N/A
- 2.00 - 6.40
- 6.41 - 12.00
- 12.01 - 21.10
- 21.11 - 36.40

0 20 40
miles
0 30 60
kilometers
March 2002

FIGURE 4-8 GIS map of infant mortality rates in Idaho, U.S. *Source:* Idaho Department of Health and Welfare, Bureau of Vital Statistics. Available at: http://inside.uidaho.edu/data/statewide/esri/idtm/atlas/infamr98_id_esri.gif. Accessed: March 31, 2003.

other places, in parts of the Los Angeles basin, and the rates for CHD tend to be low in these corresponding geographic areas. Similarly, low rates of cancer tend to be found in areas where a large proportion of the residents are Mormons, possibly because their religious beliefs advocate avoidance of stimulants, tobacco, and alcohol.

The genetic characteristics of the population may interact with the environment, suggesting a dynamic interplay between noxious environmental factors and genetic make-up. An example of gene/environment interaction is the increased prevalence of the sickle-cell gene among people who live in sections of Africa that have high malaria rates.[5] The sickle-cell trait is a genetic mutation that confers a selection advantage in areas where malaria is endemic. Tay-Sachs disease is especially common among persons of Jewish extraction and Eastern European origin. It is now more widely distributed around the world as a result of the migration of the descendants of the original carriers.

Place variations in rates of disease may reflect the influence of climate (e.g., temperature and humidity) or environmental factors (e.g., the presence of environmental carcinogens). Certain geographic areas that have mild or tropical climates permit the survival of pathogenic organisms. Trypanosomiasis (African sleeping sickness) survives only in an environment that has the tsetse fly. Yaws and Hansen's disease are found primarily in the tropics. Ectoparasites are more common in temperate climates because people wear many layers of clothing, which may harbor these organisms. Naturally occurring or human-made chemical agents in particular geographic areas may be associated with the development of cancers or other diseases. For example, the concentration of fallout from U.S. nuclear testing has elicited concerns about the health effects of exposure to ionizing radiation (discussed in more detail in Chapt. 13).

In summary, Hutt and Burkitt stated:

> The disease pattern in any country or geographical region is dependent on the constellation of environmental factors that affect each member of the population from birth to the grave. Within a particular geographical situation the response of individuals to any noxious influences may be modified by their genetic make-up. In general terms exogenous factors which play a role in the causation of disease can be categorized into one of four groups; physical agents, chemical substances, biological agents (which include all infective organisms), and nutritional factors. These are determined by the geographical features of the region, the cultural life of population groups living in the area, the socio-economic status of these groups, and, in certain situations, by specific occupational hazards. Often, the individual's or group's experience of specific factors is determined by a combination of geographical, cultural, and socio-economic influences; this particularly applies to the type and quantity of food eaten.[76(p3)]

Characteristics of Time

The temporal aspects of disease occurrence must also be critically examined. Variations in the pattern of disease associated with time may permit important insights into the pathogenesis of disease or the recognition of emerging epidemics. Just as important, when one compares measures of disease frequency between two populations or within a population over time, the timing of data collection may need to be considered if there are seasonal or cyclic variations in the rate of disease.

Cyclic Fluctuations

Cyclic fluctuations are increases and decreases in the frequency of diseases and health conditions over a period of years or within each year. For example, birth rates show a seasonal trend, increasing in the early summer, as do depressive symptoms.[90,91] Influenza, drownings, accidents, and mortality from heart attacks manifest seasonal variations within each year. Analysis of data from a community registry of heart disease found that fatal and nonfatal coronary events in an Australian population were 20% to 40% more likely to occur in winter and spring than at other times of the year.[92] Seasonal variations may be caused by seasonal changes in the behavior of persons that place them at greater risk for certain diseases, changes in exposure to infectious or environmental agents, or endogenous biologic factors.

Pneumonia-influenza deaths in the United States demonstrate cyclic fluctuations, showing both annual peaks and periodic epidemics every few years. Seasonal increases in flu begin during the cold winter months of the year, peak in February, decrease in March and April, and then reach a minimum in June. Meningococcal disease (Fig. 4-9) is another condition that varies by season, apparently peaking in the winter and declining in the late summer.

Many diseases demonstrate cyclic increases and decreases related to changes in lifestyle of the host, seasonal climatic changes, and virulence of the infectious agent for a communicable disease. Heart disease mortality peaks during the win-

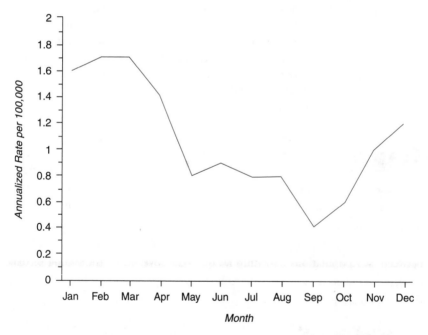

FIGURE 4-9 Seasonal variance in incidence of meningococcal disease, selected U.S. areas 1989–1991. *Source:* Reprinted from Centers for Disease Control and Prevention, Laboratory-Based Surveillance for Meningococcal Disease in Selected Areas—United States, 1989–1991, *MMWR*, vol 42, No SS-2, p 24, June 4, 1993.

ter months, when sedentary men are suddenly required to free their automobiles from the aftermath of a snowstorm. Colds increase in frequency when people spend more time indoors and are in close contact with one another, whereas accidents tend to peak during the summer, and Rocky Mountain spotted fever increases in the spring, when the ticks that carry the rickettsia become more active. Reported malaria cases in the Americas and some Asian countries show marked seasonality related to cyclic occurrence of heavy rains, leading to occasional epidemics or serious exacerbations of endemicity.[93]

Other examples of health phenomena that may show cyclic variation are responses of persons to temporary stressors. There may be an association between plasma lipid and lipoprotein levels among tax accountants during the tax season and among students at examination time. However, research has not shown such variation consistently.[94]

Point Epidemics

A point epidemic may indicate the response of a group of people circumscribed in place to a common source of infection, contamination, or other etiologic factor to which they were exposed almost simultaneously.[5] Acute infectious diseases and enteric infections sometimes manifest this type of relationship with time, as does mass illness due to exposure to chemical agents and noxious gases. Figure 4-10 illustrates time clustering of cases of *Mycoplasma pneumoniae* during an outbreak reported by the Centers for Disease Control and Prevention. Note that the most frequent day of onset was August 7, 1993, and that there was variation in the time of onset. Figure 4-10 is typical of the distribution (marked by a rapid increase and subsequent decline) of outbreaks of acute infectious disease, foodborne illness, and acute responses to toxic substances.

Secular Time Trends

Secular trends refer to gradual changes in the frequency of a disease over long time periods, as illustrated by changes in the rates of chronic diseases. For example, although heart disease was the leading cause of death in the United States from 1970 to 1988, the age-adjusted death rate for this cause declined by 34%; the decrease was 37% for white men and 24% for African-American men.[7] These trends may reflect the long-term impact of public health programs, diet improvements, and better treatment as well as unknown factors. With more women starting to smoke, especially teenagers and minority women, there has been a secular increase in lung cancer (see Fig. 4-4). Breast cancer mortality rates showed secular increases from 1973 to 1987, particularly after age 60 (Fig. 4-11).

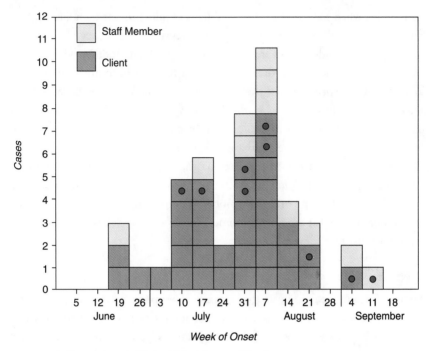

FIGURE 4-10 Cases of Mycoplasma pneumoniae among clients and staff members of a sheltered workshop, by week of onset—Ohio, June 15– September 5, 1993. *Source:* Reprinted from Centers for Disease Control and Prevention, Outbreaks of Mycoplasma Pneumoniae Respiratory Infection—Ohio, Texas and New York, 1993. *MMWR,* vol 42, p 931, December 10, 1993.

Cohort Effects

One of the consequences of long-term secular trends in exposure is a phenomenon known as cohort effects. Refer to Chapter 7 for more information on this topic.

Clustering

Case clustering refers to an unusual aggregation of health events grouped together in space or time. Examples of infectious disease clustering are the cholera epidemic in London in the 1850s (reported by John Snow) and the outbreak of Legionnaires' disease in the late 1970s. Examples of noninfectious disease clustering include the development of angiosarcoma among workers

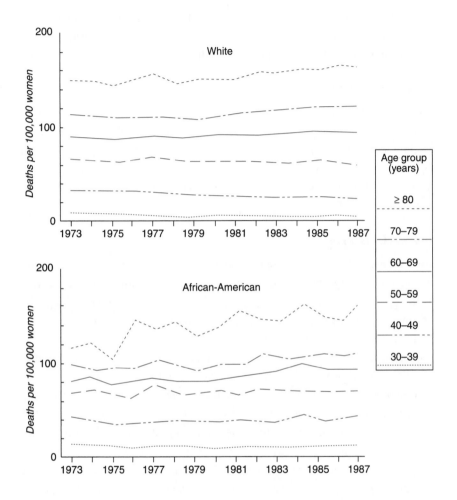

FIGURE 4-11 Breast cancer mortality rates, by age group and race—United States, 1973–1987. *Source*: Adapted from Centers for Disease Control and Prevention, Breast and Cervical Cancer Surveillance, United States, 1973–1987. *MMWR*, vol 41, No SS-2, p 11, April 24, 1992.

exposed to vinyl chloride and adenocarcinoma of the vagina among daughters whose mothers were prescribed diethylstilbestrol.[95] Other conditions that have been investigated for clustering include asthma, asbestos-related lung diseases, suicides, and leukemia and other cancers. Space and time clustering is one type of epidemiologic evidence that might suggest an association between common exposure to an etiologic agent and development of morbidity and mortality.

Among the problems surrounding the study of clusters are the fact that health events that show clustering are usually rare (e.g., certain types of cancer), producing a small number of cases, and that some clusters may occur by chance alone.

Temporal Clustering

Postvaccination reactions (adverse reactions to vaccines), such as the development of jaundice among military personnel vaccinated for yellow fever,[5] and the development of puerperal psychoses illustrate temporal clustering. Postpartum depression, ranging from the "blues" to more severe psychotic episodes, occurs in up to 80% of women within a few days after childbirth and may continue for several months or longer.[96]

Spatial Clustering

Concentration of cases of disease in a particular geographic area is the definition of spatial clustering. Hodgkin's disease, a condition of unknown etiology, is thought to have an infectious component. This possibility could be evaluated by a formal assessment of geographic and temporal variation in the incidence of Hodgkin's disease. One investigation found that, among cases of Hodgkin's disease diagnosed after 40 years of age in Washington State, there was evidence that cases lived closer together than expected as young children and teenagers.[97]

As another recent example, six childhood leukemia cases were diagnosed in a small community in northern Germany.[98] Using age-specific population and incidence data, this occurrence translated to a 460-fold standardized incidence ratio within a 5 km radius. Reports such as these can be quite alarming to the general public. Although they can be of significance, it is extremely important that they be put in perspective using appropriate epidemiologic methods. In particular, definition of the geographic area under study is critical. Drs. Julie Ross and Leslie Robison, colleagues from the University of Minnesota, liken the situation to drawing a bull's-eye around arrows that have already been shot. For example, suppose you are standing over a large enclosed circle with a jar full of 100 marbles. You dump the jar into the circle and note where the marbles land. Invariably, there will be some areas within the circle that will be dense with marbles and some areas that will be sparse. If you picked up all the marbles and repeated the process over and over again, you would note that the marble pattern would always be random and unlikely ever to appear evenly spaced. This description is analogous, perhaps, to clusters of disease, such as the childhood cancer examples. That is, marbles (cases) may fall within a small defined area (city) within a large geographic area (county, state, or country), and one could easily identify a cluster just by drawing a bull's-eye around these cases. In order to evaluate such clusters properly, one must consider the phenomena in the context of a larger geographic area and the temporal occurrence of disease.

Conclusion

This chapter covered descriptive epidemiology: person, place, and time. We have seen, for example, that age and sex are among the most fundamental attributes associated with the distribution of health and illness in populations. Secular trends are among the more important time variables. Although it is the leading cause of mortality, heart disease mortality has declined. Lung cancer mortality has shown a disturbing increase among women in the latter third of the 20th century. The data for these and other descriptive variables suggest hypotheses that can be tested in analytic epidemiologic studies. For example, particularly low or high disease rates in a circumscribed geographic area may suggest interaction between ethnicity and place variables, a hypothesis that could be followed up in etiologic research.

Study Questions and Exercises

1. Define the term *descriptive epidemiology.*
2. Describe the relevance of descriptive epidemiology to the study of disease. How do descriptive studies promote hypothesis formation? What is the relevance of Mill's canons to descriptive epidemiology?
3. Give definitions and examples of categories of descriptive epidemiology.
4. What are some examples of age associations found in epidemiologic research? What explanations have been proposed to account for them? When comparing mortality rates by age, discuss the possibility of interactions between age effects and gender effects.
5. How do mortality and morbidity differ by sex? How would you account for interactions between marital status and sex in health outcomes?
6. How do protective and selective factors increase or decrease the risk for disease based on marital status?
7. How do cultural practices and religious beliefs account for mortality and morbidity differences?
8. Describe procedures for measurement of race, ethnicity, and social class. What methodologic pitfalls are inherent in the ascertainment of these characteristics?

9. What health effects do variations in race, ethnicity, and social class have?

10. Select a health problem or disease with which you are familiar. Describe the occurrence in terms of person, place, and time.

11. To what extent are rates of common health problems similar or different across different geographic areas of the United States? How might demographic variables be linked to geographic variations in disease?

12. What are examples of the differences among international, regional (within-country), urban-rural, and localized patterns in disease? What factors may be linked to these differences?

13. Explain what is meant by a Geographical Information System (GIS). Describe the applications of GIS in epidemiology.

14. What time trends would characterize the occurrence of an influenza epidemic? How do epidemiologists account for seasonal variations in meningococcal disease and other communicable diseases, as well as for other health conditions?

15. What is meant by case clustering? Give some noteworthy examples; distinguish between temporal and spatial clustering. What considerations bear upon the interpretation of spatial clustering?

16. Complete the project found in Appendix 4 at the end of this chapter.

References

1. Suchman EA. Health attitudes and behavior. *Arch Environ Health.* 1970;20:105–110.
2. Hennekins CH, Buring JE. *Epidemiology in Medicine.* Boston, MA: Little, Brown; 1987.
3. Abramson JH. *Survey Methods in Community Medicine,* 4th ed. New York, NY: Churchill Livingstone; 1990.
4. Mill JS. *A System of Logic.* London, UK: Parker, Son & Bowin; 1856.
5. MacMahon B, Pugh TF. *Epidemiology Principles and Methods.* Boston, MA: Little, Brown; 1970.
6. National Center for Health Statistics. Advance report of final mortality statistics, 1991. *Mon Vital Stat Rep.* 1993;42(suppl 2).
7. National Center for Health Statistics. *Health, United States, 1990.* Hyattsville, MD: Public Health Service; 1991.
8. Verbrugge LM. Females and illness: recent trends in sex differences in the United States. *J Health Soc Behav.* 1976;17:387–403.
9. Waldron I. Why do women live longer than men? *Soc Sci Med.* 1976;10:349–362.
10. Johnson A. Recent trends in sex mortality differentials in the United States. *J Hum Stress.* 1977;3:22–32.
11. Kitagawa EM, Hauser PM. *Differential Mortality in the United States.* Cambridge, MA: Harvard University Press; 1973.
12. Hu YR, Goldman N. Mortality differentials by marital status: an international comparison. *Demography.* 1990;27:233–250.

13. Wenz FV. Marital status, anomie, and forms of social isolation: a case of high suicide rate among the widowed in an urban sub-area. *Dis Nerv Syst.* 1977;38:891–895.

14. Avis NE, Brambilla DJ, Vass K, McKinlay JB. The effect of widowhood on health: a prospective analysis from the Massachusetts Women's Health Study. *Soc Sci Med.* 1991;33:1063–1070.

15. Schottenfeld D. Patient risk factors and the detection of early cancer. *Prev Med.* 1972;1:335–351.

16. Cassileth BR, Lusk EJ, Miller DS, et al. Psychosocial correlates of survival in advanced malignant disease? *N Engl J Med.* 1985;312:1551–1555.

17. Syme SL. Behavioral factors associated with the etiology of physical disease: a social epidemiological approach. *Am J Public Health.* 1974;64:1043–1045.

18. Sobal J, Rauschenbach BS, Frongillo EA Jr. Marital status, fatness and obesity. *Soc Sci Med.* 1992;35:915–923.

19. McKenney NR, Bennett CE. Issues regarding data on race and ethnicity: the Census Bureau experience. *Public Health Rep.* 1994;109:16–25.

20. Krieger N. Editorial: Counting accountably: Implications of the new approaches to classifying race/ethnicity in the 2000 census. *Am J Public Health.* 2000;90(11): 1687–1689.

21. Kaufman JS, Cooper RS. Commentary: Considerations for use of racial/ethnic classification in etiologic research. *Am J Epidemiol.* 2001;154:291–298.

22. Lynberg MC, Khoury MJ. Contribution of birth defects to infant mortality among racial/ethnic minority groups, United States 1983. *MMWR CDC Surveill Summ.* 1990;39:1–12.

23. Hypertension Detection and Follow-Up Program Cooperative Group. Race, education and prevalence of hypertension. *Am J Epidemiol.* 1977;106:351–361.

24. Harburg E, Erfurt JC, Chape C, et al. Sociological stressor areas and black-white blood pressure: Detroit. *J Chronic Dis.* 1973;26:595–611.

25. Brunswick AF, Collette P. Psychophysical correlates of elevated blood pressure: a study of urban black adolescents. *J Hum Stress.* 1977;3:19–31.

26. Knowler WC, Bennett PH, Hamman RF, et al. Diabetes incidence and prevalence in Pima Indians: a 19-fold greater incidence than in Rochester, Minnesota. *Am J Epidemiol.* 1978;108:497–505.

27. Sievers ML, Nielson RG, Bennett PH. Adverse mortality experience of a southwestern American Indian community: overall death rates and underlying causes of death in Pima Indians. *J Clin Epidemiol.* 1990;43:1231–1242.

28. Yano K, Blackwelder WC, Kagan A, et al. Childhood cultural experience and the incidence of coronary heart disease in Hawaii Japanese men. *Am J Epidemiol.* 1979;109:440–450.

29. Williams CL, Berry JW. Primary prevention of acculturative stress among refugees. *Am Psychol.* 1991;46:632–641.

30. Marmot MG. Stress, social and cultural variations in heart disease. *J Psychosom Res.* 1983;27:377–384.

31. Syme SL, Marmot MG, Kagan A, Kato H, Rhoads G. Epidemiologic studies of coronary heart disease and stroke in Japanese men living in Japan, Hawaii and California: introduction. *Am J Epidemiol.* 1975;102:477–480.

32. Marmot MG, Syme SL. Acculturation and coronary heart disease in Japanese-Americans. *Am J Epidemiol.* 1976;104:225–247.

33. Matsumoto YS. Social stress and coronary heart disease in Japan: a hypothesis. *Milbank Mem Fund Q.* 1970;48:9–36.

34. Benfante R. Studies of cardiovascular disease and cause-specific mortality trends in Japanese-American men living in Hawaii and risk factor comparisons with other Japanese populations in the Pacific region: a review. *Hum Biol.* 1992;64:791–805.

35. Delgado JL, Johnson CL, Roy I, Trevino FM. Hispanic Health and Nutrition Examination Survey: methodological considerations. *Am J Public Health.* 1990;80(suppl):6–10.

36. Trevino FM, ed. Hispanic Health and Nutrition Examination Survey, 1982–84. *Am J Public Health.* 1990;80(suppl).

37. Garcia-Palmieri MR, Costas R Jr, Cruz-Vidal M, et al. Urban-rural differences in coronary heart disease in a low incidence area: the Puerto Rico Heart Study. *Am J Epidemiol.* 1978;107:206–215.

38. Hazuda HP, Haffner SM, Stern MP, Eifler CW. Effects of acculturation and socioeconomic status on obesity and diabetes in Mexican Americans. *Am J Epidemiol.* 1988;128:1289–1301.

39. Friis R, Yngve A, Persson V. Review of social epidemiologic research on migrants' health: findings, methodological cautions, and theoretical perspectives. *Scand J Soc Med.* 1998;26(3):173–180.

40. Levin JS. Religion and health: is there an association, is it valid, and is it causal? *Soc Sci Med.* 1994;38:1475–1482.

41. Fraser GE, Strahan TM, Sabate J, et al. Effects of traditional coronary risk factors on rates of incident coronary events in a low-risk population: the Adventist Health Study. *Circulation.* 1992;86:406–413.

42. Armstrong B, van Merwyk AJ, Coates H. Blood pressure in Seventh-Day Adventist vegetarians. *Am J Epidemiol.* 1977;105:444–449.

43. Phillips RL. Role of life-style and dietary habits in risk of cancer among Seventh-Day Adventists. *Cancer Res.* 1975;35:3515–3522.

44. Jarvis GK. Mormon mortality rates in Canada. *Soc Biol.* 1977;24:294–302.

45. Enstrom JE. Health practices and cancer mortality among active California Mormons. *J Natl Cancer Inst.* 1989;81:1807–1814.

46. Guralnik JM, Leveille SG. Annotation: race, ethnicity, and health outcomes—unraveling the mediating role of socioeconomic status. *Am J Public Health.* 1997;87:728–729.

47. Gregorio DI, Walsh SJ, Paturzo D. The effects of occupational-based social position on mortality in a large American cohort. *Am J Public Health.* 1997;87:1472–1475.

48. Link BG, Northridge ME, Phelan JC, et al. Social epidemiology and the fundamental cause concept: On the structuring of effective cancer screens by socioeconomic status. *Milbank Q.* 1998;76(3):375–402.

49. McDonough P, Duncan GJ, Williams D, House J. Income dynamics and adult mortality in the United States, 1972 through 1989. *Am J Public Health.* 1997;87:1476–1482.

50. Berkman LF, Syme SL. Social networks, host resistance, and mortality: a nine-year follow-up study of Alameda County residents. *Am J Epidemiol.* 1979;109:186–204.

51. Kington RS, Smith JP. Socioeconomic status and racial and ethnic differences in functional status associated with chronic diseases. *Am J Public Health.* 1997;87:805–810.

52. Blane D. Social determinants of health—socioeconomic status, social class, and ethnicity (Editorial). *Am J Public Health.* 1995;85:903–904.

53. Winkelby MA, Jatulis DE, Frank E, Fortmann SP. Socioeconomic status and health: how education, income, and occupation contribute to risk factors for cardiovascular disease. *Am J Public Health.* 1992;82:816–820.

54. Hollingshead A, Redlich F. *Social Class and Mental Illness.* New Haven, CT: Yale University Press; 1958.

55. Duncan OD. A socioeconomic index for all occupations. In: Reiss AJ Jr, Duncan OD, Hatt PK, North CC, eds. *Occupations and Social Status.* New York, NY: Free Press; 1961:109–138.

56. Dunham HW. Society, culture, and mental disorder. *Arch Gen Psychiatry.* 1976;33:147–156.

57. Mausner JS, Kramer S. *Epidemiology: An Introductory Text,* 2nd ed. Philadelphia, PA: Saunders; 1985.

58. Murphy JM, Olivier DC, Monson RR, et al. Depression and anxiety in relation to social status: a prospective epidemiologic study. *Arch Gen Psychiatry.* 1991;48:223–229.

59. Antonovsky A. Social class, life expectancy and overall mortality. *Milbank Mem Fund Q.* 1967;45:31–73.

60. Adler NE, Boyce T, Chesney MA, et al. Socioeconomic status and health: the challenge of the gradient. *Am Psychol.* 1994;49:15–24.

61. Rogot E, Sorlie PD, Johnson NJ. Life expectancy by employment status, income, and education in the National Longitudinal Mortality Study. *Public Health Rep.* 1992;107:457–461.

62. Rawlings JS, Weir MR. Race- and rank-specific infant mortality in a U.S. military population. *Am J Dis Child.* 1992;146:313–316.

63. Sorlie P, Rogot E, Anderson R, et al. Black-white mortality differences by family income. *Lancet.* 1992;340:346–350.

64. Kogevinas M, Marmot MG, Fox AJ, Goldblatt PO. Socioeconomic differences in cancer survival. *J Epidemiol Community Health.* 1991;45:216–219.

65. Songer TJ, DeBerry J, La Porte RE, Tuomilehto J. International comparisons of IDDM mortality. *Diabetes Care.* March 1992;15(suppl 1):15–21.

66. Birch HG, Richardson SA, Baird D, et al. *Mental Subnormality in the Community: A Clinical and Epidemiologic Study.* Baltimore, MD: Williams & Wilkins; 1970.

67. World Health Organization (WHO). *The World Health Report.* Geneva, Switzerland: WHO; 1977.

68. Tominaga S, Kuroishi T, Aoki K. *Cancer Statistics in 33 Countries 1953–1992.* Available at: http://publications.uicc.org/99stats/. Accessed April 8, 2003.

69. Division of Control of Tropical Diseases, World Health Organization. World malaria situation 1990. *World Health Stat Q.* 1992;45:257–266.

70. World Health Organization. Communicable disease epidemiology and control. *World Health Stat Q.* 1992;45:166–167.

71. Meslin F-X. Surveillance and control of emerging zoonoses. *World Health Stat Q.* 1992;45:200–207.

72. Diekstra RFW, Gulbinat W. The epidemiology of suicidal behaviour: a review of three continents. *World Health Stat Q.* 1993;46:56–57.

73. Korte R, Rehle T, Merkle A. Strategies to maintain health in the Third World. *Trop Med Parasitol.* 1991;42:428–432.

74. Mason TJ, McKay FW, Hoover R, et al. *Atlas of Cancer Mortality in U.S. Counties: 1950–1969.* Department of Health, Education and Welfare publication (NIH)75–780. Washington, DC: Government Printing Office; 1975.

75. Lauer K. The risk of multiple sclerosis in the USA in relation to sociogeographic features: a factor-analytic study. *J Clin Epidemiol.* 1994;47:43–48.

76. Hutt MSR, Burkitt DP. *The Geography of Non-Infectious Disease.* Oxford, UK: Oxford University Press; 1986.

77. Kappus KK, Juranek DD, Roberts JM.Results of testing for intestinal parasites by state diagnostic laboratories, United States, 1987. *MMWR CDC Surveill Summ.* 1991;40:25–30.

78. Centers for Disease Control and Prevention. Update: Influenza Activity–United States, 2002–03 Season. *MMWR.* 2003;52:224–225.

79. Chapman LE, Tipple MA, Folger SG, et al. Influenza—United States, 1988–89. *MMWR CDC Surveill Summ.*1993;42(SS-1):9–21.

80. Centers for Disease Control and Prevention. Summary of notifiable diseases, United States, 1996. *MMWR.* 1996;45(53):18.

81. Doll R. Urban and rural factors in the aetiology of cancer. *Int J Cancer.* 1991;47:803–810.

82. Keil JE, Saunders DE Jr. Urban and rural differences in cardiovascular disease in blacks. In: Saunders E, ed. *Cardiovascular Diseases in Blacks.* Philadelphia, PA: Davis; 1991:17–28.

83. Dzik AJ. Differences in cancer mortality rates in Ohio communities with respect to uraniferous geology. *Ohio Med.* 1989;85:566–568.

84. Kusiak RA, Springer J, Ritchie AC, Muller J. Carcinoma of the lung in Ontario gold miners: possible aetiological factors. *Br J Ind Med.* 1991;48:808–817.

85. Nerbrand C, Svardsudd K, Ek J, Tibblin G. Cardiovascular mortality and morbidity in seven counties in Sweden in relation to water hardness and geological settings. The project: myocardial infarction in mid-Sweden. *Eur Heart J.* 1992;13:721–727.

86. Gyllerup S, Lanke J, Lindholm LH, Scherstén B. Water hardness does not contribute substantially to the high coronary mortality in cold regions of Sweden. *J Intern Med.* 1991;230:487–492.

87. Clarke KC, McLafferty SL, Tempalski BJ. On epidemiology and geographic information systems: A review and discussion of future directions. *Emerging Infectious Diseases.* 1996;2(2):1–11. Available at: http//www.cdc.gov/ncidod/eid/. Accessed March 25, 2003.

88. Ricketts TC. Geographic information systems and public health. *Annu Rev Public Health.* 2003;24:18.1–18.6.

89. Pan American Health Organization. *Epidemiological Bulletin.* 1996;17(1):1–9. Available at: http://165.158.1.110/English/sha/be961gis.htm#use. Accessed: March 25, 2003.

90. Russell D, Douglas AS, Allan TM. Changing seasonality of birth—a possible environmental effect. *J Epidemiol Community Health.* 1993;47:362–367.

91. Maes M, Meltzer HY, Suy E, De Meyer F. Seasonality in severity of depression: relationships to suicide and homicide occurrence. *Acta Psychiatr Scand.* 1993;88: 156–161.

92. Enquselassie F, Dobson AJ, Alexander HM, Steele PL. Seasons, temperature and coronary disease. Int J Epidemiol. 1993;22:632–636.

93. Division of Control of Tropical Diseases, World Health Organization. World malaria situation, 1988. *World Health Stat Q.* 1990;43:68–79.

94. Niaura R, Herbert PN, Saritelli AL, et al. Lipid and lipoprotein responses to episodic occupational and academic stress. *Arch Intern Med.* 1991;151:2172–2179.

95. Centers for Disease Control and Prevention. Guidelines for investigating clusters of health events. *MMWR .* 1990;39(*Recomm Rep-11*):1–23.

96. Romito P. Postpartum depression and the experience of motherhood. *Acta Obstet Gynecol Scand.* 1990;69(suppl 154):7–19.
97. Ross A, Davis S. Point pattern analysis of the spatial proximity of residences prior to diagnosis of persons with Hodgkin's disease. *Am J Epidemiol.* 1990;132(suppl 1):53–62.
98. Hoffman W, Diekmann H, Schmitz-Feuerhake I. A cluster of childhood leukemia near a nuclear reactor in north Germany. *Arch Environ Health.* 1997;52:275–280.

APPENDIX
4

Project: Descriptive Epidemiology of a Selected Health Problem

Select a health problem to explore in detail by using a descriptive epidemiologic approach; for examples of health problems or diseases that might be studied, refer to Exhibit 5-4. You can also access the Internet addresses shown in Exhibit 5-1 in order to develop a reference list.

The objectives of this exercise are as follows:

- to gain experience in describing and analyzing the distribution of a health disorder in a population
- to become familiar with various sources of data for the epidemiologic description of a health disorder
- to enhance the ability to make sound epidemiologic judgments related to public health problems

Examples of sources of data:

- morbidity and mortality reports (vital statistics): World Health Organization and international reports; U.S., federal, state, and local annual and periodic reports
- current literature on the selected health problem
- reports of special surveys

Model for organization of paper:

1. Define the problem (nature, extent, significance, etc.).
2. Describe the agent.
3. Describe the condition (briefly).
4. Examine the above sources for data on morbidity and mortality in the selected health problem.
5. Summarize these data on the distribution of the selected health problem according to the following factors, using tables, graphs, or other illustrations whenever possible.

A. Host characteristics
   1. Age
   2. Sex
   3. Nativity
   4. Marital status
   5. Ethnic group

B. Environmental attributes
   1. Geographic areas
   2. Social and economic factors
      a. Income
      b. Housing
   3. Occupation
   4. Education

C. Temporal variation
   1. Secular
   2. Cyclic
   3. Seasonal
   4. Epidemic

D. Any additional characteristic that contributes to an epidemiologic description of the disease

6. Summarize any current hypotheses that have been proposed to explain the observed distribution.
7. List the principal gaps in knowledge about the distribution of the health problem.
8. Suggest areas for further epidemiologic research.
9. Critically appraise the data as a whole; consult primary sources and important original papers.

Source: Data are from an exercise distributed at the Columbia University School of Public Health during the early 1970s.

Sources of Data for Use in Epidemiology

Introduction

In Chapter 3 we learned about several measures of disease frequency that epidemiologists employ to present data on health indexes. Chapter 4 covered means to describe the occurrence of disease with respect to person, place, and time. The purpose of the present chapter is to provide in greater detail where and how the data to compute such measures are obtained. Whether one is talking about incidence, prevalence, secular trends, descriptive epidemiology, or analytic studies of disease etiology, the findings are only as good as the data upon which they are based.

As the basic methodology of public health, epidemiology necessarily deals with populations. The reasons are essentially twofold. First, because of the interest in the health of populations, data collected on entire populations (or representative samples thereof) improve the ability to generalize observations or findings beyond the group studied. Second, data on populations are needed for statistical inference, that is, for estimating parameters (incidence, prevalence, and similar measures) of health, morbidity, and mortality. For diseases that occur at low frequencies, data must be accumulated on large numbers of at-risk individuals to obtain reliable estimates. For these reasons, epidemiologic research usually requires or involves large data sets.

It would be an overwhelming task for any one person to amass the data needed for any particular measure of public health. To aid researchers, U.S. federal epidemiologic agencies compile a great deal of relevant information.[1] This chapter will inform the reader about some of the varied data sources that are available to the general public for generating indexes of morbidity and mortality. These data can be a valuable source of descriptive epidemiologic studies. However, there are a number of data sets that can be used for studies that seek to understand the etiology of disease; some of these are described also. Finally, because data collected by others may not always be perfectly suitable for all situations, this chapter covers some general issues related to primary data collection. Throughout, an attempt is made to discuss the nature of the data, their value and limitations, and the population coverage.

Criteria for the Quality and Utility of Epidemiologic Data

A number of criteria relate to the quality and utility of data:

- nature of the data
- availability of the data
- completeness of population coverage
    1. representativeness (also called external validity)
    2. thoroughness (e.g., inclusion of subclinical cases)
- value and limitations

The criterion *nature of the data* includes whether the data are from vital statistics, case registries, physicians' records, surveys of the general population, or hospital and clinic cases. The nature of the data affects the types of statistical analyses and inferences that are possible.

The criterion *availability of the data* relates to the investigator's access. Medical records and any associated data with personal identifiers are not usually available without release from the individual patient. Some data from population surveys, stripped of individually identifying characteristics, are available from government and research organizations on data tapes, compact disks, and the Internet.

The criterion *representativeness or external validity* refers to generalizability of findings to the population from which the data have been taken. For a given data set, one should assess the degree to which data are representative of the target population under study. Is there evidence for omission of major subdivisions of the population, such as low socioeconomic status individuals or minority groups? Is the population base from which the data have been taken clearly defined, or do the data encompass an unspecified mixture of different populations?

Related to the extent of population coverage is the criterion *thoroughness* with which all cases of a health phenomenon, including subclinical cases, have been identified. Do the data represent only the severe cases that have come to the attention of health authorities? Are there likely to be substantial numbers of unreported cases?

The criterion *value and limitations* denotes the utility of the data for various types of epidemiologic research, such as investigations of mortality, detection of outbreaks of infectious disease, and studies of the incidence of chronic diseases. This criterion also includes whether there are limiting factors inherent in the data, for example, incomplete diagnostic information and case duplication. Thus, value and limitations tends to overlap with the criterion of completeness of population coverage. Because the criteria are general principles, one may apply them to data sources not specifically mentioned here, and for the evaluation of published epidemiologic research.

Computerized Bibliographic Databases

A helpful starting point for both descriptive and analytic epidemiologic studies is a systematic retrieval of information from computerized bibliographic sources. Some of the basic facts relating to the distribution of diseases may be obtained by a review of the existing literature. The *Index Medicus, Psychological Abstracts, Sociological Abstracts, Education Index,* and similar volumes are a valuable starting point for gathering bibliographic citations on a health problem. In recent decades, computers have been utilized to retrieve literature citations. On-line databases include MEDLINE, TOXLINE, and DIALOG.[1] For example, the National Library of Medicine offers a free bibliographic search service that is accessible using the Internet (the URL is http://www.ncbi.nlm.nih.gov/entrez/). One enters a combination of topics or authors and receives a listing of relevant article titles, authors, complete reference citations, and, depending on the specific journal and the year it was published, an abstract. In addition, each article is followed by a prompt to request more publications similar to the one highlighted. An individual user may conduct a computerized search of this storehouse of material to compile a bibliography on a given topic. Remote searches may be accomplished through on-line services from a library, office, or other location. The Internet and World Wide Web are used as sources for bibliographic citations and for retrieval of entire articles. For example, the Health Sciences Library System at the University of Pittsburgh offers an excellent homepage to link browsers to hundreds of sources of health statistics that are available on the World Wide Web (the URL for this site is http://www.hsls.pitt.edu/. See Exhibit 5-1 for a partial list of Web sites that are relevant to epidemiology).

Confidentiality, Sharing of Data, and Record Linkage

The investigator who conducts primary or secondary analyses of epidemiologic data must maintain adequate safeguards for privacy and confidentiality of this information;

A Selection of Internet Addresses of Interest to Epidemiologists

Administration on Aging, HHS
   http://www.aoa.dhhs.gov/aoa/stats/statpage.html
Agency for Health Care Policy Research
   http://www.ahcpr.gov:80/data
American Cancer Society
   http://www.cancer.org
American Heart Association
   http://www.americanheart.org/
American Lung Association
   http://www.lungusa.org
American Public Health Association
   http://www.apha.org
British Medical Journal
   http://bmj.com/
Centers for Disease Control and Prevention
   http://www.cdc.gov
Directory of Health and Human Services Data Resources, HHS
   http://www.aspe.hhs.gov/datacncl/datadir
Emory University Health Sciences Center Library
   http://www.emory.edu/WHSCL/index.htm
Ethics in Science
   http://www.chem.vt.edu/ethics/ethics.html
The Federal Web Locator (Villanova University)
   http://www.infoctr.edu/fwl/
The Food and Drug Administration
   http://www.fda.gov
Hardin Meta Directory of Internet Health Sources, University of Iowa
   http://infotree.library.ohiou.edu/single-records/1256.html
Indiana Prevention Resource Center
   http://www.drugs.indiana.edu/drug_stats/
Journal of the American Medical Association, Archives of Internal Medicine
   http://pubs.ama-assn.org/archive_home.html

continues

EXHIBIT 5-1 *continued*

MEDLINE, National Library of Medicine (NLM)
  NLM   http://www.nlm.nih.gov/
  Pub Med®   http://ncbl.nlm.nih.gov/entrez/query
National Center for Health Statistics (NCHS)
  http://www.cdc.gov/nchs/
National Heart, Lung, and Blood Institute
  http://www.nhlbi.nih.gov/
New England Journal of Medicine
  http://www.nejm.org
Pan American Health Organization
  http://www.paho.org
U.S. Census Bureau
  http://www.census.gov
U.S. State Departments of Health
  http://www.alsna.com/usdoh.htm
University of Michigan's Monitoring the Future Study
  http://monitoringthefuture.org/index.html
The Virtual Library: Epidemiology (Biosciences and Medicine), University
of California, San Francisco
  http://www.epibiostat.ucsf.edu/epidem/epidem.html
The White House Social Statistics Briefing Room
  http://www.whitehouse.gov/fsbr/ssbr.html
World Health Organization Statistical Information System (WHOSIS)
  http://www3.who.int/whosis/menu.cfm

such privacy is legally mandated. Information that must be kept confidential is that which pertains to any personally identifiable features about a living individual; this includes information for which the research subject has not given permission for public release. Release of information regarding whether the subject participated in a study also is proscribed.[2] Information that would permit identification of a deceased person also should be kept confidential, although the guidelines for release of information about the deceased are not well established. The Privacy Act of 1974 introduced certain necessary reforms for the protection of confidential records of individuals that are maintained by federal agencies in the United States. Specifically, one of the major provisions of the Privacy Act proscribes the release of confidential data by a federal government agency or its contractors, under most circumstances, without the permission of the client whose records are to be released. On the other hand, the

Freedom of Information Act is directed toward the disclosure of government information to the public; it exempts personal and medical files, however, because release of such information would constitute an invasion of privacy. The Public Health Service Act protects the confidentiality of information collected by some federal agencies, such as the National Center for Health Statistics (NCHS). On August 21, 1996, the federal government enacted the Health Insurance Portability and Accountability Act (HIPAA). This act protects individually identifiable health information. For more information regarding the provision of the act, refer to Exhibit 5-2.

EXHIBIT 5-2

The HIPAA Privacy Rule

The Health Insurance Portability and Accountability Act of 1996 (HIPAA), Public Law 104-191, was enacted on August 21, 1996. Sections 261 through 264 of HIPAA require the Secretary of HHS to publicize standards for the electronic exchange, privacy and security of health information. . . . [The date for most covered entities to comply with the Privacy Rule was April 14, 2003.]

Protected Health Information. The Privacy Rule protects all *"individually identifiable health information"* held or transmitted by a covered entity or its business associate, in any form or media, whether electronic, paper, or oral. The Privacy Rule calls this information *"protected health information (PHI)."* . . .

"Individually identifiable health information" is information, including demographic data, that relates to:

- the individual's past, present or future physical or mental health or condition,
- the provision of health care to the individual, or
- the past, present, or future payment for the provision of health care to the individual,

and that identifies the individual or for which there is a reasonable basis to believe can be used to identify the individual. . . . Individually identifiable health information includes many common identifiers (e.g., name, address, birth date, Social Security Number).

The Privacy Rule excludes from protected health information employment records that a covered entity maintains in its capacity as an employer and education and certain other records subject to, or defined in, the Family Educational Rights and Privacy Act, 20 U.S.C. §1232g.

continues

EXHIBIT 5-2 *continued*

> **De-Identified Health Information.** There are no restrictions on the use
> or disclosure of de-identified health information. . . . De-identified health
> information neither identifies nor provides a reasonable basis to identify
> an individual. There are two ways to de-identify information; either: 1) a
> formal determination by a qualified statistician; or 2) the removal of spec-
> ified identifiers of the individual and of the individual's relatives, house-
> hold members, and employers is required, and is adequate only if the cov-
> ered entity has no actual knowledge that the remaining information could
> be used to identify the individual. . . . ■
>
> *Source:* Adapted and reprinted from USDHHS. OCR Privacy Brief: Summary of the HIPAA
> Privacy Rule. Available at: http://www.hhs.gov/ocr/hipaa/privacy.html. Accessed April 14,
> 2003.

Data sharing can greatly enhance the quality of epidemiologic research findings. Data sharing refers to the voluntary release of information by one investigator or institution to another for purposes of scientific research.[3] Illustrations of
data sharing include linkage of large data sets and the pooling of multiple studies
in meta-analyses. Data sharing may lead to enhancement of knowledge gained
from the data. One of the key scientific issues in data sharing is the primary
investigator's potential loss of control over intellectual property.

The term *record linkage* refers to joining data from two or more sources, for
example, employment records and mortality data. Record linkage has been facilitated by the advent of modern computers, which are capable of rapidly processing large amounts of data that contain common identifying features (e.g., Social
Security numbers) to connect data records on a single individual. Many of the
European countries, particularly those in Scandinavia, which have developed
extensive, nearly complete social and health records on the resident population,
have used linked data in major epidemiologic research projects. Other applications of linked records include the study of clinical outcomes associated with the
use of anti-inflammatory medications; genetic research; and planning of health
care services.[4] Record linkage systems offer a potentially rich source of information. This information may facilitate research on maternal and child concerns,
chronic disease tracking, and the natural history of specific diseases.[5]

Table 5-1 demonstrates that epidemiologic data are derived from numerous
sources, ranging from vital statistics to reports of absenteeism from work or school.
It summarizes the nature of each type of data, their availability and completeness,

Table 5-1 Overview of Epidemiologic Data Sources

Data Source	Nature of Data	Availability	Population Coverage	Value and Limitations
Mortality statistics	Data from registration of vital events	Annually, from vital registration systems and political subdivisions	Complete	Useful for studying mortality overall and by specific cause
Medical data from birth records	Data on congenital anomalies, complications of pregnancy and childbirth, birth weight, etc.	Annually, from vital registration systems and political subdivisions	Complete	Routinely available; some aspects of morbidity may be incompletely reported (e.g., etiologic factors)
Reportable disease statistics	Statistics based on physician reports, new cases of notifiable communicable diseases	Weekly reports for the United States	Complete	Useful for detection of outbreaks of infectious diseases; some conditions not completely reported
Mass diagnostic and screening surveys	Data that result from diagnostic and screening tests for specified diseases	On an ad hoc basis	Variable	Unknown completeness
Disease registries	Statistics based on existing case registries of cancer, stroke, etc.	Continuous, from national, state, and local jurisdictions	Presumably complete for selected diagnosed diseases	Useful for studying incidence of diseases such as cancer; used to select cases in a case-control study
Morbidity surveys of general population	From the U.S. Health Examination Survey (HES) and the Household Interview Survey (HIS)	Continuous, data released on computer tapes	Complete for probability sample	Useful for epidemiologic research; some HIS data may not be accurate for self-reports; HES data contain more precise diagnoses
Health insurance statistics	Cases given medical care under prepaid insurance coverage	Not generally available, although some agencies conduct research on their own insured	Covered population	Useful for health care utilization studies; research on morbidity and mortality in selected populations

Table 5-1 *continued*

Data Source	Nature of Data	Availability	Population Coverage	Value and Limitations
Life insurance statistics	Mortality data and results of physical examinations of those applying for coverage	Not generally available	Insurance policyholders	Data for selected population
Hospital inpatient statistics	Cases treated in hospital; dependent on type of hospital	Generally not available without special approval	Not determinable	Diagnostic information may be of higher quality than that from other sources; difficult to relate cases to a population denominator
Hospital outpatient statistics	Patients in clinics and outpatient divisions (OPD) of hospitals	Generally not available without special approval	Not determinable	OPDs provide a large volume of care; OPD hospital records are sometimes not well developed; diagnostic data may be incomplete
Data on diseases treated in special clinics and hospitals	Dependent on nature of clinic or hospital; essentially medical care data	Generally not available without special approval	Not determinable	Counts of patients treated; difficult to determine prevalence rates; population denominator unknown
Data from public health clinics	Data from physical examinations of clients	Generally not available without special approval	Not determinable	Possible use for identification of cases of disease and for study of health services; population denominator unknown
Data from records of physicians' practices	Medical care provided in physicians' offices	Generally not available without special approval	Not determinable	May be useful for identification of cases; records may vary in completeness and quality; duplication of cases for patients who see multiple providers

continues

Table 5-1 *continued*

Data Source	Nature of Data	Availability	Population Coverage	Value and Limitations
Absenteeism data	Frequency of absenteeism from work or school	By special arrangement with school system or industry	Probably complete for selected population groups	Nonspecific indicator of disability in selected population; useful for assessing acute disease outbreaks
Data from school health programs	Findings of physical examinations of schoolchildren	Generally not available	Elementary and secondary school population	Uneven quality and completeness of data
Statistics on morbidity in armed forces	Armed forces morbidity and hospitalization experience; results of selective service examinations	Generally available	Draftees and career military personnel	Comprehensive morbidity data on a selected population; important source for follow-up studies
Statistics on veterans	Veterans' hospitalization experience and deaths	Generally available	Hospitalization of those using Veterans Affairs hospitals; may be incomplete for veterans who use other facilities	Useful for studying case mix, demography, and hospitalization experience
Social Security statistics	Disability benefit data and Medicare statistics	Data are released on computer-readable media	Nationwide	Useful for studying disability
Labor statistics	Injuries and illnesses in industry	Routinely reported by the U.S. Bureau of Labor Statistics	Workers in various occupations and industries in the United States	Useful data for studying accidents, injuries, and occupational diseases
Census data	Counts, enumerations, and characteristics of populations by geographic location in the United States, including age, sex, race	Decennial census and annual estimates	Complete	Extremely useful for enumerating the population; some segments of the population may be undercounted, e.g., the homeless

population coverage, and value and limitations. The following sections discuss some of the data sources in more detail.

Statistics Derived from the Vital Registration System

Mortality Statistics

Data are collected routinely on all deaths that occur in the United States. Mortality data have the advantage of being almost totally complete because deaths are unlikely to go unrecorded in the United States or other developed countries. Death certificate data in the United States include demographic information about the decedent and information about the cause of death, including the immediate cause and contributing factors. The death certificate is partially completed by the funeral director. The attending physician then completes the section on date and cause of death. If the death occurred as the result of accident, suicide, or homicide, or if the attending physician is unavailable, then the medical examiner or coroner completes and signs the death certificate. Once this is done, the local registrar checks the certificate for completeness and accuracy and sends a copy to the state registrar. The state registrar also checks for completeness and accuracy and sends a copy to the NCHS, which compiles and publishes national mortality rates (e.g., in *Vital Statistics of the United States*).

Although mortality data are readily available and commonly used for indexes of public health, they are hampered also by some limitations with which one should be familiar. The first is certification of the cause of death. When an older person with a chronic illness dies, the primary cause of death may be unclear. Death certificates list multiple causes of mortality as well as the underlying cause. However, assignment of the cause of death sometimes may be arbitrary. In illustration, diabetes may not be given as the immediate cause of death; rather, the certificate may list the cause of death as heart failure or pneumonia, which could be complications of diabetes. Another factor that detracts from the value of death certificates is lack of standardization of diagnostic criteria employed by various physicians in different hospitals and settings. Yet another problem is the stigma associated with certain diseases. For example, if the decedent died as a result of acquired immune deficiency syndrome (AIDS) or alcoholism and was a long-time friend of the attending physician, the physician may be reluctant to specify this information on a document that is available to the general public.

Regardless of what the true cause of death might be, a nosologist must review the death certificate and code the information for compilation; errors in coding are possible. Furthermore, the codes that are used for the causes of death change over time. Since 1900 there has been an international classification for coding mortality. When the United Nations was formed after World War II, the World Health Organization took charge of this classification. In 1948 the 6th revision of the *International Classification of Diseases* (ICD) was published.[6] The 10th revision is now entitled *International Statistical Classification of Diseases and Related Health Problems* (ICD-10).[7] If the mortality data with which one desires to work span more than one version of the ICD, one must be especially careful, as the codes and groupings of disease change. Therefore, sudden increases or decreases in a particular cause of death may not be real, but rather a reflection of a change in coding systems. An example of a death certificate and the type of data collected are shown in Exhibit 5-3.

Birth Statistics: Certificates of Birth and of Fetal Death

Presumably, birth and fetal death statistics are nearly complete in their coverage of the general population. Although birth certificate data are needed to calculate birth rates, information also is collected about a range of conditions that may affect the neonate, including conditions present during pregnancy, congenital malformations, obstetric procedures, birth weight, length of gestation, and demographic background of the mother. Some of the data may be unreliable, reflecting possible inconsistencies and gaps in the mother's recall of events during pregnancy. It is also possible that certain malformations and illnesses affecting the neonate may not be detected at the time of birth. Many of the foregoing deficiencies of birth certificates also apply to the data contained in certificates of fetal death. In addition, variations from state to state in requirements for fetal death certificates further reduce their utility for epidemiologic studies. Birth and fetal death certificate data have been employed in studies of environmental influences upon congenital malformations. For example, these data have been used in studies that search for clusters of birth defects in geographic areas where mothers may have been exposed to teratogens, such as pesticides or industrial pollution.

Reportable Disease Statistics

By legal statute, physicians and other health care providers must report cases of certain diseases, known as reportable and notifiable diseases, to health

EXHIBIT 5-3

Sample Death Certificate

CERTIFICATE OF DEATH
STATE OF CALIFORNIA
USE BLACK INK ONLY / NO ERASURES, WHITEOUTS OR ALTERATIONS
VS-11 (REV. 1/03)

STATE FILE NUMBER

LOCAL REGISTRATION NUMBER

DECEDENT'S PERSONAL DATA

1. NAME OF DECEDENT --- FIRST (Given)
2. MIDDLE
3. LAST (Family)

AKA, ALSO KNOWN AS --- Include full AKA (FIRST, MIDDLE, LAST)

4. DATE OF BIRTH mm/dd/ccyy
5. AGE Yrs.
IF UNDER ONE YEAR Months | Days
IF UNDER 24 HOURS Hours | Minutes
6. SEX

9. BIRTH STATE/FOREIGN COUNTRY
10. SOCIAL SECURITY NUMBER
11. EVER IN U.S. ARMED FORCES? YES NO UNK
12. MARITAL STATUS (at Time of Death)
7. DATE OF DEATH mm/dd/ccyy
8. HOUR (24 Hours)

13. EDUCATION --- Highest Level/Degree (see worksheet on back)
14/15. WAS DECEDENT SPANISH/HISPANIC/LATINO? (If yes, see worksheet on back) YES NO
16. DECEDENT'S RACE --- Up to 3 races may be listed (see worksheet on back)

17. USUAL OCCUPATION --- Type of work for most of life. DO NOT USE RETIRED
18. KIND OF BUSINESS OR INDUSTRY (e.g., grocery store, road construction, employment agency, etc.)
19. YEARS IN OCCUPATION

USUAL RESIDENCE

20. DECEDENT'S RESIDENCE (Street and number or location)

21. CITY
22. COUNTY/PROVINCE
23. ZIP CODE
24. YEARS IN COUNTY
25. STATE/FOREIGN COUNTRY

INFORMANT

26. INFORMANT'S NAME, RELATIONSHIP
27. INFORMANT'S MAILING ADDRESS (Street and number or rural route number, city or town, state, ZIP)

SPOUSE AND PARENT INFORMATION

28. NAME OF SURVIVING SPOUSE --- FIRST
29. MIDDLE
LAST (Maiden Name)

31. NAME OF FATHER --- FIRST
32. MIDDLE
33. LAST
34. BIRTH STATE

35. NAME OF MOTHER --- FIRST
36. MIDDLE
37. LAST (Maiden)
38. BIRTH STATE

FUNERAL DIRECTOR/ LOCAL REGISTRAR

39. DISPOSITION DATE mm/dd/ccyy
40. PLACE OF FINAL DISPOSITION

41. TYPE OF DISPOSITION(S)
42. SIGNATURE OF EMBALMER
43. LICENSE NUMBER

44. NAME OF FUNERAL ESTABLISHMENT
45. LICENSE NUMBER
46. SIGNATURE OF LOCAL REGISTRAR
47. DATE mm/dd/ccyy

SAMPLE

EXHIBIT 5-3 *continued*

PLACE OF DEATH

101. PLACE OF DEATH

102. IF HOSPITAL, SPECIFY ONE
IP □ ER/OP □ DOA □

103. IF OTHER THAN HOSPITAL, SPECIFY ONE
Hospice □ Nursing Home/LTC □ Decedent's Home □ Other □

104. COUNTY

105. FACILITY ADDRESS OR LOCATION WHERE FOUND (Street and number or location)

106. CITY

CAUSE OF DEATH

107. CAUSE OF DEATH

IMMEDIATE CAUSE (A)
(Final disease or condition resulting in death)

Enter the chain of events --- diseases, injuries, or complications --- that directly caused death. DO NOT enter terminal events such as cardiac arrest, respiratory arrest, or ventricular fibrillation without showing the etiology. DO NOT ABBREVIATE.

Sequentially, list conditions, if any, leading to cause on Line A. Enter UNDERLYING CAUSE (disease or injury that initiated the events resulting in death) LAST

(B)

(C)

(D)

Time Interval Between Onset and Death
(AT)
(BT)
(CT)
(DT)

108. DEATH REPORTED TO CORONER?
YES □ NO □
REFERRAL NUMBER

109. BIOPSY PERFORMED?
YES □ NO □

110. AUTOPSY PERFORMED?
YES □ NO □

111. USED IN DETERMINING CAUSE?
YES □ NO □

112. OTHER SIGNIFICANT CONDITIONS CONTRIBUTING TO DEATH BUT NOT RESULTING IN THE UNDERLYING CAUSE GIVEN IN 107

113. WAS OPERATION PERFORMED FOR ANY CONDITION IN ITEM 107 OR 112? (If yes, list type of operation and date)

SAMPLE

PHYSICIAN'S CERTIFICATION

114. I CERTIFY THAT TO THE BEST OF MY KNOWLEDGE DEATH OCCURRED AT THE HOUR, DATE, AND PLACE STATED FROM THE CAUSES STATED.
Decedent Attended Since   Decedent Last Seen Alive
(A) mm/dd/ccyy   (B) mm/dd/ccyy

115. SIGNATURE OF ATTENDING CERTIFIER ►

116. LICENSE NUMBER

118. TYPE ATTENDING PHYSICIAN'S NAME, MAILING ADDRESS, ZIP CODE

117. DATE mm/dd/ccyy

113A. IF FEMALE, PREGNANT IN LAST YEAR?
YES □ NO □ UNK □

CORONER'S USE ONLY

119. I CERTIFY THAT IN MY OPINION DEATH OCCURRED AT THE HOUR, DATE, AND PLACE STATED FROM THE CAUSES STATED.

MANNER OF DEATH Natural □ Accident □ Homicide □ Suicide □ Pending Investigation □ Could not be determined □

120. INJURED AT WORK?
YES □ NO □ UNK □

121. INJURY DATE mm/dd/ccyy

122. HOUR (24 Hours)

123. PLACE OF INJURY (e.g., home, construction site, wooded area, etc.)

124. DESCRIBE HOW INJURY OCCURRED (Events which resulted in injury)

125. LOCATION OF INJURY (Street and number, or location, and city, and ZIP)

126. SIGNATURE OF CORONER / DEPUTY CORONER ►

127. DATE mm/dd/ccyy

128. TYPE NAME, TITLE OF CORONER / DEPUTY CORONER

STATE REGISTRAR

A □ B □ C □ D □ E □

FAX AUTH. #

CENSUS TRACT

authorities. The diseases are usually infectious and communicable ones that might endanger a population; examples are the sexually transmitted diseases, rubella, tetanus, measles, plague, and food-borne disease. Individual states may elect to maintain reports of communicable and noncommunicable diseases of local concern also.

The process of reporting diseases is known as public health surveillance, which denotes ". . .the ongoing systematic collection, analysis, interpretation, and dissemination of health data."[8(p290)] Health care providers and related workers send reports of diseases to local health departments, which in turn forward them on to state health departments and then to the CDC. The CDC reports the occurrence of internationally quarantinable diseases, e.g., plague, cholera, and yellow fever, to the World Health Organization. The method of reporting diseases in the United States (the information cycle) is illustrated in Figure 5-1.

Supplementing the notifiable disease surveillance system, the CDC operates a surveillance system for a few diseases of interest, such as salmonellosis, shigellosis, and influenza. For example, reports of influenza are tracked from October through May. The CDC collects information from four sources as shown in Figure 5-2: laboratories across the United States, influenza mortality reports from 121 U.S. cities, sentinel physicians (a network of 150 family practice physicians), and state epidemiologists. For more information on surveillance systems for reporting notifiable disease statistics, refer to Centers for Disease Control and Prevention (*Principles of Epidemiology,* 2nd ed. Atlanta, GA; 1998). The present text provides more information on surveillance of environmental health problems in Chapter 13.

FIGURE 5-1 The information cycle. *Source:* Centers for Disease Control and Prevention. *Principles of Epidemiology.* 2nd ed. Atlanta, GA: CDC; 1998, p 305.

FIGURE 5-2 Four different surveillance systems for influenza. *Source:* Centers for Disease Control and Prevention. *Principles of Epidemiology.* 2nd ed. Atlanta, GA: CDC; 1998, p 309.

A detailed list of reportable diseases is shown in Exhibit 5-4. Some of the diseases and conditions are reportable in some states only; others are reportable in all states. For information regarding United States and state requirements, refer to "Mandatory Reporting of Infectious Diseases by Clinicians, and Mandatory Reporting of Occupational Diseases by Clinicians," a publication of the Centers for Disease Control and Prevention.[9]

The major deficiency of this category of data for epidemiologic research purposes is the possible incompleteness of population coverage. First of all, not every person who develops a disease that is on this list of notifiable conditions may seek medical attention; this would be especially likely for asymptomatic and subclinical cases. For example, an active case of typhoid fever will go unreported if

EXHIBIT 5-4

Infectious Diseases Designated as Notifiable at the National Level— United States

Acquired immune deficiency
  syndrome (AIDS)
Anthrax
Botulism
Brucellosis
Chancroid
Chlamydia trachomatis,
  genital infections
Cholera
Coccidioidomycosis
Cryptosporidiosis
Diphtheria
Encephalitis, California serogroup
Encephalitis, eastern equine
Encephalitis, St. Louis
Encephalitis, western equine
Escherichia coli O157:H7
Gonorrhea
Haemophilus influenzae,
  invasive disease
Hansen's disease (leprosy)
Hantavirus pulmonary syndrome
Hemolytic uremic syndrome,
  postdiarrheal
Hepatitis A
Hepatitis B
Hepatitis, C/non-A, non-B
HIV infection, pediatric
Legionellosis
Lyme disease

Malaria
Measles
Meningococcal disease
Mumps
Pertussis
Plague
Poliomyelitis, paralytic
Psittacosis
Rabies, animal
Rabies, human
Rocky Mountain spotted fever
Rubella
Rubella, congenital syndrome
Salmonellosis
Shigellosis
Streptococcal disease, invasive,
  Group A
Streptococcus pneumoniae,
  drug-resistant, invasive disease
Streptococcal toxic shock
  syndrome
Syphilis
Syphilis, congenital
Tetanus
Toxic shock syndrome
Trichinosis
Tuberculosis
Typhoid fever
Yellow fever

Source: Reprinted from p 2 of the article, Case definitions for infectious conditions under public health surveillance, *MMWR Recomm Rep.* vol 46, 1–55, 1997, Centers for Disease Control and Prevention.

the affected individual is unaware that he or she has the disease. Another factor associated with lack of complete population coverage is the occasional failure of physicians to fill out the required reporting forms. This can occur if they do not keep up to date on the frequently changing requirements for disease reporting in a local area. As discussed earlier in this chapter, the physician may also be unwilling to risk compromising the confidentiality of the physician-patient relationship. There is much concern and controversy about reporting cases of diseases that carry social stigma. For example, there has been concern about the completeness of AIDS reporting because of the potential sensitivity of the diagnosis.[2] It is the experience of Robert Friis, who was previously associated with a local health department, that widespread and less dramatic conditions such as streptococcal pharyngitis sometimes are unreported. More severe and unusual diseases, such as diphtheria, are usually reported.

Screening Surveys

Screening surveys are often conducted on an ad hoc basis to identify individuals who may have infectious or chronic diseases. It is common practice for community health agencies to set up neighborhood screening clinics for hypertension or breast cancer. Another example is the health fair that may be organized by civic groups. The clientele for the screening programs are highly selected because they consist primarily of individuals who are sufficiently concerned about the disease to participate in screening. Epidemiologic studies might utilize the data yielded from screening programs of this type for research purposes; nevertheless, it would be difficult to generalize the results obtained to any other setting because of the nonrepresentative nature of the sample.

Many large corporations and other employers have set up multiphasic screening programs for their employees. In this type of screening, the employees of an entire large plant may be surveyed. Through the possible early detection of health problems, complications from chronic diseases may be reduced and the life of the employee extended. Because of the ongoing nature of multiphasic screening programs for employees as well as the possible coverage of a total working population, it may be fruitful to utilize data that have been collected for epidemiologic research. These data could be utilized in incidence studies and for research on occupational health problems. One negative feature of the data would be biases resulting from worker attrition and turnover. High loss to follow-up would compromise the validity of the study. A second difficulty is that such data may not contain etiologic information required for a specific analysis.

Disease Registries

A registry is a centralized database for collection of information about a disease. Registries are widely used for the compilation of statistical data on cancer, prominent examples being the Connecticut Tumor Registry, the California Tumor Registry, and a New York State cancer registry. There are many other types of registries devoted to conditions as divergent as mental retardation, strokes, accidents, and enteric diseases. The completeness of population coverage depends upon the ability of the registry staff to secure the cooperation of agencies and medical facilities that would submit data about diseases. If agencies that come into contact with new cases of disease do not report them to the registry, population coverage will be incomplete. The success of a registry is often dependent upon the conscientiousness of the staff and adequate funding. Nonreporting biases are also likely to occur as public concern grows about the confidentiality of medical data; patients may not want their personal records to be released to an outside agency by the service provider. It is necessary to maintain some personal identifiers from a medical record when it is released to a registry to permit record linkage or follow-up investigations. This has been accomplished by using coding algorithms that create a unique identifier for each medical record.

There are several noteworthy applications of registries, such as patient tracking, development of information about trends in rates of disease, and the conduct of case-control studies. For example, registries have been used to facilitate regular follow-up of patients with cancer and to study the natural history of infectious and chronic diseases. Population-based cancer registries, such as those incorporated in the Surveillance, Epidemiology, and End Results (SEER) program, have provided unique data on cancer survival, incidence, and treatment[10] (Exhibit 5-5).

Morbidity Surveys of the General Population

Morbidity surveys collect data on the health status of a population group. Typically, they use a scientifically designed representative sample of a population. The purposes of morbidity surveys are to determine the frequency of chronic and acute diseases and disability, to collect measurements of bodily characteristics, to conduct physical examinations and laboratory tests, and to probe other health-related characteristics of specific concern to those directing the survey. Morbidity surveys strive to gather more comprehensive information than would be available from routinely collected data.[10] The U.S. National

The SEER Program

"The National Cancer Act of 1971 mandated the collection, analysis, and dissemination of all data useful in the prevention, diagnosis, and treatment of cancer. The act resulted in the establishment of the National Cancer Program under which the Surveillance, Epidemiology, and End Results (SEER) Program was developed. A continuing project of the National Cancer Institute (NCI), the SEER Program collects cancer data on a routine basis from designated population-based cancer registries in various areas of the country. Trends in cancer incidence, mortality and patient survival in the United States, as well as many other studies, are derived from this data bank.

"The geographic areas comprising the SEER Program's data base represent an estimated 13.9% of the United States population. The data base contained information on 1.7 million *in situ* and invasive cancers diagnosed between 1973 and 1991; approximately 120,000 new cases are accessioned yearly in 9 areas including the states of Connecticut, Iowa, New Mexico, Utah, Hawaii and the metropolitan areas of Detroit, San Francisco, Seattle-Puget Sound, and Atlanta." ■

Source: Reprinted from *SEER Program: Surveillance, Epidemiology and End Results,* National Cancer Institute, National Institutes of Health, Publication No 94-3074, October 1993.

Health Survey is a notable example.[11] The survey was authorized under the National Health Survey Act of 1956 to obtain information about the health status of the U.S. population. Various components of the survey probe the amount, distribution, and effects of illness and disability in the United States and the services received for or because of such conditions. It also is used for the development and improvement of survey and other methods for obtaining health-related data.

The National Health Survey consists of three separate and distinct programs that are conducted by NCHS: the National Health Interview Survey (NHIS, a household health interview survey), the Health Examination Survey (HES), and a family of surveys of health resources.

National Health Interview Survey

According to NCHS, the NHIS is a:

> General household health survey of the U.S. civilian noninstitutionalized population using a multistage probability design that permits continuous sampling throughout the year. The sample is designed in such a way that the sample of households interviewed each week is representative of the target population and that weekly samples are additive over time. Independent samples are selected each year. Interviews have been conducted annually since 1957 with approximately 111,000 persons living in about 42,000 households. The sample has ranged in magnitude from a high of about 134,000 persons in some 44,000 households in 1972 to a low of about 62,000 people in approximately 35,000 households in 1986. The 1986 sample represented only one-half of the new sample, which was redesigned in 1985. About 123,000 persons in 1987 and about 122,000 persons in 1988 and 1989 were interviewed in approximately 47,000 households each year.[12(p26)]

The range of conditions studied is comprehensive and includes diseases, injuries, disability, and impairments. Because the survey relies on reports of medical conditions by a principal respondent reporting for everyone in the household, the results should be interpreted with caution. These responses may be even less accurate than self-reports, which are known to reflect inadequately certain chronic illnesses.[10]

Health Examination Survey

The HES is the second of the three different programs operated by NCHS as part of the National Health Survey.[11] Data are collected from a sample of the civilian, noninstitutionalized population of the United States. Although the HIS provides data on self-reports of morbidity, the HES provides more direct information about morbidity through examinations, measurements, and clinical tests to yield data on unrecognized and untreated diseases. It is felt that these are the best sources of information about standardized clinical, physiologic, and physical data. The HES is conducted in a series of cycles that are limited to a specific segment of the U.S. population. Through the various tests and measurements that are taken, information is obtained about diagnosed conditions that the person fails to report in an interview or about previously undiagnosed conditions. One of the uses of these data is to provide baseline measurements on physical, physiologic, and psychologic characteristics not previously available for a defined population.

The HES has been amalgamated with the National Nutrition Surveillance Survey and renamed as the Health and Nutrition Examination Survey (HANES). HANES surveys include the first National Health and Nutrition

Examination Survey (NHANES I). Turczyn and Drury stated that the purpose of NHANES I was to conduct a:

> survey of the U.S. civilian noninstitutionalized population ages 1-74 years, using a multistage, clustered probability sample stratified by geographic region and population size. Interviews and examinations with about 21,000 persons were conducted from 1971 through 1974. This sample was augmented with approximately 3,000 persons ages 25-74 in 1974 and 1975. . . . Data on all examined persons include household and demographic information; nutrition information; medical, dental, dermatological, and ophthalmological examinations; anthropometric measurements; hand-wrist X-rays (ages 1-17 only); and a variety of laboratory tests.[12(p13)]

Related surveys and data collected by the National Center for Health Statistics include NHANES II and HHANES (Exhibit 5-6). Several health care surveys also are conducted as part of the National Health Survey:

- National Hospital Discharge Survey
- National Ambulatory Medical Care Survey
- National Nursing Home Survey

In addition, there are several vital statistics surveys:

- National Natality Survey
- National Fetal Mortality Survey
- National Mortality Followback Survey

For more information regarding the data from these sources, refer to the articles by Rice[13] and Gable.[1]

Insurance Data

Social Security, health insurance, and life insurance statistics are all examples of insurance data that have been used widely in epidemiologic studies. One of the major problems inherent in the data is that they do not provide any information about people who are not insured and thus may not accurately represent all segments of society.

Some of the types of information provided by insurance statistics are as follows. Social Security statistics yield data on recipients of disability benefits and participants in Medicare programs. Both types of data may be used in studies of the frequency and severity of disabling conditions. Health insurance statistics contain information about individuals receiving medical care through a prepaid medical program. Some notable examples of these programs are the Health Insurance

EXHIBIT 5-6

Hispanic Health and Nutrition Examination Survey (HHANES), 1982–1984

From 1982 to 1984, the HHANES was conducted by NCHS to obtain data on the health and nutritional status of three Hispanic groups:

1. Mexican Americans from Texas, Colorado, New Mexico, and California
2. Cuban Americans from Dade County, Florida
3. Puerto Ricans from the New York City area

In the Mexican-American portion, 9,894 persons were sampled, of whom 8,554 were interviewed and 7,462 were examined. In the Cuban-American portion, 2,244 persons were sampled, of whom 1,766 were interviewed and 1,357 were examined. In the Puerto Rican portion, 3,786 persons were sampled, of whom 3,369 were interviewed and 2,834 were examined. Respondents, whose ages ranged from 6 months to 74 years, were selected by using a multistage, clustered probability sample. Approximately 76% of the Hispanic origin population of the United States resides in the sampled areas. Interviews, conducted in the household or in a mobile examination clinic, included basic demographic, health history, and health practices information. A variety of tests and medical examinations were performed in the mobile clinics. The survey focused on two major aspects of health: certain important chronic conditions (e.g., heart disease, diabetes, hypertension, and depression) and nutrition status. An extensive database ($n \cong 12,000$) was collected from English or Spanish interviews. The data are available for analysis from a public use data tape. ■

Source: Adapted from JL Delgado, CL Johnson, I Roy, FM Trevino. Hispanic Health and Nutrition Examination Survey: Methodological Considerations, *American Journal of Public Health,* vol 80, Supplement, pp 6–10, American Public Health Association, © 1990.

Plan of New York and the Kaiser Medical Plan. These plans, as well as health maintenance organizations, are proliferating as the emphasis on cost containment and primary prevention of disease grows. A number of investigators have employed data from these programs for epidemiologic studies. Data from prepaid plans may be valuable for long-term studies of chronic disease, especially incidence studies, because data collection is often continued over a number of years for each patient; special questionnaires may be added as needed. In contrast to health insurance statistics, life insurance statistics provide data on causes of mortality among insured groups and also on the results of physical examinations for those applying for insurance policies. Health and life insurance statistics may contain an overrepresentation of healthier individuals because unhealthy individuals may not be allowed to hold life insurance policies and because an ongoing health insurance program may result in a healthier population among insured individuals than among the noninsured. Findings derived from those populations may not necessarily be representative of the overall population of the United States.

Hospital Data

Hospital statistics consist of both inpatient and outpatient data that are routinely collected when a patient enrolls in a hospital or an outpatient treatment program. These categories of data may be deficient for purposes of epidemiologic research because the individuals included do not represent any specific population but rather are collected on an ad hoc basis. Patients who are treated in the hospital setting, especially those in large metropolitan hospitals, may be drawn from all over the metropolitan area or even from other countries. Furthermore, there is often a lack of standardization in the types of information collected on each patient and the diagnostic procedures that are used by the attending physicians. There also may be variation from one physician to another in the completeness with which information is collected. Hospital data, those derived from inpatient and outpatient divisions and specialized clinics, are limited with respect to the socioeconomic composition of patients who may be treated. The majority of patients at certain specialized clinics and the renowned hospitals in urban areas may represent the upper socioeconomic strata of our society. Hospital emergency departments and outpatient clinics may contain large proportions of lower socioeconomic individuals in some of the urban areas because some indigent patients use the hospital emergency department and related clinics of public hospitals as their primary source of medical care.

Diseases Treated in Special Clinics and Hospitals

As is true of data from hospitals in general, these data cannot be generalized readily to a reference population because the patients of a special clinic by definition are a highly selected group. Case-control studies might be conducted with patients who present with rare and unusual diseases, but it would not be possible to determine incidence and prevalence rates of disease without making assumptions about the size of the denominator.

An exception to the general rule about special clinics and hospitals is work done by investigators at the Mayo Clinic in Rochester, Minnesota. The Rochester Epidemiology Project provides a capability for population-based studies of disease causes and outcomes that is unique in the United States, if not the world.[14] This ability is due to a medical records linkage system that has afforded access to details of the medical care provided to residents of Rochester and Olmsted County, Minnesota, since the turn of the century. This project exists, in part, because the Mayo Clinic is geographically isolated from other urban centers. Although best known as a tertiary referral center, the Mayo Clinic has always provided primary and secondary care, as well as tertiary care to local residents. Because Mayo offers care in every medical and surgical specialty and subspecialty, local residents are not obliged to seek providers throughout a large region, but are able to obtain most of their medical care within the community. Indeed, in a comprehensive survey of community residents, 90% of those who sought medical assessment received care at the Mayo Clinic, the Olmsted Medical Group, or one of their affiliated hospitals, and 96% selected one of these providers when they had a major medical problem. This unusually close correspondence between a circumscribed geographic population and its health care providers comprises a natural laboratory for population-based studies.

The Rochester Epidemiology Project studies are facilitated by the Mayo unified medical record system, wherein all data about a specific patient are contained in a single file linked to a unique Mayo identification number. Today the dossiers for each of the more than 5 million patients who have ever been seen at Mayo Clinic Rochester are maintained in a central repository and tracked by computerized bar codes. Fewer than 500 histories have been lost since the records were initiated 90 years ago. In 1966, indexes were created for the records of the other providers of medical care to Rochester and Olmsted County residents. The result is linkage of medical data from almost all sources of medical care available to, and used by, the local population in and near Rochester. These sources include the Mayo Clinic and its affiliated hospitals (Saint Mary's and Rochester Methodist), the Olmsted Medical Group and its affiliated Olmsted Community Hospital, the University of Minnesota hospitals and the Department of Veterans Affairs Medical Center, located in Minneapolis, as well as other medical institutions in the region. During the past several decades, the Rochester Epidemiology Project has successfully provided the data and facilities to complete over 1,000 reports on the epidemiology of acute and chronic diseases. Several of these investigations have been descriptive studies of disease incidence or prevalence, especially long-term trends. Each year, more than half of the Olmsted County population is examined at one of the Mayo facilities, and most local residents have at least one Mayo contact during any specific three-year period. Thus, the Rochester Epidemiology Project records-linkage system provides what is essentially an enumeration of the population. Therefore, samples from this system should approximate samples of the general population. This assertion was validated in a survey in which every subject contacted through a random-digit dialing telephone sample or by residence in a local nursing home or senior citizens complex was found to have a medical record in the community.

Data From Physicians' Practices

The records from private physicians' medical practices would seem to be a logical source of information about health and illness. In practice, however, this source of information may have limited application in epidemiologic research. Because of professional codes of confidentiality and privacy, physicians may be either reluctant or prohibited to release any information about their patients without written informed consent. The patients of private physicians are also a highly select group that can afford the higher cost of private medical care, making them unrepresentative of the total population. Finally, little effort has been made to standardize the kinds of information collected about each individual patient, making it difficult to carry out a prevalence study or an incidence study without a considerable degree of missing or incomplete data. The records of physicians in private practice are likely to be highly idiosyncratic documents that cannot be readily linked to other data sources.

Although data exclusively from physicians' records may be insufficient to generate reliable measures of disease frequency, they nonetheless represent a valuable supplement to analytic epidemiologic studies. For example, suppose you are interested in assembling a population of women at risk for breast cancer. The plan is to measure usual dietary intake, follow the women for the development of disease, and determine whether dietary exposures measured at baseline were associated with incidence. In this situation, it would be important to exclude women who had developed cancer previously because cancers that developed among this subset would not be first cancers. Although such cancer history data could be collected by self-report, a more precise characterization of the cohort at risk could be obtained by verifying self-reported cancers with medical records. It also would be reasonable to take a sample of women who reported themselves free from cancer and verify self-reports against medical records.

Physicians' records may be an important source of exposure data also. Continuing with the hypothetical breast cancer study, suppose one decided to collect detailed information about oral contraceptive use. Again, although this information could be obtained by self-report from the subjects themselves, because the use of oral contraceptives requires a physician's prescription more detailed information about age at first use, duration of use, and formulation might be obtained from the medical record.

Absenteeism Data

Another kind of data that may be used for epidemiologic research is the records of absenteeism from work or school. This type of data, unfortunately, is subject to a host of possible deficiencies. First of all, these data omit populations that neither work nor attend school. Second, not all people who are absent have an illness. Third, not all people who are ill take time off from work or school. In spite of these deficiencies, the data are probably useful for the study of respiratory disease outbreaks and other rapidly spreading conditions, such as epidemics of influenza, that may be reflected in massive school absenteeism.

School Health Programs

The administration office and school nurse maintain records on the immunization history of pupils in school, findings of required physical examinations, and self-reports of previous illness. Detailed information may be retained about cognitive and other tests. The health-related data from this source are probably sporadic and incomplete, although there are exceptions to this general caveat. School health data have been used in studies of intelligence and mental retardation. For studies of disease etiology, there are some well-known examples where data routinely collected on students have proven to be extremely valuable. Paffenbarger et al.[15] used historical records on college students to identify causes of common chronic diseases. They studied nearly 45,000 men and women who attended the University of Pennsylvania from 1931 through 1940 or Harvard University from 1921 through 1950. Standardized case taking by physicians in student health services provided data on medical, social, and psychologic histories and an extensive physical examination. Although the methods of data collection varied slightly between universities and complete data were not obtained on all students, valuable measures were taken on such factors as vital capacity, pulse rise after exercise, urinalysis, and electrocardiogram. Information was obtained about mortality through the college alumni office, and causes of death were determined from official state or federal sources. The detailed medical, physiologic, and lifestyle information plus the data on mortality afford an efficient analysis of precursive and causative factors. We will revisit this example in Chapter 7.

Morbidity in the Armed Forces: Data on Active Personnel and Veterans

The types of information collected under this heading include reported morbidity among active armed forces personnel and veterans, results of routine physical examinations, military hospitalization records, and results of selective service examinations. The last of these were, at one time, universally required of all qualified men upon reaching 18 years of age. With the abolition of the draft, physical examinations are given selectively to volunteers for military service. Thus, this source of epidemiologic data, which tends to be representative primarily of volunteer groups, is not particularly useful for estimates of disease frequency for the general population.

Nonetheless, records on military personnel may be quite useful for studies of disease etiology. For example, the National Academy of Sciences-National Research Council assembled a large panel of twins to help sort out the influences of "nature and nurture" on the pathogenesis of disease.[16] The twin panel comprised approximately 16,000 white male twin pairs born between 1917 and 1927. Both members of each twin pair served in the U.S. military during the Korean War or World War II. Zygosity was determined by blood typing for 806 pairs, by fingerprinting for 1,947 pairs, and by questionnaire for 10,732 pairs. Several investigators have used these data to examine the role of genetic factors in human obesity.[17,18] Weight and height, measured during the induction physical examination, were available for 5,884 monozygotic (identical) and 7,492 dizygotic (fraternal) pairs. A comparison of the degree of similarity in various measures of obesity suggested that the identical twins were more alike than the nonidentical twins, an expectation consistent with genetic influences.[17]

Other Sources of Data Relevant to Epidemiologic Studies

The U.S. Bureau of the Census provides much information of value to epidemiologic research, for example, general, social, and economic characteristics of the U.S. population. The U.S. Census is administered every 10 years to the entire population of the nation. The decennial census attempts to account for every person and his or her residence and to characterize the population according to sex, age, family relationships, and other demographic variables.[19] Beginning with the 1940 census, a more detailed questionnaire has also been administered to representative samples of the population. The Census Bureau also makes annual estimates of the number of persons in the population. Some of the publications developed by the Bureau of the Census include the following:

- *Statistical Abstract of the United States*
- *County and City Data Book*
- *Decennial Censuses of Population and Housing*
- *Historical Statistics of the United States, Colonial Time to 1957*

Two other examples of important terminology utilized by the U.S. Bureau of the Census have particular relevance to epidemiology: metropolitan statistical areas (MSAs) and census tracts. MSAs (formerly known as standard metropolitan statistical areas) are geographic areas of the United States established by the Bureau of the Census to provide a distinction between metropolitan and nonmetropolitan areas by type of residence, industrial concentration, and population concentration. According to the NCHS, "The general concept of a metropolitan area is one of a large population nucleus together with adjacent communities that have a high degree of economic and social integration with that nucleus."[20(p3)] To be defined as an MSA, an area must include one of the following:

- one city with a population of 50,000 or more
- an area that is defined by the U.S. Bureau of the Census, using various criteria, as urbanized; such an area would have a total MSA population of at least 100,000 (75,000 in New England)

Census tracts are small geographic subdivisions of cities, counties, and adjacent areas. The average tract has about 4,000 residents and is designed to provide a degree of uniformity of population economic status and living conditions within each tract.

Conclusion

This chapter covered a variety of types and sources of data used in epidemiologic research. A central concern of epidemiologists is how to find the best quality of data to describe the distribution of morbidity and mortality in a population or to conduct studies of disease etiology. To assess the potential utility of data, one needs to consider the nature, availability, representativeness, and completeness of the data. The criterion *nature of the data* includes whether the data are from vital statistics, case registries, physicians' records, surveys of the general population, or hospital and clinic cases. The criterion *availability of the data* relates to the investigator's ability to gain access to the data. The criterion *representativeness* or *external* validity refers to generalizability of findings to populations other than the one from which the data have been obtained. Related to the extent of population coverage is the criterion *completeness of the data,* which refers to the thoroughness of identification of all cases with a particular health phenomenon, including subclinical cases.

Some of the diverse sources of epidemiologic data include statistics compiled by government, industry, or organizations such as the United Nations. Much progress has been made in the development of computerized databases and the Internet; a helpful starting point for epidemiologic research studies is a systematic retrieval of information from computerized bibliographic sources. Epidemiologic data are derived from the vital registration system, reports of absenteeism from work or school, disease registries, morbidity surveys of the general population, hospital statistics, and census tracts, to cite a few examples. Epidemiologic data from these sources have many useful applications, including development of descriptive studies of trends in disease and analytic studies of disease etiology.

Study Questions and Exercises

1. Are you able to define the following?
   a. disease registry
   b. National Health Survey
   c. NHANES I and HHANES
2. What is likely to be the best routinely available data source for each of the following kinds of studies?
   a. incidence of influenza in the U.S.
   b. cancer morbidity

     c. congenital malformations

     d. prevalence of selected disabling conditions

     e. work-related accidents

     f. precursive factors for heart disease among college graduates

     g. ethnic differences in mortality

3. Death certificates are an important source of information for epidemiologic studies. In the United States, death certificates have which of the following advantages (circle all that apply):

     a. There is a uniform national system of collection and coding.

     b. The cause of death is usually confirmed by autopsy.

     c. The international coding system for cause of death has remained constant for the last 50 years.

     d. Data collection is comprehensive; virtually no deaths go unrecorded.

     e. The decedent's personal physician always completes the form and can add his or her own knowledge of past illnesses.

4. Which of the following data sources are best able to provide numerator data for the calculation of incidence of death by gunshot?

     a. hospital discharge survey

     b. autopsy or coroners' records

     c. National Health Survey

     d. disease registries

     e. prepaid group practice insurance programs

5. An abrupt drop in mortality due to a specific cause is observed from one year to the next. Identify at least three reasons for such a change.

6. Pick up the local paper and search for an article on a recent medical finding or public health issue. Conduct a Medline search to find relevant published articles on the same topic.

7. Access the University of Pittsburgh "Guide to Locating Health Statistics" on the Internet. Determine five vital statistics on your city or county: income, education, health care, land, and mortality rates.

8. State funding for a childhood injury prevention program has just become available. To gather baseline data on childhood injuries, the staff is discussing whether to conduct a survey or establish a surveillance system. Discuss the advantages and disadvantages of these two approaches.

9. During the previous 6 years, 1–3 cases per year of Kawasaki syndrome had been reported by a state health department. During the past 3 months, 17 cases have been reported. All but two of these cases have been reported from one county. The local newspaper carried an article about

one of the first reported cases, a young girl. Describe the possible causes of the increase in reported cases.

10. You have recently been hired by a state health department to run surveillance activities, among other tasks. All surveillance data are entered into a personal computer and transmitted to CDC each week. The state, however, has never generated its own set of tables for analysis. What three tables might you want to generate by computer each week?

11. [Suppose that] Last week, the state public health laboratory diagnosed rabies in 4 raccoons that had been captured in a wooded residential neighborhood. This information will be duly reported in the tables of the monthly state health department newsletter. Is this sufficient? Who needs to know this information?

Source (Questions 8–11): Centers for Disease Control and Prevention. *Principles of Epidemiology.* 2nd ed. Atlanta, GA: CDC; 1998:332–334.

References

1. Gable CB. A compendium of public health data sources. *Am J Epidemiol.* 1990;131:381–394.
2. Feinleib M. The epidemiologist's responsibilities to study participants. *J Clin Epidemiol.* 1991;44(suppl I):73S–79S.
3. Hogue CJR. Ethical issues in sharing epidemiologic data. *J Clin Epidemiol.* 1991;44(suppl I):103S–107S.
4. Lilienfeld DE, Stolley PD. *Foundations of Epidemiology.* 3rd ed. New York, NY: Oxford University Press; 1994.
5. Timmreck TC. *An Introduction to Epidemiology.* Boston, MA: Jones & Bartlett; 1994.
6. World Health Organization (WHO). *International Classification of Diseases,* 6th rev. Geneva, Switzerland: WHO; 1948.
7. World Health Organization (WHO). *International Statistical Classification of Diseases and Related Health Problems:* ICD-10, 10th rev. Geneva, Switzerland: WHO; 1992.
8. Centers for Disease Control and Prevention. *Principles of Epidemiology,* 2nd ed. Atlanta, GA: 1998.
9. Chorba TL, Berkelman RL, Safford SK, Gibbs NP, Hull HF. Mandatory reporting of infectious diseases by clinicians, and mandatory reporting of occupational diseases by clinicians. *MMWR Recomm Rep.* 1990;39(RR-9):1–17.
10. Mausner JS, Kramer S. *Epidemiology: An Introductory Text.* 2nd ed. Philadelphia, PA: Saunders; 1985.
11. Miller HW. *Plan and Operation of the Health and Nutrition Examination Survey: United States—1971–1973* (Vital and Health Statistics ser 1, no 10a). Department of Health, Education and Welfare publication (PHS)79–1310. Hyattsville, MD: National Center for Health Statistics; 1978.

12. Turczyn KM, Drury TF. *An Inventory of Pain Data from the National Center for Health Statistics.* Department of Health and Human Services publication (PHS)92–1308. Hyattsville, MD: National Center for Health Statistics; 1992.

13. Rice DP. Data needs for health policy in an aging population (including a survey of data available in the United States of America). *World Health Stat Q.* 1992;45:61–67.

14. Melton LJ III. History of the Rochester Epidemiology Project. *Mayo Clin Proc.* 1996;71:266–274.

15. Paffenbarger RS Jr, Notkin J, Kreuger DE, et al. Chronic disease in former college students, II. methods of study and observations on mortality from coronary heart disease. *Am J Public Health.* 1966;56:962–971.

16. Jablon S, Neel JV, Gershowitz H, et al. The NAS-NRC twin panel: methods of construction of the panel, zygosity diagnosis, and proposed use. *Am J Hum Genet.* 1967;19:133–161.

17. Stunkard AJ, Foch TT, Hrubec Z. A twin study of human obesity. *JAMA.* 1986;256:51–54.

18. Selby JV, Newman B, Quesenberry CP Jr, et al. Evidence of genetic influence on central body fat in middle-aged twins. *Hum Biol.* 1989;61:179–193.

19. U.S. Bureau of the Census. *Statistical Abstract of the United States: 1990,* 110th ed. Washington, DC: U.S. Bureau of the Census; 1990.

20. Collins JG, Hendershot GE. *Health Characteristics of Large Metropolitan Statistical Areas: United States, 1988–89.* Department of Health and Human Services publication (PHS)93–1515. Hyattsville, MD: National Center for Health Statistics; 1993.

Study Designs: Ecologic, Cross-Sectional, Case-Control

LEARNING OBJECTIVES

By the end of this chapter the reader will be able to:

- define the basic differences between observational and experimental epidemiology
- identify an epidemiologic study design by its description
- list the main characteristics, advantages, and disadvantages of ecologic, cross-sectional, and case-control studies
- calculate and interpret an odds ratio

CHAPTER OUTLINE

Introduction

An arsenal of study design options is available to the epidemiologist. The selection of a particular technique from this arsenal and its application to the study of health issues will be a central theme of this chapter. The discussion will demonstrate that the choice of a study design is, to a certain extent, dependent on the amount of information that is already known about a particular health issue proposed for investigation. When relatively little is known, the investigator should not commence a costly and lengthy study. Rather, a more prudent approach would be to employ, if possible, a study design that uses existing data, is quick and easy to conduct, and is economical. As knowledge increases, and the complexity of the research questions increases, then more rigorous study designs may be merited.

The preceding paragraph, although an oversimplification, previews some of the factors involved in the full decision process of selecting a particular study design. This chapter is the first of three that will provide a more complete picture of the factors involved by presenting the various study designs in sequence from simpler, faster, and less expensive to more complex, time consuming, and expensive. Chapter 6, which introduces study designs, explores three varieties of observational studies (ecologic, cross-sectional, case control); Chapter 7 completes observational studies by covering cohort studies; and Chapter 8 focuses on quasi-experimental and experimental designs. An attempt will be made to justify the added expense (in time, resources, and money) of each new design over its predecessors.

The chapter will demonstrate that the major study designs differ from one another in several respects:

- *Number of observations made:* In some cases, observations on subjects may be made only once, whereas in others two or more examinations may be made.
- *Directionality of exposure:* The directionality of exposure measurement relative to disease varies. The investigator may elect to start with subjects who already have a disease and ask them retrospectively about previous exposures that may have led to the outcome under study, or he or she may start with a disease-free group for which exposures are determined first. The latter group would then be followed prospectively for development of disease.
- *Data collection methods:* Some methods require almost exclusive use of existing, previously collected data, whereas others require collection of new data.
- *Timing of data collection:* If long periods of time have elapsed between measurement of exposure and disease, questions might be raised about the quality and applicability of the data.

- *Unit of observation:* For some studies the unit of observation is an entire group, whereas for others the unit of observation is the individual.
- *Availability of subjects:* Certain classes of subjects may not be available for epidemiologic research as a result of a number of considerations, including ethical issues.

In defining and characterizing the more common study designs used in epidemiology, the chapter will place particular emphasis on the following key points: how study subjects are selected, how each design fits into the spectrum of design options, and how each design has inherent strengths and weaknesses. The discussion will not belabor the points about each type of design, but rather will provide a sense of how they differ from one another and how they are applied.

Observational Versus Experimental Approaches in Epidemiology

A basic typology of epidemiologic research will help put the various study designs in proper perspective.[1] Consider two basic facets of research designs:

1. Manipulation of the study factor (M) means that the exposure of interest is controlled by the investigator, a government agency, or even nature, not by the study subjects. For example, local water treatment plant personnel may have chlorinated the water supply. Water consumers are exposed to chlorine and byproducts of the chlorination process because of the water treatment regulations, not necessarily because of their own free choice.

2. Randomization of study subjects (R) refers to a process in which chance determines the likelihood of subjects' assignment to exposure conditions. Thus, by the flip of a coin, for example, an individual may be designated to receive either an intensive, experimental smoking cessation program or the current standard of care.

The various permutations of these two factors, M and R, produce three different study types: experimental, quasi-experimental, and observational (Table 6-1). We shall learn in Chapter 8 that an experimental study involves both M and R, and that a quasi-experimental study involves M but not R. An observational study involves neither M nor R.

Table 6-1 Typology of Epidemiologic Research

M	R	Study Type
Yes	Yes	Experimental
Yes	No	Quasi-experimental
No	No	Observational

Overview of Study Designs Used in Epidemiology

In order to compare and contrast the main types of study designs used in epidemiology, we will provide a brief summary of each type: experimental, quasi-experimental, and observational.

Experimental Studies

Experimental studies (in comparison to quasi-experimental and observational studies) maintain the greatest control over the research setting; the investigator both manipulates the study factor and randomly assigns subjects to the exposed and nonexposed groups. From the perspective of epidemiology, one common experimental design is a clinical trial, used primarily in research and teaching hospitals for several purposes: to test the efficacy of new therapies, surgical procedures, or chemopreventive agents; to test etiologic hypotheses and estimate long-term effects; and to study the effect of interventions to modify health status. For example, dietary modification of fat intake may be tested within the context of a controlled clinical trial to determine acceptability, potential problems, and sources of dissatisfaction or confusion; clinical trials thus may help demonstrate the feasibility of a large-scale population intervention. The number of subjects who can be included may limit the conclusions from clinical trials. Large trials are indeed conducted, but their considerable expense limits their use.

Community interventions are types of experimental designs that greatly enhance the potential to make a widespread impact on a population's health. Typical community interventions are oriented toward education and behavior change at the population level. Examples of issues addressed are smoking cessation, control of alcohol use, weight loss, establishment of healthy eating behaviors, and encouragement of increased physical activity. Community interventions also focus upon persons at high risk of disease within a particular population.

Finally, successful community interventions may suggest public health policies, such as mandatory seat belt use or proscription of alcohol consumption by pregnant women.

Quasi-Experimental Studies

Table 6-1 indicates that quasi-experimental studies involve manipulation of the study factor but not randomization of study subjects; thus, in some respects they may be thought of as natural experiments. Before federal law mandated seat belt use in the United States, individual states varied in seat belt legislation; some states had seat belt laws, and others did not. Residents in the various states did not determine their own "exposure" to seat belts; rather, state politicians who enacted the seat belt laws were responsible for assignment of the "exposure." A comparison of traffic fatalities in states with and without seat belt laws represents a quasi-experimental design.

By contrasting appropriate indices before and after public health programs are implemented, the quasi-experimental design can be used to evaluate the extent to which the programs meet public health goals. For example, researchers wanted to evaluate a statewide West Virginia intervention program's efficacy in reducing neonatal mortality. They compared pre- and postprogram neonatal mortality.[2] Other applications for the quasi-experimental approach are to compare programs to determine reasons for success or failure of an intervention, to compare costs and benefits, and to suggest changes in current health policies or programs. For example, the 1987 Omnibus Budget Reconciliation Act included regulation of antipsychotic drug use in nursing homes. An analysis of drug use in all Medicare- and Medicaid-certified nursing homes in Minnesota revealed that the rates of antipsychotic drug use declined by more than a third in apparent anticipation of, and as a result of, the legislation.[3] Thus, the legislation appeared to achieve its intended effect.

Observational Studies

In some instances an experiment would be impractical; in others, unethical. Accordingly, much of epidemiologic research is relegated to observational studies, which, as shown in Table 6-1, entail neither manipulation of the study factor nor randomization of study subjects. Rather, observational studies make use of careful measurement of patterns of exposure and disease in populations to draw inferences about etiology. There are two main subtypes of observational studies:

1. Descriptive studies, covered in Chapter 4, include case reports, case series, and cross-sectional surveys. They are used to depict individuals' health characteristics (e.g., morbidity from specific diseases or mortality) with respect to person, place, and time and to estimate disease frequency and time trends. Although descriptive studies may be used for health planning purposes and allocation of resources, they are used also to generate etiologic hypotheses.

2. Analytic studies include ecologic studies, case-control studies, and cohort studies. These designs are employed to test specific etiologic hypotheses, to generate new etiologic hypotheses, and to suggest mechanisms of causation. As a body of knowledge builds regarding likely etiologic factors for a disease, it becomes possible to generate preventive hypotheses and to suggest and identify potential methods for disease prevention.

The 2 by 2 Table

The foregoing concludes the brief overview of three types of epidemiologic research designs: experimental, quasi-experimental, and observational. The remainder of the chapter will define and illustrate one group of observational studies more fully. When thinking about study designs, it is helpful for the reader to visualize how the study groups are assembled in the context of the 2 by 2 table. The reader should bear in mind an important caveat, however: The model tends to underestimate the complexity of the potential linkage between exposure and disease. It was previously mentioned (see Chapt. 2) that exposures do not always fall neatly into the categories of exposed and nonexposed. Hence, the notion of one exposure–one disease is admittedly naive. Nevertheless, a comprehension of this rather simplistic model leads one to an understanding of more complex issues, such as a single exposure with multiple levels or more than one exposure.

Figure 6-1 depicts the 2 by 2 table, an important tool in evaluating the association between exposure and disease. Note that the columns represent disease status or outcome (yes or no) and that the rows represent exposure status (yes or no). To avoid confusion, remember that the first column always should refer to those with the disease and the first row should refer to those with the exposure of interest. Although this recommended standard is not critical to representation of data, consistency in usage will establish a common frame of reference for comparison of study designs and will reduce the likelihood of errors when one is calculating measures of effect.

		Disease Status		
		Yes	No	Total
	Yes	A	B	A + B
Exposure Status				
	No	C	D	C + D
		A + C	B + D	N

FIGURE 6-1 The 2 by 2 table

The table cross-classifies exposure status and disease status. Thus, the total number of individuals with disease is A + C, and the total number free from disease is B + D. The total number exposed is A + B, and the total number not exposed is C + D. These four totals are referred to as the marginal totals. The entries (or cells) within the table represent the cross-classification of exposure and disease. Thus, the entry labeled A reflects the number of subjects who had both exposure and disease, B reflects the number of subjects with exposure but no disease, C represents subjects with disease but without exposure, and D is the number of individuals who have neither disease nor exposure. For most study design options, the joint classification (or distribution) of exposure and disease for each subject is known.

One means for keeping track of the different observational study designs is to think of each in terms of the point of reference for selection of the study groups. Inspection of Figure 6-1 reveals several options. For example, one could start by selecting a sample (N) and then determining each subject's exposure and disease status. The results would be tabulated and entered into the four cells of the table (A, B, C, and D). The marginal totals would be determined afterward. This approach is a cross-sectional study. Alternatively, one could start with the marginal totals of exposed (A + B) and nonexposed (C + D) subjects and follow them for the development of disease. The interior cells of the table would be filled at the conclusion of the period of follow-up. This approach represents a cohort study design. The third option would be to start with the column totals

A + C (disease) and B + D (no disease) and determine exposures to complete the interior cell totals. This approach is called a case-control study. Note that for each of these study designs information is known about each subject's exposure and disease status. That is, it is possible to cross-classify each subject with respect to exposure and disease and thereby fill in each of the interior cells of the 2 by 2 table. In the fourth category of observational studies, the ecologic study, the interior cell counts are not known, as will be discussed in the following section.

What is an ecologic study?

An ecologic study is one that examines a group as a unit of analysis. The ecologic approach differs from most study designs, which use an individual as the unit of analysis.

Example: A study of mortality from lung disease in different cities that are known to have differing levels of air pollution would comprise an ecologic study. The unit of analysis is a city.

Uses of ecologic studies: They can be used for generating hypotheses, and also in analytic studies.

Limitations: The ecologic fallacy

Refer to the text for more details.

Ecologic Studies

As just mentioned, for cross-sectional, case-control, and cohort studies, data on exposure and disease are known at the level of the individual. In ecologic studies, the unit of analysis is the group. Here is an example: in the southern California (U.S.) basin, a geographic area that spans more than 200 miles (330 km) from the California border with Mexico to Santa Barbara, concentrations of air pollutants vary greatly. The highest concentrations are in urban centers, such as central Los Angeles and sections of Long Beach near oil refineries; conversely, air pollution levels are lowest in the coastal areas that are farthest from heavy industry. Suppose data were available on the average mortality and average particulate levels (one of the components of air pollution) during the year for each census tract in the basin. We could then assess the association between particulate pollution and mortality by

Table 6-2 Examples of Questions Investigated by Ecologic Studies

- Is the ranking of cities by air pollution levels associated with the ranking of cities by mortality from cardiovascular disease, adjusting for differences in average age, percent of the population below poverty level, and occupational structure?
- Have seat belt laws made a difference in motor vehicle fatality rates? This question could be addressed by comparing the motor vehicle fatality rates from years before and years after seat belt laws were passed.
- Are daily variations in mortality in Boston related to daily variations in particle air pollution, adjusting for season of year and temperature?
- What are the long-term time trends (1950–1995) for mortality from the major cancers in the United States, Canada, and Mexico?

Source: Adapted from *ERIC Notebook,* April 2000, Issue 12, pp. 1–2. Department of Veterans Affairs, Epidemiologic Research and Information Center at Durham, NC. Available at: http://www.sph.unc.edu/courses/eric/notebooks. Accessed: June 11, 2003.

plotting the mortality levels within each census tract. This hypothetical example illustrates one of the typical schemas for an ecologic study, which in this case uses a census tract, rather than individuals, as the unit of analysis. Refer to Table 6-2 for additional examples of questions asked by ecologic studies.

Referring to Figure 6-2, you can see that the number of exposed persons (preferably the rate of exposure) and the number of cases (preferably the rate of disease) are known, but the number of exposed cases is not known. The number of nonexposed persons and noncases may be inferred also. Thus, the marginal

Disease Status

Exposure Status	Yes	No	Total
Yes	A	B	A + B
No	C	D	C + D
	A + C	B + D	N

FIGURE 6-2 Illustration of sample selection for an ecologic study

totals are known, but the interior cells are not. As shown in Figure 6-2, the known information is surrounded by boxes.

This text will cover two major types of ecologic studies: ecologic comparison studies and ecologic trend studies. **Ecologic comparison studies** (sometimes called cross-sectional ecologic studies) involve an assessment of the correlation between exposure rates and disease rates among different groups or populations *over the same time period;* usually there are more than 10 groups or populations. (Note that the term cross-sectional is defined in the next section.) The data on disease may include incidence rates, prevalence, or mortality rates for multiple, defined populations. Data on rates of exposure must also be available on the same defined populations. Examples of exposure data include:

- measures of economic development (e.g., per capita income and illiteracy rate)
- environmental measures (mean ambient temperature, levels of humidity, annual rainfall, and levels of mercury or microbial contamination in water supplies)
- measures of lifestyle (smoking prevalence, mean per capita intake of calories, annual sales of alcohol, and number of memberships in health clubs)

The important characteristic of ecologic studies is that the level of exposure for each individual in the unit being studied is unknown. Although one may have to do considerable work to amass the data needed for such studies, ecologic studies generally make use of secondary data that have been collected by the government, some other agency, or other investigators. Thus, in terms of cost and duration, ecologic studies are clearly advantageous.

A second type of ecologic study, **the ecologic trend study,** involves correlation of changes in exposure and changes in disease *over time* within the same community, country, or other aggregate unit. For example, within the United States there has been a consistent downward trend in the incidence of and mortality from coronary heart disease (CHD). The exact reasons for the decline are unknown. A cynic, however, might assert that some organizations that have worked hard to achieve such results may find it desirable to claim responsibility (to ensure continued funding). Ecologic correlation data could be generated to support the claim that the downward trends reflect increased prescription of antihypertension medications or the number of coronary bypass surgeries performed.

A classic example of an ecologic correlation is the association between breast cancer and dietary fat.[4] Rates of breast cancer mortality and estimates of per capita dietary fat intake were collected for 39 countries. When presented graphically, the data led to a striking observation: Countries with high per capita intakes of dietary fat tended to be the same countries with high rates of breast cancer mortality (Fig. 6-3).

A second example is a study of childhood lead poisoning in Massachusetts.[5] More than 200,000 children from birth through four years of age were screened at physicians' offices, hospitals, and state-funded screening sites, through nutritional supplementation programs, and by door-to-door screening in high-risk areas. Blood samples were drawn and analyzed for lead levels using standard procedures. Communities were the unit of analysis, the value for each being the proportion of screened children with high blood levels of lead. The severity of blood lead poisoning was correlated with indexes from U.S. census data. Community rates of lead poisoning were positively associated with a poverty index, the percentage of houses built before lead-based paints were banned, and the percentage of the community that was African American. Median per capita income was inversely associated with lead poisoning. This example was an ecologic study because the outcomes were measured on groups (summary rates of lead poisoning by community) and the exposures were measured on groups (based on census data). By identifying factors in communities associated with high rates of lead poisoning, this study provided data that may be relevant to the identification of high-risk communities where funding for screening may not be available.

Our third example of an ecologic study explores the unexpected inverse relationship found in the Seven Countries Study between mean systolic blood pressure levels and stroke mortality rates.[6] (An inverse relationship is the converse of a direct relationship: in a direct relationship, when a risk factor increases the outcome increases also; in an inverse relationship, the outcome decreases when the risk factor increases.) Thus, in the Seven Countries Study, investigators expected stroke mortality rates to increase as mean blood pressures levels increased, but the opposite relationship was found. Investigators obtained stroke mortality rates in a 25-year follow-up of 16 cohorts of men aged 40 to 59 in the United States, several European countries, and Japan. All age-eligible men in the targeted countries were followed from 1958 to 1964. At the population (ecologic) level, the association between mean entry-level blood pressure levels and mortality due to strokes over 25 years was inverse and strong. When the analyses were repeated at the individual level within cohorts, the association was strongly positive among most of the cohorts examined. Although the findings for the group level seemed to contradict those for the individual level analysis, this study provided an excellent example of the ecologic approach in which countries are the unit of analysis.

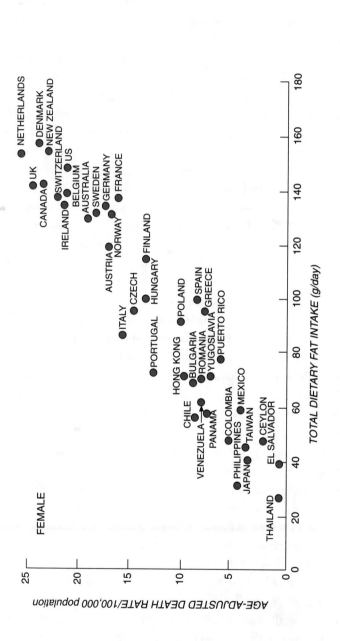

FIGURE 6-3 Ecologic correlation of breast cancer mortality and dietary fat intake. *Source:* Reprinted with permission from KK Carroll, Experimental Evidence of Dietary Factors and Hormone-Dependent Cancers. *Cancer Research,* vol 35, p 3379, © 1975, American Association for Cancer Research.

In summary, the ecologic approach has applications in a wide variety of situations. Some additional examples: the effect of fluoridation of the water supply on hip fractures,[7] the association of naturally occurring fluoride levels and cancer incidence rates,[8] and the relationship between neighborhood or local area social characteristics and health outcomes.[9]

The preceding examples reveal some of the applications and merits of ecologic studies; the following discussion presents some of their disadvantages. One of these is known as the **ecologic fallacy,** a term that will be defined subsequently. Let us begin with a hypothetical illustration. For the sake of argument, suppose that we found the mortality rates for emphysema to be lower in central Los Angeles, California (a highly industrialized area), than they were in the desert resort of Palm Springs, California (a less industrialized area). We might conclude erroneously that areas with lower air pollution levels have higher emphysema mortality rates than do areas with higher air pollution levels. How could we explain this apparently contradictory finding? The answer lies in differentiating between lifelong residents and in-migrants (Fig. 6-4).

After spending their working years in central Los Angeles, which is a major employment setting, some people migrate to Palm Springs during their retirement years, especially if they are afflicted with pulmonary difficulties. This retirement haven is also a magnet for in-migrants from northern industrialized cities throughout the United States. As Figure 6-4 shows, when we examine the composite emphysema mortality data (which do not disclose length of residence in

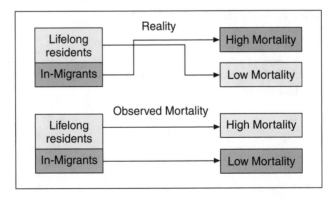

FIGURE 6-4 Example of ecologic fallacy. *Source:* Adapted from *ERIC Notebook*, April 2000, Issue 12, p. 1. Department of Veterans Affairs, Epidemiologic Research and Information Center at Durham, NC. Available at: http://www.sph.unc.edu/courses/eric/notebooks/. Accessed: June 11, 2003.

Palm Springs), we may be misled into reaching an erroneous conclusion about the association between exposure and disease (refer to the bottom panel of the figure). This incorrect observation results from the ecologic fallacy: individuals' levels of exposure to air pollution have not been specified. When degree of exposure is differentiated at the individual level by comparing in-migrants and life-long residents of Palm Springs, the correct exposure and disease relationships become apparent (top panel of the figure). When those who have had long-term exposure to air pollution (in-migrants) are compared to lifelong residents with respect to emphysema mortality, the former have higher mortality.

We have seen that ecologic studies, which by definition use observations made at the group level, may not represent the exposure-disease relationship at the individual level. Hence, the term **ecologic fallacy** is defined as "The bias that may occur because an association observed between variables on an aggregate level does not necessarily represent the association that exists at the individual level."[10]

To give a second illustration, consider the association between wearing hats and protection against sunburn, an example that can be viewed from the perspective of the individual and the group. Suppose that among a sample of 10 individuals there are 7 (70%) who have sunburned foreheads and 6 (60%) who wear hats when they go outside. At this point, we do not specify at the individual level who wore hats and who were sunburned. We specify only the overall percent who wore hats and the percent who were sunburned, just as we would in an ecologic study. The similar proportion of hats and sunburns suggests that there is an association between the exposure (wearing hats) and disease (sunburn). The conclusion is illusory, however (Table 6-3).

Table 6-3 Hypothetical Ecologic Relationship Between Hats and Sunburn

Person	Hat Wearer	Sunburned Head
1	Yes	Yes
2	Yes	Yes
3	Yes	Yes
4	No	Yes
5	Yes	No
6	No	Yes
7	Yes	No
8	No	Yes
9	Yes	No
10	No	Yes

To verify the error in this conclusion, note that among the six persons who wore hats outside, three were sunburned (50%). Among the remaining four persons who did not wear hats, however, all four (100%) had sunburned foreheads. Thus, the conclusion based on the association between hats and sunburns at the group level was incorrect.

The reader may infer from the hat-sunburned head example that aggregate data on populations may not apply to individuals. To cite still another example, although rates of breast cancer tend to be higher in countries in which fat consumption is high than in those in which fat consumption is low, one cannot be certain that the breast cancer cases had high fat intakes. One could draw a similar correlation between the number of cars in a country and breast cancer rates, yet few would be willing to provide it as evidence of a cause-effect relationship. Thus, more rigorous study designs in which data on exposure and disease are collected on individuals are desirable as further support.

Other limitations of the ecologic study also must be acknowledged. Imprecision in the measurement of exposure and disease makes accurate quantification of the exposure-disease associations difficult. The ability to adjust for the influence of extraneous variables is limited by the availability of such data and the analytic approaches for incorporating them.

In summary, despite the problems of the ecologic fallacy and other limitations, ecologic studies have earned a well-deserved place in epidemiologic research. They are quick, simple to conduct, and inexpensive. Thus, when little is known about the association between an exposure and disease, an ecologic study is a reasonable place to start if there are suitable data available. If the investigator's hypothesis is not supported, then few resources have been invested. In addition, when a disease is of unknown etiology, ecologic analyses represent a good approach for generating hypotheses.

Cross-Sectional Studies

The cross-sectional study, or prevalence study, is the first design to be covered in this chapter in which exposure and disease measures are obtained at the level of the individual. One starts by selecting a sample of subjects (N) and then determining the distribution of exposure and disease. Note that it is not imperative that a cross-sectional study include assessment of both exposure and disease. Some studies may be designed to provide only a measure of the burden of disease in a population, whereas others may focus exclusively on the distribution of certain exposures.

The features of this type of study design include a single period of observation (Figure 6-5). Exposure and disease histories are collected simultaneously but may include assessment of history of disease or exposures. The unit of observation and analysis in cross-sectional studies is the individual. The majority of data are collected for the first time, primarily for the purpose of the study, although they may be supplemented with secondary data, such as school records and medical records. Data from national surveys by the U.S. government are frequently used.

As mentioned earlier in this chapter, cross-sectional studies are typically descriptive in nature. Primarily, they provide quantitative estimates of the magnitude of a problem, but do not measure the temporal ordering of cause and effect.[10] One could take two basic approaches to provide a measure of the severity of a public health problem: Collect data on each member of the population (i.e., a census, used frequently in prevalence studies); or take a sample of the population and draw inferences to the remainder. The more common method, however, is the second: In a shorter period of time, and much less expensively, one could derive reasonable estimates of the extent of a health problem through a survey on a subset of the population.

Sampling schemes for cross-sectional studies comprise two main types: probability samples and nonprobability samples. They are defined as follows[11(p15)]:

> A *probability sample* has the characteristic that every element in the population has a nonzero probability of being included in the sample. A *nonprobability sample* is one based on a sampling plan that does not have that feature.

Examples of probability samples include simple random samples, systematic samples, and stratified samples. Simple random samples refer to a type of sample in which each individual in the population (or other group) has an equal probability of being selected. Simple random samples require enumeration of all potential subjects before sampling, an expensive process that may not be feasible to implement. A systematic sample is "The procedure of selecting according to some simple, systematic rule, such as all persons whose names begin with specified alphabetical letters, born on certain dates, or located at specified points on a master list."[10(p151)] Construction of a systematic sample does not necessarily require prior knowledge of the total number of sampling units. A sampling unit refers to "that element or set of elements considered for selection in some stage of sampling."[12(p198)] In epidemiologic research, a sampling unit is usually a specific

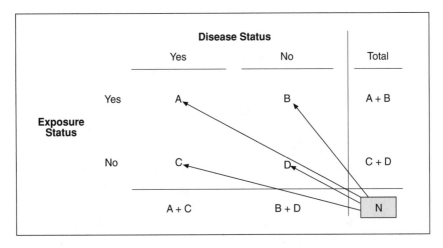

FIGURE 6-5 Illustration of subject selection in a cross-sectional study

person selected for the study. It is possible to perform systematic sampling at the same time as the sampling frame is being constructed, a feature that makes systematic sampling the most widely used of all sampling procedures.[11] ("A sampling frame is the actual list of sampling units from which the sample or some stage of the sample is selected."[12(p198)])

Suppose one wishes to derive estimates of the magnitude of a health problem in a relatively small subset of the population. Simple random samples and systematic samples will not ensure that sufficient numbers of this subgroup will be represented for meaningful estimates to be derived. A stratified sampling approach requires that the population be divided into mutually exclusive and exhaustive strata; sampling is then performed within each stratum (strata are "distinct subgroups according to some important characteristic, such as age or socioeconomic status."[10(p151)])

Nonprobability samples include quota samples and judgmental samples. An example of a quota sample design is one that requires interviewers to obtain information from a fixed number of subjects with particular characteristics regardless of their distribution in the population. A judgmental sample selects subjects on the basis of the investigator's perception that the sampled persons will be representative of the population as a whole. Nonrandom samples are not appropriate for cross-sectional studies because the reliability of the estimates derived from such samples cannot be evaluated.[11] Details on how to determine sample sizes and parameter estimates are beyond the scope of this book. The reader is referred to any of several excellent textbooks on the subject.[11,13]

Some examples of cross-sectional studies are now presented. Murray et al.[14] surveyed smokeless tobacco use among ninth graders in four school districts representative of the Minneapolis-St. Paul metropolitan area of Minnesota. A questionnaire was administered in the classroom during the fall of 1985 to estimate the prevalence of usage and to identify correlates of usage that might predict those teenagers who were at greater risk than their peers of using smokeless tobacco. The study revealed that nearly 63.0% of boys and 24.0% of girls had ever used smokeless tobacco, but only 18.5% of boys and 2.4% of girls had used it in the past week. Ethnicity also was associated with prevalence of usage, especially among boys. Self-reported prevalence ranged from a low among Asians and African Americans (21.0% and 22.0%, respectively), medium (45.5%) among whites, and high (60.8%) among Native Americans. The prevalence among boys from a two-parent household was 42.1%, 41.3% if only the mother lived at home, and 54.5% if the boy came from a father-only household. The smokeless tobacco use was much more common among cigarette smokers than among nonsmokers. Only 6.0% of nonsmoking girls reported using smokeless tobacco, in contrast to 16.4% of girls who smoked. A similar magnitude of difference was observed among the boys: 34.5% versus 56.1% for nonsmokers and smokers, respectively. Additional analyses revealed a clustering of unhealthy behaviors. For example, prevalence of smokeless tobacco use among subjects who did not drink, smoke cigarettes, or smoke marijuana was 6.9%. In contrast, the prevalence of smokeless tobacco use among respondents who drank alcoholic beverages, smoked cigarettes, and smoked marijuana was 50.8%, more than 7 times higher.

The preceding example was based on a survey of schoolchildren from a single major metropolitan area. Prevalence studies may also be done with a much broader sampling frame. For example, a national survey of urology, general surgery, and family practice physician practices was conducted to estimate the annual number of vasectomies performed in the United States in 1991.[15] Possible health risks associated with vasectomy have generated considerable medical and scientific interest. The prevalence study permitted an estimate of the number of vasectomies performed (~493,500), the rate of vasectomies (10.3 procedures per 1,000 men aged 25 through 49), the specialist most likely to perform the procedure (urologist), and regional variation in the surgical approach. The prevalence survey generated several important questions to be answered in future studies, including the effectiveness of the various methods of sterilization and characteristics of men who elect to have the procedure performed.

Prevalence studies provide a fertile source of hypotheses for more detailed etiologic studies. Since the mid-1980s, pregnancy among American teenagers has been a significant problem. Of an estimated 11% of females between the ages of 15 and 19 who become pregnant, half will go on to deliver a live infant.[16] Data from the California Birth Defects Monitoring Program for 1983 through 1988 were used to determine the prevalence of congenital malformations across the maternal age spectrum and to determine specific malformations that contributed to overall prevalence among mothers under the age of 20 years.[17] Results suggested a general J-shaped prevalence with maternal age: highest at young and old ages, and lowest at middle ages (Figure 6-6).

Curiously, when examined by the race/ethnicity of the mother, the pattern was not apparent for African Americans. The investigators raised the question as to "whether the increased risk of malformations among young mothers is due to behavioral or developmental factors and when, relative to conception, these factors may be etiologically important."[17(p713)]

Prevalence surveys are useful for planning interventions. The historical neglect of the health needs of minority populations has begun to show signs of reversal. Hispanics (a term used to describe many diverse cultural subgroups, such as

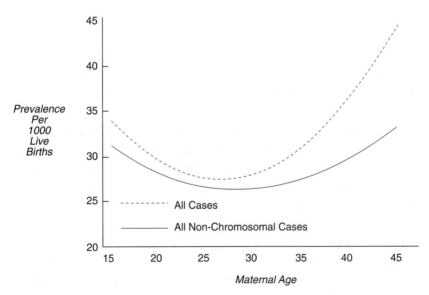

FIGURE 6-6 Prevalence of congenital malformations across maternal age: California, 1983–1986. *Source:* Reprinted from LA Croen and GM Shaw, Young Maternal Age and Congenital Malformations: A Population-Based Study. *American Journal of Public Health,* vol 85, p 711, with permission of the American Public Health Association, © 1995.

Mexican Americans, Cuban Americans, and Puerto Ricans) represent the second largest minority group in the United States.[18] Data from the Hispanic Health and Nutrition Examination Survey and the second National Health and Nutrition Examination Survey were used to compare energy and macronutrient intakes among adult Mexican Americans, Cuban Americans, mainland Puerto Ricans, and non-Hispanics.[19] Important differences were identified among the major ethnic groups, suggesting that efforts to reduce the occurrence of chronic disease must incorporate the development of dietary recommendations and interventions targeted to each Hispanic group.

Repeated cross-sectional surveys can be used to examine trends in disease or risk factors that can vary over time. The Centers for Disease Control and Prevention used data on persons 12 through 19 years of age from the National Household Surveys on Drug Abuse (NHSDA), High School Seniors Surveys, and National Health Interview Surveys (NHIS) to examine the prevalence of cigarette smoking among U.S. adolescents.[20] Data were available from 1974 (1976 for the High School Seniors Surveys), 1980, 1985, and 1991. The results (Fig. 6-7) suggest that overall smoking levels declined at all survey periods, but that there was notable variation by race, sex, and time period.

In general, the decline of smoking was most rapid between 1974 and 1980; the decline was faster for females than males and greater for African Americans than whites. The authors of the report concluded that the slowing of the trend toward lower smoking prevalence was evidence of the success of increased tobacco advertising and promotional activities aimed at adolescents or inadequate antitobacco educational efforts.

These examples have been selected to illustrate a number of important applications of the cross-sectional study design. Perhaps the greatest utility of such studies is for collecting data to describe the magnitude and distribution of a health problem, data essential for planning health services and administering medical care facilities. The survey of smokeless tobacco use among ninth graders provided evidence that usage was quite common even at this early age, representing a significant public health problem. The foregoing example also demonstrated that cross-sectional studies permit determination of various characteristics of a population, which may help target appropriate interventions and educational materials. An example of such a characteristic would be the prevalence of single-parent households. The survey of vasectomies in the United States revealed that urologists perform most of the surgical procedures and that local anesthesia is typically used. Sometimes, repeated cross-sectional surveys examine quantitative factors that vary over time. Finally, prevalence studies may generate new etiologic hypotheses that can be tested in future studies.

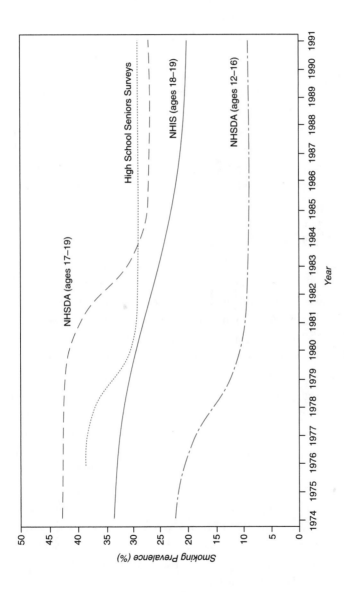

FIGURE 6-7 Overall weighted estimates of current smoking prevalence among adolescents in the United States, by survey, 1974–1991. *Source:* Reprinted from DE Nelson, et al., Trends in Cigarette Smoking among US Adolescents, 1974–1991. *American Journal of Public Health*, vol 85, p 36, with permission of the American Public Health Association, © 1995.

The limitations of cross-sectional designs stem mainly from their relative lack of utility for studies of disease etiology. First, prevalent cases represent survivors: The study of prevalent cases makes it difficult to sort out factors associated with risk of disease from factors associated with survival, such as treatment and severity. For diseases in which onset is difficult to determine (e.g., mental disorders), however, prevalence is an acceptable substitute for incidence. In other situations, the study of existing cases is the only feasible and affordable strategy to test etiologic hypotheses. The second major limitation applies to the ability to study diseases of low frequency. Recall from Chapter 3 that the prevalence of disease in a population is proportional to the incidence of the disease times its duration. Therefore, even a large survey may yield but few cases of rare diseases or diseases with short duration. Third, because exposure and disease histories are taken at the same time in a cross-sectional study, one must be careful about the temporality issue (i.e., whether exposure or disease came first), making assertions about any apparent cause-effect relationship tenuous.

Case-Control Studies

The basic premise of analytic epidemiology is that disease does not occur randomly but rather in describable patterns that reflect the underlying etiology. This rationale certainly applies to case-control studies. Consider two groups, one in which everyone has the disease of interest (cases) and a comparable one in which everyone is free of the disease (controls). The case-control study seeks to identify possible causes of the disease by finding out how the two groups differ. That is, because disease does not occur randomly, the case group must have been exposed to some factor, either voluntarily (e.g., through diet, exercise, or smoking) or involuntarily (through such factors as cosmic radiation, air pollution, occupational hazards, or genetic constitution), that contributed to the causation of their disease. Therefore, a comparison of the frequency of exposure among cases and controls may permit inferences as to the basis for the difference in disease status. Case-control studies are a mainstay of epidemiologic research. From the standpoint of selection of study groups for research into disease etiology, one is going from effect to cause. In Figure 6-8, the column totals, denoted by boxes, represent the presence (i.e., cases) or absence (i.e., controls) of disease. In recent years, the case-control design has proven to be useful and efficient for evaluation of vaccine effectiveness,[21] treatment efficacy,[22] evaluation of screening programs,[23] and outbreak investigations.[24]

The number of observation points for a case-control study is only one. Cases and controls are selected, and data are collected about past exposures that may have contributed to disease. As is true also of cross-sectional studies, the unit of

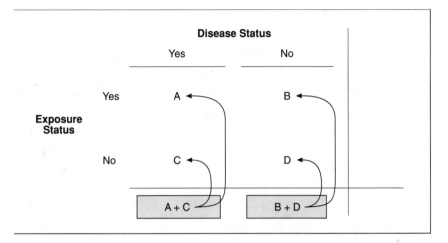

FIGURE 6-8 Illustration of selection in a case-control study

observation and the unit of analysis are the individual. The method of data collection typically involves a combination of both primary and secondary sources. Usually the data on exposure are collected by the investigators, although one can easily imagine situations where valuable information might be obtained from medical, school, and employee records. Data on disease are often collected by someone other than the investigator, especially if one is making use of special registries or surveillance systems for case identification. In some situations, however, the investigator might conduct a population screening survey to identify suitable cases. Notice that Figure 6-8 does not include the marginal totals A + B, C + D, or a total N. Because one is taking only a subset of the total population, namely the cases and some number of controls, these marginal totals are meaningless.

Selection of Cases

Two tasks are involved in case selection: defining a case conceptually, and identifying a case operationally.[25] The definition of a case is influenced by a number of factors, including whether there are standard diagnostic criteria, the severity of the disease, and whether the criteria to diagnose the disease are subjective or objective. At issue is misclassification. If the criteria are broad, the case group is more likely to include individuals who truly do not have the disease. Conversely, overly restrictive criteria may limit the number of subjects available for study. Although the selection criteria need to be weighed for each individual study, there is some evidence that the benefits of a more restrictive definition of a case outweigh the benefits of being overly inclusive.[26]

Sources of Cases

Once a case has been defined conceptually, one can then proceed to develop a strategy for case identification. The researcher's goal "is to ensure that all true cases have an equal probability of entering the study and that no false cases enter."[25(p8)] The ideal situation is to identify and enroll all incident cases in a defined population in a specified time period. For example, a tumor or disease registry or Vital Statistics Bureau may provide a complete listing of all available cases. The advantage of using incident cases is that, when all cases in a population are identified, there can be little question of their representativeness. In the real world, however, logistics or the lack of a suitable disease registry may restrict case selection to one or a few medical facilities. The main caveat in the selection of cases is the representativeness of the cases derived from special care facilities. Such institutions may receive only the most severe cases, ones in which the distribution of risk factors is atypical. Per the discussion in the last section on cross-sectional designs, prevalent cases make it difficult to separate characteristics that are causal or consequential. Additional benefits of studying incident (as opposed to prevalent) cases include subjects' better recall of past exposures and a reduced likelihood that exposure has changed as a consequence of the disease.

Selection of Controls

Suppose you have a strong and justified hypothesis about a new risk factor for a disease and wish to conduct a case-control study. How should the controls be selected? To determine whether this risk factor is truly associated with the disease—not indirectly or incorrectly associated because of some third (confounding) factor—the ideal controls should have the same characteristics as the cases (except for the exposure of interest). That is, if the controls were equal to the cases in all respects other than disease and the hypothesized risk factor, one would be in a stronger position to ascribe differences in disease status to the exposure of interest. Taking this example one step further, imagine a study of childhood vaccination and an adult chronic disease in which the cases and controls were all the same age, the same sex, and the same race, worked at the same job, ate the same foods, were educated at the same schools, and had the same leisure activities. Speculate that the cases and controls were identical in every respect except for vaccinations in childhood; all of the cases were exposed and none of the controls was exposed. This situation would provide the most clear-cut evidence that an exposure was indeed a risk factor for the disease. Clearly, such an ideal selection of cases and controls is extremely unlikely to occur, but the point should be obvious: Cases are presumed to have a given disease because of an excess (or deficiency) of an exposure. To identify whether the exposure patterns of a group of cases are excessively high or excessively low, the investigator needs to know what exposure pattern should normally be expected. Selection of a group of disease-free individuals (controls) supposedly will reveal what a normal or expected level of exposure should be in the absence of disease.

Note, however, that controls are neither always nor necessarily disease free; to examine the specificity of an exposure-disease association, one might identify controls with a different disease, assuming that the illness has a different etiologic basis from the disease of interest. For example, a review of 106 cancer case-control studies identified nine that used controls who had a type of cancer that was different from that of the cases.[27]

The epidemiologist needs to be able to isolate the effect of the risk factor on the outcome from influences that emanate from the controls. For example, suppose that the cases and controls differ in demographic characteristics, such as age or socioeconomic status. These demographic factors could operate as rival explanations to account for observed outcomes. That is, the researcher would be unable to distinguish the effects of the risk factor from the influence of demographic factors. To overcome the potential impact of systematic case-control differences in demographic and other characteristics upon the outcome, the investigator can use matching. Two methods of matching are the use of matched pairs (individual matching) and frequency matching (group matching). Refer to Chapter 10 (section entitled "Three Prevention Strategies to Control Confounding") for an extended discussion of matching.

In addition to the problem of **how** to select the controls, a second issue is the number of controls to select. Estimating the number of controls is an aspect of statistical power (ability to identify a significant difference), a topic that is beyond the scope of this text. (For more information, refer to Chernick and Friis, 2003[28]). However, here is a rule of thumb: epidemiologic researchers sometimes use an equal number of cases and controls (one-to-one ratio), a perfectly acceptable procedure. Preferably, researchers may select more controls than cases (up to a three-to-one or four-to-one ratio). When the ratio of controls to cases is at about a four-to-one ratio, statistical power of the design is maximal. A single case-control study also may use more than one control group, as in the case of hospital controls for hospitalized cases as well as community controls who represent a less selected group than do the controls from a hospital.

Sources of Controls

The general concept guiding the selection of controls is that they should come from the same population at risk for the disease or condition as the cases being studied. That is, one should ask, if a "control" had developed the outcome under investigation, would he or she have been ascertained as a case? Moreover, suitable controls should have the potential to become a case. For example, if you are conducting a study of ovarian cancer, women who have had bilateral oophorectomy (removal of their ovaries) would not be eligible as controls, since they could not develop ovarian cancer. Table 6-4 provides a guide for selection of controls who are comparable to the cases. Several options are available to the investigator regarding sources of controls. Each option has inherent strengths and weaknesses, advantages and disadvantages. The more common sources of controls are described below.

Population-based Controls

Perhaps the best way to ensure that the distribution of exposure among the controls is representative of the exposure levels in the population is to select population-based controls. A method to identify such controls is to obtain a list that contains names and addresses of most residents in the same geographic area as the cases. For example, a driver's license list would include most people between the ages of 16 and 65, and a roster from The Centers for Medicare and Medicaid Services (the former Health Care Financing Administration) would be a good source for subjects over the age of 65. Tax lists, voting lists, and telephone directories may be useful, provided that their coverage of the population is complete

Table 6–4 Guide for Selection of Comparable Cases and Controls

Example	Cases	Controls
1	All cases diagnosed in the community	Sample of the general population in a community
2	All cases diagnosed in a sampled population	Noncases, in a sample of the general population, or a specified subgroup
3	All cases diagnosed in all hospitals in the community	Sample of persons who reside in the same neighborhood as cases
4	All cases from one or more hospitals	Sample of patients in one or more hospitals in the community who do not have the same or related diseases being studied
5	All cases from a single hospital	Sample of noncases from the same hospital
6	Any of the above	Spouses, relatives, or associates of cases

or nearly complete. One then could randomly select controls from the total list, making sure to verify that selected persons met all exclusion criteria. Another method would be to select controls matched to the cases on variables such as age or sex. An approach that historically worked well in countries where most households have a telephone is random-digit dialing.[29] This technique uses a computer to generate randomly the last two to four digits of a telephone number for potential controls who have the same three-digit telephone prefix as the cases. The procedure is repeated until a suitable control is found. There is some evidence, however, that controls selected by random-digit dialing are better educated and more likely to be employed than survey controls.[30] In addition, increasing use of caller identifications (IDs) on home telephones and inundation by telemarketers has decreased the yield of this approach.

In comparison to other methods for selection of controls, the use of population-based controls is most likely to result in a control group that is representative of the exposure rate in the general or target population. Controls selected from the general population may have little incentive to participate in a research study, producing low participation rates and the need to contact more individuals to find an eligible control willing to participate. Consequently, the study becomes more expensive. Another consequence of low participation is that individuals who do ultimately agree to participate may be systematically different in the frequency of exposure than the target population they are intended to represent.

Patients from the Same Hospital as the Cases

For the reasons noted, a preferred approach is to conduct case-control studies in which both study groups are population based. When selection of population-based study groups is not feasible, however, cases may need to be derived from one or more major hospitals. Although hospital-based studies are inherently subject to greater potential for errors than population-based studies, their use is certainly justified when little information has been reported about a particular exposure-disease association or when a population-based case registry is not available. After the decision has been made to select cases from hospitals, it is perfectly appropriate to select hospital controls.

There are several practical advantages to using hospital controls. The study personnel who are already in the hospital to interview cases may achieve time efficiency by also interviewing controls. This time saving, plus the fact that hospital controls may be more likely than population controls to participate, ultimately equates to cost savings.

Perhaps the main difficulty of using hospital controls is trying to decide the diagnostic categories from which to select the controls. A second major limitation of hospital controls is that they may not be representative of the true exposure rates in the target population; after all, they were ill enough to require medical attention and motivated enough to seek it. Taken to the extreme, a possible category of controls is deceased persons. If cases were defined as individuals who had died from a particular cause, dead controls would permit testing of hypotheses regarding exposures and each cause of death.[25]

Relatives or Associates of Cases

Earlier in this chapter it was stated that the ideal control is a person free of the outcome of interest and similar in every respect to the case except for the exposure of interest. This objective is not only difficult to achieve, but also difficult to evaluate. One approach to control indirectly for factors that will not be measured directly as part of the study is to select relatives, associates, or neighbors of cases as the control group. This strategy tends to be a good method to control for possible differences in socioeconomic status, education, or other characteristics assumed to be determinants of friendship or neighborhood.[25] At the same time, use of this category of controls is not without some disadvantages. Compared with the use of hospital controls, the method is more expensive and time consuming. Although one might intuitively expect "friend" controls to be highly cooperative, several investigators have noted that cases may be unwilling to provide the name of a friend to fill this role.[31,32] A greater problem is that one may end up controlling for an important (unidentified) risk factor that could no longer be evaluated.

Measure of Association

The objective of case-control studies is to identify differences in exposure frequency that might be associated with one group having the disease of interest and the other group not having it. Although several measures of association between exposure and disease can be calculated (covered in Chapt. 9), at this point we will introduce the most frequently calculated measure of effect. The guiding principle is to determine how much more (or less) likely the cases are to be exposed than the controls.

In Figure 6-9, first consider only the cases. The proportion of the cases exposed is $A/(A + C)$. The proportion of cases not exposed is $C/(A + C)$. The odds of exposure, given that an individual is a member of the case group, are simply the ratio of these two proportions: $[A/(A + C)] \div [C/(A + C)]$. To simplify this expression,

FIGURE 6-9 Distribution of exposures in a case-control study

one inverts the second term and multiplies it by the first: $[A/(A + C)][(A + C)/C]$. The terms $(A + C)$ cancel out, and one is left with A/C; this term represents the odds of exposure among the case group. Repeating the same calculations, one determines that the odds of exposure among the control group are B/D. To evaluate whether the odds of exposure for the case group are different from the odds of exposure for the control group, we create a ratio of these two odds, or an odds ratio (OR): $(A/C) \div (B/D)$. Note that this can be more conveniently expressed as $(AD)/(BC)$, which is the cross-product of the cells from our 2 by 2 table. A calculation example is shown in Exhibit 6-1.

The OR literally measures the odds of exposure of a given disease. An OR of 1.0 implies that the odds of exposure are equal among the cases and controls and suggests that a particular exposure is not a risk factor for the disease in this study. An OR of 2.0 indicates that the cases were twice as likely as the controls to be exposed. The implication of this OR, given proper consideration to the issues of causality, is that this particular exposure is a risk factor for the disease. More specifically, an OR of 2.0 implies that this particular exposure is associated with twice the risk of disease. Not all risk factors increase risk; a factor that is associated with lower risk of disease (i.e., a protective factor) would manifest as an OR of less than 1.0.

The reader is advised to interpret the OR with caution. The case-control study is retrospective in nature with only one period of observation. Therefore, rates (and consequently risk, which can be determined only from prospective studies) cannot be directly determined. The reason for this inability to determine rates and risks

EXHIBIT 6-1

Sample Calculation of an Odds Ratio

Those of us who have a predilection for spicy foods have wondered about the health hazards associated with consumption of chili peppers. López-Carrillo et al.[33] conducted a population-based case-control study in Mexico City of the relationship between chili pepper consumption and gastric cancer risk. They reported that consumption of chili peppers was significantly associated with high risk for gastric cancer (age- and sex-adjusted OR = 5.49). Subjects for the study consisted of 220 incident cases and 752 controls randomly selected from the general population. Interviews produced information regarding chili consumption. In the present example, the data from this study are abstracted to illustrate how to calculate the OR.

Chili pepper consumption	Cases of gastric cancer	Controls
Yes	A = 204	B = 552
No	C = 9	D = 145

The OR (unadjusted for age and sex) is:

$$\frac{AD}{BC} = \frac{(204)(145)}{(552)(9)} = 5.95$$

Source: Data from L López-Carrillo, MH Avila, and R Dubrow, Chili Pepper Consumption and Gastric Cancer in Mexico: A Case-Control Study, *American Journal of Epidemiology,* vol 139, pp 263–271, Johns Hopkins University, School of Hygiene and Public Health, © 1994.

centers upon the way the study groups are assembled. Referring back to Figure 6-8, one notices that groups (A + B) and (C + D) do not represent the total populations exposed and not exposed to the factor. That is, there are no appropriate denominators for the population at risk, and one therefore cannot directly determine disease rates. Under certain conditions, however, as noted below, the OR provides a good approximation of the risk associated with a given exposure:

- *The controls are representative of the target population.* The key issue is that the controls are representative of the target population in the frequency of the exposure of interest.

- *The cases are representative of all cases.* Cases should be typical with respect to severity and diagnostic criteria.
- *The frequency of the disease in the population is small.* Algebraically, the formula for relative risk approximates that of the OR when the number of cases is small relative to the population at risk. There is some debate over whether this assumption is necessary, however.

Table 6-5, which summarizes examples of case-control studies presented in this chapter, highlights the many uses of the case-control approach in such diverse areas as research on cancer, birth defects, heart disease, and infectious disease. (This list is by no means exhaustive.) Note that several of the research studies cited in Table 6-5 deal with cancer etiology. Many forms of cancer have unknown causation and low prevalence in the general population; for this reason, case-control studies are used frequently to investigate cancer etiology. For example, the association between green tea consumption and lung cancer was the focus of a case-control study conducted in Shanghai, People's Republic of China.[34] A total of 649 incident cases of primary lung cancer diagnosed among women between early 1992 and early 1994 were selected from the Shanghai Cancer Registry. Investigators matched the cases to 675 control women selected at random and reported a significantly reduced risk of lung cancer (OR = 0.94) among women who consumed green tea and also did not smoke. The association was not significant among women who smoked.

To give another example from cancer etiology, we note that the case-control method is well suited to explore in greater detail unusual clinical observations based on a small number of cases. A classic historical example is exposure of

---

Table 6-5 Examples of Research Conducted with Case-Control Studies

Cancer reseasrch
    Young women's cancers resulting from in utero exposure to diethylstilbestrol
    Smoking and invasive cervical cancer
    Chili pepper consumption and gastric cancer
    Green tea consumption and lung cancer
    Parental smoking and childhood cancer
    Efficacy of colonoscopic screening
    Cigarette tar yield and risk of upper digestive tract cancers

Birth defects research
    Maternal anesthesia and fetal development of birth defects

Heart disease research
    Passive smoking at home and risk of acute myocardial infarction

Infectious disease research
    Household antibiotic use and antibiotic resistant pneumococcal infection

female fetuses in utero to diethylstilbestrol (DES) and the development of vaginal adenocarcinoma as young women.[35] A sudden increase in the number of vaginal cancers of a rare histologic type at an atypical age led to a small case-control study that successfully identified maternal exposure to DES as the cause.

The preceding example may give the erroneous impression that case-control studies examine only a single exposure or a series of related exposures. In fact, especially when one is exploring a disease for which relatively little is known about the etiology, the exposure data being collected can cover a broad range of known and suspected factors. Consider the case-control study conducted by Brinton et al.[36] on cervical cancer. The cases included 480 patients with invasive cervical cancer diagnosed at 24 hospitals in five U.S. cities: Birmingham, Chicago, Denver, Miami, and Philadelphia. All patients were between the ages of 20 and 74 years. A total of 797 population controls were identified through random-digit dialing. Two controls were matched to each case by using the variables of telephone exchange, race, and five-year age group. Women who had a previous hysterectomy were excluded. Data on cases and controls were collected through extensive home interviews that included questions on a variety of known and hypothesized risk factors, including smoking, sexual behavior, pregnancy history, menstrual history and hygiene practices, oral contraceptive use, medical history, diet, marital status, and family history.

A history of ever having smoked cigarettes was reported by 256 cases (61.4%) and 383 controls (48.1%). The corresponding OR was 1.7; when examined by currency of smoking, the ORs were 1.4 for ever-smokers and 1.9 for current smokers. There was evidence for a dose-response relationship: Compared with never-smokers, the ORs for those who smoked fewer than 10, 10 to 19, 20 to 29, and 30 or more cigarettes per day were 1.2, 1.6, 1.7, and 3.2, respectively.

Case-control studies have explored the relationship between tobacco use and cancers at various cites. Smoking is a risk factor for oral and throat (upper digestive tract) cancers; risk of these forms of cancer is thought to be associated with the concentration of tars in cigarettes. A case-control study conducted in Italy and Switzerland (with 749 cases and 1770 controls) confirmed an association between cigarette consumption and upper digestive tract neoplasms.[37] Investigators reported a direct relationship between the tar yield of cigarettes and such cancers. The ORs between current smokers and never-smokers were 6.1 for cigarettes with lower tar concentrations and 9.8 for cigarettes with higher tar concentrations.

The United Kingdom Childhood Cancer Study examined parental smoking behavior as a risk factor for childhood cancers[38] The study included 3838 children with cancer and 7629 control children. Cancers were classified into four major groups: leukemia, lymphomas, central nervous system tumors, and other solid tumors. Information was collected on self-reported smoking habits of parents. Statistical analyses adjusted for factors such as parental age. In general, the study did not demonstrate that parental smoking was a significant risk factor for childhood cancers, although risk of one form of cancer (hepatoblastoma) was significant when both parents smoked (OR = 4.74).

Case-control studies have evaluated the efficacy of cancer screening programs.[39] The efficacy of colonoscopic screening and polypectomy for preventing colorectal cancer (CRC) was assessed in a small-scale case-control study. The cases consisted of 40 asymptomatic persons diagnosed with CRC and 160 normal controls. Researchers selected subjects from a high-risk population of first-degree relatives of CRC patients. It was found that cases and controls varied in frequency of screening procedures, with procedures such as screening colonoscopy occurring less frequently among the cases than among the controls.

The remainder of this section will illustrate the use of case-control studies to investigate conditions other than cancer (e.g., heart disease, birth defects, infectious disease). For example, exposure to side-stream cigarette smoke has been hypothesized to be a risk factor for heart disease. A study conducted in Argentina examined the risk associated with passive smoking and acute myocardial infarction (AMI).[40] Both cases (*n* = 336) and controls (*n* = 446) consisted of never-smokers admitted to the same network of hospitals. Cases were patients with AMI; controls were patients admitted with acute disorders unrelated to smoking or known to be risk factors for AMI. Trained interviewers administered a structured questionnaire that contained items on smoking by close relatives, such as children and spouses. The risk of AMI was significantly associated with passive smoking; the ORs ranged upward of 1.68 depending on the contrast category (e.g., numbers of relatives who smoked and the number of cigarettes smoked).

Regarding the use of case-control studies to explore risk of birth defects, an example is the report based on a record linkage of Swedish health care registries. This research identified six infants with neural tube defects (NTDs) born to mothers who had undergone surgery in the first trimester of pregnancy when only 2.5 were expected.[41] The observation was evaluated in more detail by investigators at the Centers for Disease Control and Prevention.[42] Cases were infants with major central nervous system defects, including NTDs (anencephaly, spina bifida, and encephalocele), microcephaly, and hydrocephaly ascertained through the population-based surveillance system known as the Metropolitan Atlanta Congenital Defects Program. Controls were a 1% random sample of infants born in the same geographic region over the same time period. Trained interviewers, blinded to the case-control status of the infant, collected data from the mothers by telephone. (See Chapter 8 for information on blinding.) Maternal anesthesia exposure immediately before becoming pregnant or during the first three months of gestation was ascertained. Data were collected from the mothers of 694 case infants and the mothers of 2,984 control infants. There were no differences between mothers of the cases and controls with respect to mean age, parity, smoking status, use of alcohol-containing beverages, weight gain during pregnancy, or education. Maternal exposure to general anesthesia during the first trimester, however, was reported by 1.7% of case mothers versus only 1.1% of control mothers. This equates to an OR of 1.7, with a 95% confidence interval (CI) of 0.8 to 3.3. Because the 95% CI includes the null value of 1.0, the results are consistent with the hypothesis of no association. Further analysis of the data revealed that a stronger association was evident for one subtype of defect, hydrocephalus (OR, 3.8; 95% CI, 1.6 to 9.1). Thus, the mothers of infants with hydrocephalus were nearly four times as likely to have reported early exposure to general anesthesia as mothers of infants without congenital malformations, an association that does not appear to be due to chance alone. When multiple defects were considered, stronger associations were identified. For example, there were eight infants with both hydrocephalus and eye defects. Three of the mothers of these eight infants (37.5%) reported general anesthesia exposure, an odds of exposure 39.6 times greater (95% CI, 7.5 to 209.2) than among control mothers. These intriguing data warrant additional research to determine why the surgeries were performed as well as the types of surgeries, premedications for surgery, and use of general anesthesia and whether there were complications during or after the surgery.

Case-control studies are often the method of choice in infectious disease research. Outbreaks of new and unusual diseases, such as toxic shock syndrome, anthrax, and even occurrence of antibiotic-resistant organisms, may be explored fruitfully by applying case-control methods. A case-control study examined the issue of whether a person's risk of antibiotic-resistant infection is increased if a member of that person's family is exposed to antibiotics.[43] The data were derived from patients enrolled in health maintenance organizations in western Washington State and northern California. The study outcome was affliction with penicillin non-susceptible pneumococcal disease (143 cases) versus penicillin susceptible disease (79 controls). A significant association between antibiotic use within two months prior to diagnosis and antibiotic resistance was found. Use of antibiotics by other family members within four months prior to diagnosis was not related to antibiotic resistance.

Summary of Case-Control Studies

In this section we have indicated the numerous attractive features of case-control studies. Compared with large-scale surveys or prospective studies, case-control studies tend to be smaller in size: hundreds to thousands of subjects versus thousands to tens of thousands. As such, they are relatively quick and easy to complete as well as cost effective. The smaller sample size increases the likelihood that a case-control study will be repeated. In fact, because consistency is critical to epidemiologic research, it is highly desirable that several investigators repeat studies of a particular outcome in different populations. Although progression from case-control studies to a cohort study may be a logical pursuit, prospective studies are not feasible for some exposures and outcomes; a meaningful cohort study of a rare disease would require a large study group, a long period of follow-up, or both. In comparison with cohort studies, case-control studies are particularly useful for investigations into the etiology of rare diseases.

Limitations of the case-control design include the uncertainty of the exposure-disease time relationship and the inability to provide a direct estimate of risk. It is frequently difficult to determine the representativeness of the cases and controls selected for study, and there is a real possibility of introduction of errors in selection of subjects, measurement of exposures, and analysis. If the exposure is rare in the population, then case-control studies may be inefficient. That is, despite a large number of cases, one may still end up with few exposed cases. For a more detailed coverage of case-control studies, the reader is referred to the textbook by Schlesselman.[44] An entire issue of *Epidemiologic Reviews* was devoted to this topic.[45]

Conclusion

Chapter 6 provided an overview of major study designs that are used in epidemiology. The authors noted that study designs differ in a number of key respects, including the unit of observation, the unit of analysis, the timing of exposure data in relation to occurrence of disease end point, complexity, rigor, and amount of resources required. Some studies are designed to infer etiology; others are designed to affect parameters of health. Study designs differ with respect to control over exposure and the ability to assign subjects to study conditions. There are two major categories of study designs: observational and experimental. Chapter 6 presented three major types of observational designs: ecologic, cross-sectional, and case-control. The measure of effect used in case-control studies, odds ratio (OR), was illustrated. Chapter 7 will provide information on the other major observational design used in epidemiology—the cohort study—and its corresponding measure of effect, relative risk. Chapter 8 will cover the use of experimental designs in public health. Chapter 9 will expand on the two measures of effect used in observational study designs and will present several ways to summarize the results of epidemiologic studies.

Study Questions and Exercises

1. Define in your own words the following terms:
   a. ecologic study
   b. ecologic comparison study
   c. ecologic trend study
   d. ecologic fallacy
   e. cross-sectional study
   f. case-control study
2. Compare ecologic, cross-sectional, and case-control studies with respect to their strengths and weaknesses, and advantages and disadvantages.
3. The following question lists examples of observational studies. Indicate the type of study design that is being described.
   a. A study of the effect of hormone replacement therapy on cancer identified cancer cases by using a cancer registry in northern California. Controls were selected from a random sample of Bay Area cities.
   b. Data from the Behavioral Risk Factor Survey were used in a secondary data analysis to examine the effect of income inequality and race on preventive health practices.
   c. The level of unemployment was used as a measure of economic distress in Germany. Researchers examined the association between distress and general anxiety syndrome across states (e.g., Saxony) in Germany.
4. What are the differences between probability and non-probability samples used in cross-sectional designs?
5. You are interested in conducting a case-control study of childhood leukemia and exposure to environmental toxins in utero. Describe how you would select cases and controls for this study and how you would define exposure and outcome factors. How could the same problem be investigated using an ecologic study design?

6. Describe the advantages and disadvantages of each of the following types of controls in a case-control study:
   a. Population-based
   b. Hospital cases
   c. Relatives
7. Calculate the OR for the following 2 by 2 table:

	Outcome	
	Yes	No
Factor		
Yes	37	68
No	24	121

8. An investigator wanted to determine whether vitamin deficiency was associated with birth defects. By reviewing the birth certificates during a single year in a large U.S. county, the researcher located 189 infants born with neural tube defects (NTDs). A total of 600 other births were selected at random from the certificates. Mothers were given a dietary questionnaire. Among mothers who gave birth to an infant with an NTD, 84 reported no use of supplementary vitamins; a total of 137 control mothers did not use a vitamin supplement. Construct the appropriate 2 by 2 table and calculate the OR between vitamin use and NTDs.

9. The association between job-related exposure to welding fumes and chronic obstructive pulmonary disease (COPD) was explored in a case-control study. The following data were reported for 399 COPD patients: (37 currently employed as welders; the remainder had no occupational exposure). Among 800 controls, 48 were employed as welders. Set up a 2 by 2 table and calculate the OR.

10. Suppose you hypothesize that cell phone (mobile telephone) use by drivers is related to fatal automobile accidents. Design a hypothetical case-control study, giving attention to the following points: definition of the outcome, selection of controls, and difficulties in conducting such a study.

11. Why would you exclude as controls in a case-control study of gynecologic cancer women who cannot develop the disease?

12. The following ORs are reported for several hypothetical examples. Give your interpretation of the results, assuming all results are statistically significant unless otherwise specified.

    a. OR (low-fat diet and colon cancer) = 0.6

    b. OR (aerobic exercise and dental caries) = 1 (not significant)

    c. OR (exposure to side-stream cigarette smoke and lung cancer) = 1.3

    d. OR (infectious disease of the pelvis and ectopic (tubal) pregnancy) = 3.0

13. A random-digit dialed survey conducted in the City of Long Beach, California, reported that a greater proportion of non-smokers endorsed a ban on smoking in alcohol-serving establishments than did smokers. What type of study design was this?

14. Case-control studies allow the investigator to examine only one outcome at a time, but they permit examination of several different exposures at a time. Select a disease or other health outcome with which you are familiar and see how many potential exposures you can identify.

15. How would you design an ecologic study to investigate the following problems? How might the ecologic fallacy come into play in each situation?

    a. lung disease and air pollution

    b. birth defects and hazardous waste

    c. cancer and radiation leakage from a power plant

References

1. Kleinbaum DG, Kupper LL, Morgenstern H. *Epidemiologic Research: Principles and Quantitative Methods.* Belmont, CA: Lifetime Learning; 1982.

2. Myerberg DZ, Carpenter RG, Myerberg CF, Britton CM, Bailey CW, Fink BE. Reducing postneonatal mortality in West Virginia: a statewide intervention program targeting risk identified at and after birth. *Am J Public Health.* 1995;85:631–637.

3. Garrard J, Chen V, Dowd B. The impact of the 1987 federal regulations on the use of psychotropic drugs in Minnesota nursing homes. *Am J Public Health.* 1995;85: 771–776.

4. Carroll KK. Experimental evidence of dietary factors and hormone-dependent cancers. *Cancer Res.* 1975;35:3374–3383.

5. Sargent JD, Brown MJ, Freeman JL, Bailey A, Goodman D, Freeman DH. Childhood lead poisoning in Massachusetts communities: its association with sociodemographic and housing characteristics. *Am J Public Health.* 1995;85:528–534.

6. Menotti A, Blackburn H, Kromhout D, et al. The inverse relation of average population blood pressure and stroke mortality rates in the seven countries study: A paradox. *Eur J Epidemiol.* 1997;13:379–386.

7. Jacobsen SJ, O'Fallon WM, Melton LJ 3rd. Hip fracture incidence before and after the fluoridation of the public water supply, Rochester, Minnesota. *Am J Public Health.* 1993;83:743–745.

8. Steiner GG. Cancer incidence rates and environmental factors: An ecological study. *J Environ Pathol Toxicol Oncol.* 2002;21:205–212.

9. Pickett KE, Pearl M. Multilevel analyses of neighbourhood socioeconomic context and health outcomes: A critical review. *J Epidemiol Community Health.* 2001;55: 111–122.

10. Last JM, ed. *A Dictionary of Epidemiology,* 3rd ed. New York, NY: Oxford University Press; 1995.

11. Levy PS, Lemeshow S. *Sampling for Health Professionals.* Belmont, CA: Lifetime Learning; 1980.

12. Babbie E. *The Practice of Social Research,* 6th ed. Belmont, CA: Wadsworth; 1992.

13. Kish L. *Survey Sampling.* New York, NY: Wiley; 1965.

14. Murray DM, Roche LM, Goldman AI, Whitbeck J. Smokeless tobacco use among ninth graders in a North-Central metropolitan population: cross-sectional and prospective associations with age, gender, race, family structure, and other drug use. *Prev Med.* 1988;17:449–460.

15. Marquette CM, Koonin LM, Antarsh L, Gargiullo PM, Smith JC. Vasectomy in the United States, 1991. *Am J Public Health.* 1995;85:644–649.

16. Ventura SJ, Taffel SM, Mosher WD, Henshaw S. Trends in pregnancies and pregnancy rates, United States, 1980–1988. *Mon Vital Stat Rep.* 1992;41(suppl): 93–1120. Available at: http://cdc.gov/nchs/products/pubs. Accessed: June 1, 2003.

17. Croen LA, Shaw GM. Young maternal age and congenital malformations: a population-based study. *Am J Public Health.* 1995;85:710–713.

18. U.S. Bureau of the Census. U.S. population estimates, by age, sex, race and Hispanic origin: 1980 to 1991. In: *Current Population Reports.* Washington, DC: Government Printing Office; 1993:P25–P1095.

19. Loria CM, Bush TL, Carroll MD, et al. Macronutrient intakes among adult Hispanics: a comparison of Mexican Americans, Cuban Americans, and Mainland Puerto Ricans. *Am J Public Health.* 1995;85:684–689.

20. Nelson DE, Giovino GA, Shopland DR, Mowery PD, Mills SL, Eriksen MP. Trends in cigarette smoking among U.S. adolescents, 1974 through 1991. *Am J Public Health.* 1995;85:34–40.

21. Comstock GW. Evaluating vaccination effectiveness and vaccine efficacy by means of case-control studies. *Epidemiol Rev.* 1994;16:77–89.

22. Selby JV. Case-control evaluations of treatment and program efficacy. *Epidemiol Rev.* 1994;16:90–101.

23. Weiss NS. Application of the case-control method in the evaluation of screening. *Epidemiol Rev.* 1994;16:102–108.

24. Dwyer DM, Strickler H, Goodman RA, Armenian HK. Use of case-control studies in outbreak investigations. *Epidemiol Rev.* 1994;16:109–123.

25. Lasky T, Stolley PD. Selection of cases and controls. *Epidemiol Rev.* 1994;16:6–17.

26. Brenner H, Savitz DA. The effects of sensitivity and specificity of case selection on validity, sample size, precision, and power in hospital-based case–control studies. *Am J Epidemiol.* 1990;132:181–192.

27. Linet MS, Brookmeyer R. Use of cancer controls in case-control studies. *Am J Epidemiol.* 1987;125:1–11.

28. Chernick MR, Friis RH. *Introductory Biostatistics for the Health Sciences: Modern Applications Including Bootstrap.* Hoboken, NJ: John Wiley & Sons, Inc.; 2003.

29. Hartge P, Brinton LA, Rosenthal JF, et al. Random digit dialing in selecting a population-based control group. *Am J Epidemiol.* 1984;120:825–833.

30. Olson SH, Kelsey JL, Pearson TA, et al. Evaluation of random digit dialing as a method of control selection in case-control studies. *Am J Epidemiol.* 1992;135:210–222.

31. Shaw GL, Tucker MA, Kase RG, et al. Problems ascertaining friend controls in a case-control study of lung cancer. *Am J Epidemiol.* 1991;133:63–66.

32. Jones S, Silman AJ. Re: "Problems ascertaining friend controls in a case-control study of lung cancer." *Am J Epidemiol.* 1991;134:673–674.

33. López-Carrillo L, Avila MH, Dubrow R. Chili pepper consumption and gastric cancer in Mexico: a case-control study. *Am J Epidemiol.* 1994;139:263–271.

34. Zhong L, Goldberg MS, Gao Y-T, et al. A population-based case-control study of lung cancer and green tea consumption among women living in Shanghai, China. *Epidemiology* 2001;12:695–700.

35. Herbst AL, Scully RE. Adenocarcinoma of the vagina in adolescence. *Cancer.* 1970;25:745–757.

36. Brinton LA, Schairer C, Haenszel W, et al. Cigarette smoking and invasive cervical cancer. *JAMA.* 1986;255:3265–3269.

37. Gallus S, Altieri A, Bosetti C, et al. Cigarette tar yield and upper digestive tract cancers: Case-control studies from Italy and Switzerland. *Ann Oncol.* 2003;14:209–213.

38. Pang D, McNally R, Birch JM. Parental smoking and childhood cancer: Results from the United Kingdom Childhood Cancer Study. *Br J Cancer.* 2003;88:373–381.

39. Niv Y, Dickman R, Figer A, et al. Case-control study of screening colonoscopy in relatives of patients with colorectal cancer. *Am J Gastroenterol.* 2003;98:486–489.

40. Ciruzzi M, Pramparo P, Esteban O, et al. Case-control study of passive smoking at home and risk of acute myocardial infarction. *J Am Coll Cardiol.* 1998;31:797–803.

41. Kallen B, Mazze RI. Neural tube defects and first trimester operations. *Teratology.* 1990;41:717–720.

42. Sylvester GC, Khoury MJ, Lu X, Erickson JD. First-trimester anesthesia exposure and the risk of central nervous system defects: a population-based case-control study. *Am J Public Health.* 1994;84:1757–1760.

43. Kwan-Gett TS, Davis RL, Shay DK, et al. Is household antibiotic use a risk factor for antibiotic-resistant pneumococcal infection? *Epidemiol Infect.* 2002;129:499–505.

44. Schlesselman JJ. *Case-Control Studies: Design, Conduct, Analysis.* New York, NY: Oxford University Press; 1982.

45. Armenian HK, ed. Applications of the case-control method. *Epidemiol Rev.* 1994;16(1).

CHAPTER 7

Study Designs: Cohort Studies

LEARNING OBJECTIVES

By the end of this chapter the reader will be able to:

- differentiate cohort studies from other epidemiologic study designs
- list the main characteristics, advantages, and disadvantages of cohort studies
- describe at least three research questions that lend themselves to cohort studies
- calculate and interpret a relative risk

CHAPTER OUTLINE

Introduction

The previous chapter provided an overview of types of epidemiologic study designs, as well as key features of each type, and distinctions between the experimental and observational approaches. In addition, the chapter covered three observational study designs in detail: ecologic, cross-sectional, and case-control designs.

The authors indicated that a distinguishing feature of each type of study design—whether observational or experimental—was the **temporality** of data collection with respect to exposure and disease. The term *temporality* referred to the timing of information about cause and effect, i.e., whether the information about cause and effect referred to the same point in time or whether information about the cause was garnered before or after the information about the effect.

Cross-sectional and case-control study designs (and many types of ecologic study designs) are premised upon exposure information and disease information that are collected at the same time. Although this strategy is efficient for generating and testing hypotheses, the strategy does lead to almost unavoidable challenges regarding interpretation of results. In particular, cross-sectional studies present difficulties in distinguishing the *causes* (e.g., certain exposures) from the *consequences* (e.g., certain outcomes) of the disease, especially if the outcome marker is a biological or physiological parameter. Similarly, case-control studies may raise concerns that recall of past exposures differs between the cases (i.e., those study participants who have the disease or outcome of interest) and the controls (those study participants who do not). In addition, although investigators may query subjects about exposures that took place many years in the past, there has been no actual lapse of time between measurement of exposure and disease. Chapter 10 (in the section titled "Factors That Contribute to Systematic Errors") will present more information regarding these issues. Finally, none of the designs discussed in Chapter 6 is especially well suited for exposures that are uncommon in the population. Chapter 7 will elaborate on one of the most powerful epidemiologic designs, the cohort study, which overcomes many of the foregoing problems associated with temporality of data collection and rare exposures.

Cohort Studies Defined

Cohorts and Cohort Effects

A *cohort* is defined as a population group, or subset thereof (distinguished by a common characteristic), that is followed over a period of time. The term *cohort* is said to originate from the Latin *cohors*, which referred to one of ten divisions of an ancient Roman legion. The common characteristic may be either that the group members experience an exposure associated with a specific setting (e.g., an occupational cohort or a school cohort) or that they share a non-specific exposure associated with a general classification (e.g., a birth cohort—being born in the same year or era). For example, people who belong to the same birth cohort may be exposed to similar environmental and societal changes, whereas those who belong to different birth cohorts may grow up exposed to differing environmental conditions that are reflected in differences in health outcomes. The influence of membership in a particular cohort is known as a cohort effect.

The term *cohort analysis* refers to "The tabulation and analysis of morbidity or mortality rates in relationship to the ages of a specific group of people (cohort) identified at a particular period of time and followed as they pass through different ages during part or all of their life span."[1] Wade Hampton Frost helped to draw attention to the method of cohort analysis, even though he did not originate this methodology.[2] Table 7-1 reproduces Frost's data. "To illustrate cohort

Table 7-1 Death Rates per 100,000 from Tuberculosis, All Forms, for Massachusetts, 1880 to 1930, by Age and Sex, with Rates for Cohort of 1880 Indicated

Age	1880	1890	1900	1910	1920	1930
Male						
0–4	760	578	309	209	108	41
5–9	43	49	31	21	24	11
10–19	126	115	90	63	49	21
20–29	444	361	288	207	149	81
30–39	378	368	296	253	164	115
40–49	364	336	253	253	175	118
50–59	366	325	267	252	171	127
60–69	475	346	304	246	172	95
70+	672	396	343	163	127	95
Female						
0–4	658	595	354	162	101	27
5–9	71	82	49	45	24	13
10–19	265	213	145	92	78	37
20–29	537	393	290	207	167	92
30–39	422	372	260	189	135	73
40–49	307	307	211	153	108	53
50–59	334	234	173	130	83	47
60–69	434	295	172	118	83	56
70+	584	375	296	126	68	40

Source: Reproduced with permission. WH Frost. The Age Selection of Mortality from Tuberculosis in Successive Decades. *Am J Epidemiol,* 1995, vol 141, p 95. ©The Johns Hopkins University School of Hygiene and Public Health.

analysis, Frost first arranged tuberculosis mortality rates from Massachusetts, . . . in a table with age on one axis and year of death on the other. . . . Arranged in this way, one could quickly see the age-specific mortality for each of the available years on one axis, and the time trend for each age group on the other. What proved to be most interesting in this instance were the rates in the cells of the table that lay on the diagonals, starting with the youngest ages and earliest years. These 'diagonal rates' were analogous to tuberculosis mortality rates . . . experienced by each cohort of persons as they simultaneously aged and passed through time."[2(p9-10)] Referring to Table 7-1, you will note that the 1880 mortality rates from tuberculosis were high among males aged zero to four and five to nine years—the highest rates occurring among the cohort aged zero to four years—when compared to mortality for the cohort as it aged. You can confirm this observation by tracing along the diagonal shown in the table. With respect to 1890 and subsequent decades, the groups that were zero to four and five to nine years of age in 1880 are combined as one moves along the diagonal. In comparison to 1880, mortality rates for that same cohort were lower during subsequent points of observation; however, during 1900 and 1910 they were higher than in 1890 and then declined again. The mortality pattern was similar for the female cohort that was aged zero to four years and five to nine years in 1880.

We offer as another example of a cohort effect the use of tobacco products in the United States (Fig. 7-1). A low proportion (less than 5%) of the population smoked cigarettes around the turn of the 20th century. As a result of widespread distribution of free cigarettes to the troops during World War I, however, the prevalence of smoking in the population began to increase gradually, reaching a peak in the 1960s.[3] When smoking first became popular, the age at which the habit was initiated varied greatly; that is, there were considerable differences according to age, sex, and education levels.

Although some people began smoking as young adults, a large number of people adopted the habit much later in life. Over the years, more and more people began to smoke and began smoking earlier in life. This trend is depicted graphically in Figure 7-2. One of the net effects was a shift in the distribution of the age of onset of lung cancer.[4] Consider, for example, the birth cohort of 1850. If smoking prevalence in this cohort was similar to that of the general population, then most individuals did not begin smoking until around 1915, when the average cohort member was in his or her 60s. Because there is a delay between the onset of smoking and the development of cancer, these individuals would not develop cancer for 10 years or more, perhaps around the age of 70. In contrast, individuals born in 1890 were only 20 when smoking became popular. As a result, a greater proportion of this age cohort would have started smoking at an earlier age, and the distribution of the entire age at onset curve for lung cancer would be shifted toward earlier ages. The more traditional approach of examining trends through repeated cross-sectional surveys leads to a distorted impression of

FIGURE 7-1 United States per capita tobacco consumption for adults aged 18 and older (1900–1990). *Source:* Reprinted from *Strategies to Control Tobacco Use in the United States: A Blueprint for Public Health Action in the 1990s.* Washington, DC: National Cancer Institute, National Institutes of Health; Publication No 92-3316. 1992:75.

FIGURE 7-2 Changes in prevalence of cigarette smoking among successive birth cohorts of U.S. men, 1900–1987. *Source:* Reprinted from *Strategies to Control Tobacco Use in the United States: A Blueprint for Public Health Action in the 1990s*, Washington, DC: National Cancer Institute, National Institutes of Health; 1992: p 82. Publication No 92-3316.

the smoking-cancer association. In particular, it leads to an underestimation of the past smoking behavior of the older segments of the current population. That is because smoking behavior (age at initiation and total duration) is greatly influenced by the calendar year of birth.

Table 7-2 demonstrates a final example of a cohort effect, this time for lung cancer death rates in the United Kingdom and the United States.[5] The table presents the midpoint of birth cohorts on the Y-axis (left side) and the midpoint of five-year age groups on the X-axis (across the top). From the table, one is able to

Table 7-2 Lung Cancer Death Rate per 100,000 for the United Kingdom and United States

Age (Midpoint of 5-year Age Group)
United Kingdom

Midpoint of Birth Cohort	32.5	37.5	42.5	47.5	52.5	57.5	62.5	67.5	72.5	77.5	82.5
1873											167.30
1878										243.01	259.83
1883									305.25	377.48	391.85
1888								329.25	431.62	506.16	509.23
1893							289.47	428.10	538.81	650.73	679.95
1898						219.13	353.38	512.62	662.33	764.63	812.65
1903					126.17	232.18	374.27	528.11	682.74	796.69	832.76
1908				59.72	125.16	228.23	369.44	514.73	655.69	756.35	767.28
1913			24.87	57.76	120.75	215.69	344.15	479.32	616.24	678.27	669.39
1918		9.78	25.00	55.08	111.60	202.32	316.22	437.96	553.20	592.54	
1923	3.76	9.47	22.38	53.96	106.37	184.94	294.74	402.30	475.24		
1928	3.53	9.06	21.01	46.80	92.11	158.66	245.40	326.52			
1933	2.80	6.29	16.30	36.15	69.26	122.78	184.53				
1938	2.49	5.90	12.96	29.62	59.51	102.18					
1943	2.24	4.97	11.24	26.26	49.74						
1948	1.56	4.07	9.72	20.74							
1953	1.09	3.13	8.02								
1958	0.77	2.13									
1963	0.65										

United States

Midpoint of Birth Cohort	32.5	37.5	42.5	47.5	52.5	57.5	62.5	67.5	72.5	77.5	82.5
1873											116.80
1878										138.60	176.30
1883									148.90	199.60	222.60
1888								157.80	232.20	268.30	325.40
1893							135.50	219.70	302.60	380.60	431.60
1898						95.90	180.70	277.30	371.00	464.00	477.70
1903					58.20	114.92	199.88	306.95	418.93	502.80	543.33
1908				30.40	68.71	127.55	228.01	329.42	458.80	546.20	584.96
1913			11.60	31.79	76.79	152.13	244.30	359.11	470.70	565.40	580.60
1918		4.90	13.99	38.61	84.32	150.01	255.74	367.06	485.89	529.90	
1923	1.70	5.73	17.26	44.03	90.91	162.93	262.46	374.07	470.90		
1928	1.97	7.05	21.54	47.86	95.28	167.41	268.18	359.60			
1933	2.00	7.34	19.30	45.44	86.59	159.35	233.60				
1938	2.03	6.15	17.43	40.26	80.52	132.70					
1943	1.80	5.29	15.19	34.64	66.10						
1948	1.12	4.32	11.63	26.20							
1953	0.98	3.85	9.50								
1958	1.16	3.30									
1963	1.20										

Source: Adapted from National Cancer Institute. *Risks Associated with Smoking Cigarettes with Low Machine-Measured Yields of Tar and Nicotine,* p 128. Smoking and Tobacco Control Monograph No. 13, NIH Pub. No. 02-5074. Bethesda, MD: U.S. Department of Health and Human Services, National Institutes of Health, National Cancer Institute; October 2001.

infer cohort effects as a particular cohort ages and also is able to compare mortality between the two regions. For example, the respective lung cancer death rates per 100,000 of the 1923 cohort at age 32.5 years are 3.76 and 1.70. The cohort effect can be traced along a diagonal: the respective rates at the intersection of year 1928 and age 37.5 years are 9.06 and 7.05. The overall trend shown in the table is for age-specific lung cancer death rates to start at lower levels in the United States but then show more rapid increases than in the United Kingdom, perhaps due to differences in age of initiation of smoking, particularly among males.

Life Table Methods

According to Chernick and Friis, "Life tables give estimates for survival during time intervals and present the cumulative survival probability at the end of the interval."[6(p339)] We are able to construct life tables in order to portray the survival times of patients in clinical trials. (Clinical trials are discussed in Chapt. 8.) For the population of the United States, the National Center for Health Statistics produces life tables known as periodic life tables.[7] Two major types of life tables exist: cohort life tables and period (or current) life tables. A cohort life table shows the mortality experience of all persons born during a particular year, such as 1900. A period life table gives an overview of the present mortality experience of a population and shows projections of future mortality experience. With respect to a year of interest (e.g., 2000), a period life table enables us to project the future life expectancy of persons born during the year as well as the remaining life expectancy of persons who have attained a certain age. Table 7-3 in Exhibit 7-1 shows an abridged life table for the total U.S. population in 2000. From the table, you can see (column e_x) that the life expectancy at birth (0–1 years) was 76.9 years and at age 79–80 years was 9.1 years. For more information about life table methods, refer to Chernick and Friis.[6]

Survival Curves

In addition to life tables, one of the methods for portraying survival times is to use **survival curves.** Take the case of a small-scale clinical study; in order to construct a survival curve, the following information would be required about each subject: time of entry into the study, time of death (or other outcome), and status of the patient at that time (either dead or censored—meaning, perhaps, that the patient is lost to follow-up).

Consider a simple example in which 15 subjects were followed over 36 months and all entered the study at the same time.[8] (Refer to Fig. 7-3.) A total of nine subjects died at different points during the study. Each step of the curve indicates the death(s) of one or more patients. The steep drop at 19 months is

Illustration of a Life Table

EXHIBIT 7-1

Table 7-3 Life Table for the Total Population: United States, 2000 (Abridged)

Age	Probability of dying between ages x to x+1	Number surviving to age x	Number dying between ages x to x+1	Person-years lived between ages x to x+1	Total number of person-years lived above age x	Expectation of life at age x
	q_x	l_x	d_x	L_x	T_x	e_x
0–1	0.006930	100,000	693	99,392	7,686,810	76.9
1–2	0.000517	99,307	51	99,281	7,587,418	76.4
2–3	0.000347	99,256	34	99,238	7,488,137	75.4
3–4	0.000243	99,221	24	99,209	7,388,898	74.5
4–5	0.000202	99,197	20	99,187	7,289,689	73.5
5–6	0.000189	99,177	19	99,168	7,190,502	72.5
6–7	0.000177	99,158	18	99,150	7,091,334	71.5
7–8	0.000167	99,141	17	99,132	6,992,185	70.5
8–9	0.000154	99,124	15	99,117	6,893,052	69.5
9–10	0.000137	99,109	14	99,102	6,793,936	68.6
10–11	0.000125	99,095	12	99,089	6,694,833	67.6
11–12	0.000130	99,083	13	99,077	6,595,744	66.6
12–13	0.000170	99,070	17	99,062	6,496,668	65.6
13–14	0.000253	99,053	25	99,041	6,397,606	64.6
14–15	0.000366	99,028	36	99,010	6,298,565	63.6
15–16	0.000491	98,992	49	98,968	6,199,555	62.6
16–17	0.000607	98,943	60	98,913	6,100,587	61.7
17–18	0.000706	98,883	70	98,848	6,001,674	60.7
18–19	0.000780	98,814	77	98,775	5,902,826	59.7
19–20	0.000833	98,736	82	98,695	5,804,051	58.8
20–21	0.000888	98,654	88	98,610	5,705,355	57.8
67–68	0.018933	79,406	1,503	78,655	1,305,916	16.4
68–69	0.020701	77,903	1,613	77,097	1,227,262	15.8
69–70	0.022663	76,290	1,729	75,426	1,150,165	15.1
70–71	0.024673	74,561	1,840	73,641	1,074,739	14.4
71–72	0.026741	72,722	1,945	71,749	1,001,098	13.8
72–73	0.029042	70,777	2,056	69,749	929,349	13.1
73–74	0.031663	68,721	2,176	67,633	859,600	12.5
74–75	0.034588	66,545	2,302	65,395	791,966	11.9
75–76	0.037675	64,244	2,420	63,034	726,571	11.3
76–77	0.040886	61,823	2,528	60,560	663,538	10.7
77–78	0.044437	59,296	2,635	57,978	602,978	10.2
78–79	0.048530	56,661	2,750	55,286	545,000	9.6
79–80	0.053313	53,911	2,874	52,474	489,714	9.1

continues

EXHIBIT 7-1 *continued*

Explanation of the columns of the life table

Column 1—Age (x to x + 1): This column shows the age interval between the two exact ages indicated. For instance, "20–21" means the 1-year interval between the 20th and 21st birthdays.

Column 2—Probability of dying (q_x): This column shows the probability of dying between the ages x to $x + 1$. For example, in the age interval 20–21 years, the probability of dying is 0.000888. The "probability of dying" column forms the basis of the life table; all subsequent columns are derived from it.

Column 3—Number surviving (l_x): This column shows the number of persons from the original cohort of 100,000 live births, who survive to the beginning of each age interval. For information regarding how this cohort is constructed, refer to the original document. Thus, out of 100,000 persons born alive, 99,307 will complete the first year of life and enter the second; 99,095 will reach age 10; 98,654 will reach age 20; and 53,911 will live to age 79.

Column 4—Number dying (d_x): This column shows the number dying in each successive age interval out of the original 100,000 live births. For example, out of 100,000 persons born alive, 693 will die in the first year of life; 88 between ages 20 and 21; and 2,874 will die between ages 79 and 80. Each figure in column 4 is the difference between two successive figures in column 3.

Column 5—Person-years lived (L_x): This column shows the number of person-years lived by the life table cohort within an age interval x to $x + 1$. Each figure in column 5 represents the total time (in years) lived between two indicated birthdays by all those reaching the earlier birthday. Thus, the figure 98,610 for the total population in the age interval 20–21 is the total number of years lived between the 20th and 21st birthdays by the 98,654 (column 3) persons who reached their 20th birthday out of 100,000 persons born alive.

Column 6—Total number of person-years lived (T_x): This column shows the total number of person-years that would be lived after the beginning of the age interval x to $x + 1$ by the life table cohort. For example, the figure 5,705,355 is the total number of years lived after attaining age 20 by the 98,654 persons reaching that age.

Column 7-Expectation of life (e_x): The expectation of life at any given age is the average number of years remaining to be lived by those surviving to that age on the basis of a given set of age-specific rates of dying. Thus, the average remaining lifetime for persons who reach age 20 is 57.8 years.

For more information regarding how the numbers shown in the table are calculated, refer to the original source. ■

Source: Adapted from E. Arias. United States Life Tables, 2000, *National Vital Statistics Reports,* vol 51, No 3, pp 2–3, 7–8, 2002, National Center for Health Statistics.

caused by the death of two patients. The foregoing section provided an extremely simplified example of a survival curve. In practice, the process of constructing survival curves may be much more complicated. Survival curves have numerous applications in research on infectious diseases, clinical trials, occurrence of psychiatric disorders, and many other situations. For more detailed information, consult Chernick and Friis.[6]

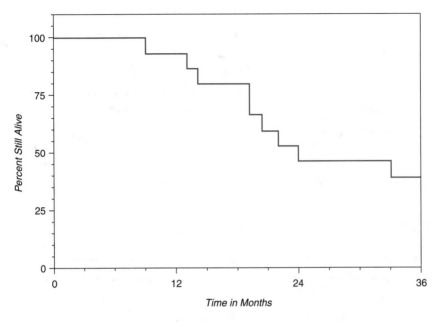

FIGURE 7-3 A simple survival curve. *Source:* Reprinted with permission from H Motulsky, *Intuitive Biostatistics.*New York, NY: Oxford University Press, Inc, 1995. Available at: http://www.graphpad.com/www/book/ survive.htm. Accessed March 17, 2003.

Cohort Studies

The bases for forming a cohort are almost limitless with regard to the unifying feature, but the rationale for studying a particular cohort should be guided by the scientific question of interest, rather than mere availability of a group for study. Also known as a prospective or longitudinal study, a cohort study is distinguished from other observational research designs by the fact that it starts with a group of subjects who lack a positive history of the outcome of interest and are at risk for the outcome. From the standpoint of selecting study groups, cohort studies can be thought of as going from cause to effect. That is, the exposure(s) of interest is/are determined for each member of the cohort at baseline or time of study; then the group is followed through time to document the incidence of an outcome among the exposed and nonexposed members. Possible outcome measures include the incidence of disease (cohort studies measure disease incidence directly); mortality, health status, and certain biological parameters, which are examined for changes that occur as a result of exposure to a risk factor.

In contrast to other observational designs, an additional characteristic of cohort studies is that they include at least two observation points: one to determine exposure status and eligibility and a second (or more) to determine the number of incident cases that developed during follow-up. This feature (i.e., two or more observation points) permits the calculation of disease rates, which cannot be obtained with only a single time point of observation. In cohort studies, the individual forms the unit of observation and the unit of analysis, as is also true of cross-sectional studies and case-control studies. Cohort studies almost always involve the collection of primary data, although secondary data sources are used sometimes for both exposure and disease assessment.

Sampling and Cohort Formation Options

Although all cohort studies share certain common features, such as measurement of exposure before disease onset and at least two periods of observation, some types of cohort studies differ from one another. We make note of these differences now, as they have implications for the measures of association that can be calculated with the data generated. (The measures of association used in cohort studies will be discussed in more detail in Chapt. 9.) One of the differences is the sampling strategy used to define the cohort; these two strategies are population-based samples and exposure-based samples.

Population-Based Cohort Studies

In **population-based cohort studies,** the cohort includes either an entire population or a representative sample of the population. As illustrated in Figure 7-4, a population-based cohort study starts with N; the total of exposed (A + B) and nonexposed (C + D) subjects is determined as part of the research process. Population-based cohorts have been used in studies of coronary heart disease (CHD). Perhaps the best known cohort study of CHD was initiated in 1949 in Framingham, Massachusetts.[9] When the study commenced, the town had a population of 28,000; the study design called for a random sample of 6,500 from the targeted age range of 30 to 59 years. This sample, representative of the population, was followed subsequently for changes in risk factors and incidence of disease.

An example of a cohort based on an entire population comes from the city of Tecumseh, Michigan, which was selected to examine the contribution of environmental and constitutional factors to the maintenance of health and the origins of illness. Begun in 1959–1960, the Tecumseh study successfully enrolled 8,641 persons, 88% of the community residents.[10] For some applications,

FIGURE 7-4 Illustration of sample selection in a one-sample cohort study

cohort studies may be larger than a given community. The Iowa Women's Health Study, described earlier in Chapter 3, included a random sample of 41,836[11] women between the ages of 55 and 69 in 1986 in the entire state.

The important point to remember is that these cohorts—Framingham, Tecumseh, and Iowa—were not heterogeneous in terms of their exposures; they were not selected because of a particular exposure (or risk factor) for disease. Consequently, the frequency of the exposures within the cohort was expected to be representative of the target population. Thus, in a population-based cohort study the proportion of the population exposed can be determined either directly (when the entire population has been selected) or indirectly (when a known fraction of the population has been selected). Let us explain how exposure could be determined.

With a population-based cohort, exposures are unknown until the first period of observation when exposure information is collected. For example, after administration of questionnaires, collection of biologic samples, clinical examinations, or physiologic testing, the cohort can be divided into two or more exposure categories as a result of what is learned from the subjects. For a simple dichotomy (i.e., exposed versus nonexposed), the nonexposed subjects become an internal comparison group. Sometimes, exposure may be categorized along a continuum, called a continuous variable. (Blood pressure measurements represent a continuous variable, whereas the designation of exposed/nonexposed forms a dichotomy.) For a continuous variable, such as dietary intake or blood pressure, one typically constructs multiple levels of exposure. A statistical procedure is used to subdivide the exposure variable into quantiles, which are divisions of a distribution into equal, ordered subgroups[1] (e.g., quartiles or quintiles). These subdivisions are then used to define the levels of exposure. Subjects in one of the extreme categories, such as the upper or lower quintile, serve as the comparison (or referent) category. The incidence rate among this referent category becomes the expected rate of disease occurrence.

Exposure-Based Cohort Studies

One often hears about the touted superiority of *population-based studies.* Indeed, this sampling feature has benefits regarding generalizability of results and the measures of effect that can be estimated. However, population-based cohort designs (or case-control studies, for that matter) are not efficient for rare exposures. This assertion can be best illustrated with an example. Suppose that experiments with animals provided evidence that exposure to lead causes long-term neurologic toxicity. The amounts of lead used were much greater than those found in most human exposures. Certain occupational groups, however, such as those involved in battery production, might have sufficient occupational exposure to incur significant health risks. Although one could consider using a case-control study, because the proportion of the population employed in the battery manufacturing industry is low, there would likely be few cases or controls with exposure in the study sample. An alternative approach might be to assemble an *exposure-based cohort* of employees in battery production factories, quantify levels of exposure using job titles and assignments, and determine incidence rates of neurotoxicity.

Comparison (Nonexposed) Group

Cohort studies involve the comparison of disease rates between exposed and nonexposed groups. Continuing with our example of neurotoxicity and lead exposure among workers in the battery manufacturing industry, there are essentially three options in defining the comparison group. First, it may be that certain workers within the industry have no exposure to lead. For example, sales staff, secretaries, and management may have significantly less (or more) exposure to lead than factory workers. Thus, an internal comparison would be possible (exposed vs. nonexposed) within the factory or factories under investigation. However, consider the situation in which everyone in the factory or industry is exposed to lead, and a nonexposed group could not be identified. The second option would therefore be the construction of a nonexposed group from a separate industrial cohort, similar in demographics and geography to the battery factory, but without lead exposure. A third option would be to compare disease rates among workers in the battery manufacturing industry with available population rates. Because population rates are summary rates, however, perhaps only specific to age-, sex-, and race-defined subgroups, they may have limited utility in some situations.

Consider the example of a cohort study of lung cancer among uranium ore miners. Careful attention is paid to collection of data on other exposures that contribute to lung cancer risk, including use of tobacco products and diet. In fact, in this population a high percentage of the cohort consists of current smokers. Population rates of lung cancer, however, are based on the entire population. They are not adjusted for smoking, nor are smoking status-specific rates available. In this situation, because of the smoking levels alone, comparison of lung cancer rates among the miners with population lung cancer rates would not be instructive.

Except in certain circumstances, the use of special exposure groups to form study groups precludes determination of the proportion of the target population exposed; as a result this design limits the public health inferences (generalization to a larger population). As shown in Figure 7-5, such designs typically involve select subgroups with known exposures, for example an exposed cohort (A + B) and a nonexposed, comparison cohort (C + D). Thus, in most situations the cohort members are *homogeneous* with respect to exposure, and because of the selection procedure, the frequency of exposure in the population cannot be determined.

		Disease Status		Total
		Yes	No	
Exposure Status	Yes	A	B	A + B
	No	C	D	C + D

FIGURE 7-5 Illustration of sample selection in a multisample cohort study

Additional examples of exposure-based cohorts include:

- Prepaid medical care plans, such as Kaiser Permanente or Group Health of Puget Sound, keep detailed medical information about a potentially large number of readily accessible subjects and maintain regular contact for follow-up information. In this case, the cohort is defined by insurance membership and the exposure of interest may be some medical condition or test recorded in the medical record.

- Physicians, nurses, and other health professionals have been the focus of several cohort studies. Because these individuals typically belong to national organizations (e.g., the American Medical Association), they are often easier to follow over the long term than other occupational groups. Their knowledge of disease makes them good respondents for surveys; they can be expected to report previous medical conditions and recent diagnoses reliably.

- Childhood cancer survivors are becoming increasingly common, due mainly to remarkable improvements in therapy. The Childhood Cancer Survivor Study[12] represents the largest (>14,000 five-year survivors initially diagnosed between 1970 and 1986 from 25 centers) and most extensively characterized cohort of childhood and adolescent cancer survivors in North America. It serves as a resource for addressing important issues, such as risk of second malignancies, endocrine and reproductive outcome, cardiopulmonary complications, and psychosocial implications, among this unique and ever-growing population.

- Veterans, because of the benefits they receive from the U.S. government, usually remain in contact with the relevant agency, making long-term follow-up feasible.

- College graduates are a final example of special resource groups that have been investigated in several noteworthy epidemiologic studies (later in this chapter we will cover in detail findings from a longitudinal study of Harvard alumni[13]).

Outcome Measures in Cohort Studies

In a previous section, we mentioned that although many cohort studies gather information on the incidence of disease as the principal outcome measure, several other types of outcomes may be assessed. Table 7-4 illustrates types of outcomes used for cohort studies and lists three categories of outcomes: discrete events, levels of disease markers, and changes in disease markers.[14] Discrete

Table 7-4 Types of Outcomes for Cohort Studies

Discrete events
    Single events
        Mortality
        First occurrence of a disease or health-related outcome
            Incidence (density)
            Cumulative incidence (risk)
            Ratios (incidence density and cumulative incidence)
    Multiple occurrences:
        Of disease outcome
        Of transitions between states of health/disease
        Of transitions between functional states

Level of a marker for disease or state of health

Change in a functional/physiologic/biochemical/anatomical marker for disease or health
    Rate of change
        Patterns of growth and/or decline
        "Tracking" of markers of disease/health
    Change in level with time (age)

Source: Adapted with permission from IB Tager. Outcomes in cohort studies. *Epidemiologic Reviews.* 1998, vol 20, p 16.

events cover single events and multiple occurrences, an example of the former being death and the first occurrence of a disease such as cancer, and the latter referring to repeated occurrence of disease such as recurrent heart disease (heart attacks) or strokes. Examples of discrete measures include the age-standardized annual death rate, annual age-specific death rates, and the cumulative incidence of disease of specific time intervals (e.g., five years).

Cohort studies that include multiple occurrences outcomes involve the repeated assessment of these outcomes over time. The multiple occurrences can involve discrete events, as in the case of repeated heart attacks or changes in status of outcome markers. Research questions may address the association between changes in risk markers over time and health status, studies of the effects of aging on the natural history of disease, and transitions of health status, such as the shift to functional disability among some elderly persons.

Temporal Differences in Cohort Designs

Although the basic feature of all cohort studies is measurement of exposure and follow-up for disease, there are several variations in cohort designs that depend on the timing of data collection on exposure and outcomes. These variations are prospective and retrospective cohort studies.

Prospective Cohort Studies

A **prospective cohort study** is purely prospective in nature and is characterized by determination of exposure levels at baseline (the present) and follow-up for occurrence of disease at some time in the future (Fig. 7-6). The sampling strategy may be population-based or defined by a special exposure of interest. There are numerous advantages to prospective studies:

- Prospective cohort studies enable the investigator to collect data on exposures; the collection of exposure information at baseline may result in the most direct and specific test of the study hypothesis. Examples include assessment of diet, physical activity, alcohol use, occupation, coping skills, and quality of life, each of which can be assessed with a few specific items or a comprehensive battery of items.
- The size of the cohort to be recruited is under greater control by the investigators than is the size of a retrospective cohort (see next section). Cohort studies that rely on historical records are sometimes fixed in size.
- Biological and physiological assays can be performed with decreased concern that the outcome will be affected by the underlying disease process. Examples include measures of serum factors, or nutrient levels and medical examinations (e.g., specific functional tests, antibody titers, or cholesterol levels).
- Direct measures of the environment (e.g., indoor radon levels, electromagnetic field radiation, cigarette smoke concentration, or chlorination byproducts in the water supply) can be made in order to define exposures precisely.

DESIGN	PAST	PRESENT	FUTURE
Prospective		E ⟶	D
Retrospective	E ⟶	D	
Historical prospective	E ⟶	E ⟶	D

FIGURE 7-6 Cohort design options on timing of data collection. E, exposure; D, disease

Retrospective Cohort Study

Despite the substantial benefits of prospective cohort studies, investigators must wait for cases to accrue while conducting such a study. Depending upon the size of the cohort and the prevalence of a disease in the population, several years could elapse before meaningful analyses are feasible. An alternative is a **retrospective cohort study** that makes use of historical data to determine exposure level at some baseline in the past; "follow-up" for subsequent occurrences of disease between baseline and the present is performed. A design that makes use of both retrospective (to determine baseline exposure) and prospective (to determine disease incidence in the future) features is the **historical prospective cohort study** (also known as an **ambispective cohort study**).

There are several advantages to retrospective cohort studies:

- In a relatively short period of time a significant amount of follow-up may be accrued. For example, Sellers et al.[15] performed a follow-up beginning in 1991 of a cohort of 426 families originally ascertained between 1944 and 1952 at the Dight Institute of Genetics at the University of Minnesota. Three-generation pedigrees were constructed at baseline with data collected from mothers, aunts, sisters and daughters of breast cancer patients. Records of breastfeeding, reproductive history, and validated occurrences of cancer were stored. Thus, when the family members were recontacted and interviewed regarding subsequent occurrences of cancer, almost 50 years of follow-up was completed during a five-year period of funding.

- The amount of exposure data collected can be quite extensive, and can be available to the investigator at minimal cost. For example, Hartmann and colleagues[16] at the Mayo Clinic, using an index of surgical procedures, were able to construct a cohort of women who received prophylactic mastectomy between 1963 and 1986. Details were available in the medical record on type of surgery, age at surgery, family history of cancer, and complications following surgery. Follow-up through 1997 was performed to identify subsequent occurrences of breast cancer. Analyses based on a median 14 years of follow-up were possible, even though the actual study took less than five years to complete.

Many beginning epidemiology students find the distinction between case-control studies and retrospective cohort studies difficult to grasp. The nuances may be subtle, but noteworthy. Recall that case-control studies begin with ascertainment of study subjects on the basis of disease status. Data are then collected regarding exposures that occurred prior to disease onset. Because there is only one time point of observation, there is no longitudinal component and disease rates cannot be computed. Retrospective cohort studies begin with exposure, although these measurements occurred sometime in the past. The subsequent occurrence of disease, perhaps supplemented with additional exposure assessments, is the primary focus of research activity.

Practical Considerations

Given the considerable advantages of cohort studies over other observational study designs, some readers may wonder why cohort studies are not the only designs used. In this next section we will provide a brief answer, under the unifying theme of practical considerations. Such considerations include availability of exposure data, size and cost of the cohort used, data collection and data management, follow-up issues, and sufficiency of scientific justification.

Availability of Exposure Data

Although development of prospective cohort studies may leverage data collected for other reasons besides the cohort study itself, the quality and extent of historical exposure data are absolutely essential for retrospective cohort studies. In most situations investigators will find themselves trying to weigh the trade-offs between a retrospective study design—with the associated benefits of more immediate follow-up time—versus the value of collecting the primary exposure data in the most ideal manner in a prospective cohort design. There are no simple rules to guide this decision, which must be carefully evaluated for each particular research question.

Size and Cost of the Cohort

From a scientific standpoint there is little question that the larger the size of the cohort, the greater the opportunity to obtain answers in a timely manner. For a fixed rate of disease or outcome, only by increasing the denominator can the number of cases be increased during an interval. Of course, there is a direct relationship between size and cost, and resource constraints typically influence design decisions. One approach to design cohorts with the greatest future value is to focus initial development on the collection of risk factor data and biological samples, with subsequent (future) or parallel (nested studies) grants to obtain funding for analyses of the samples. For example, Zheng and colleagues[17] obtained funding to establish the Shanghai Women's Cohort Study of 75,000 women by limiting activities during the first five years to collection of diet and risk factor data, blood samples, tissue blocks, and urine samples. To keep costs within funding limits, initial aims did not focus on assays of the biological specimens. Subsequent renewal of the funding for that study was obtained to begin testing hypotheses related to hormone metabolism (urine), growth factor levels (serum), and genetic polymorphisms (DNA from lymphocytes in the blood).

Data Collection and Data Management

An axiom of epidemiologic research design is that larger studies necessarily are more demanding than smaller ones with regard to challenges in data collection and data management. Coordination of activities in the field is especially complex when multiple sites are necessary for recruitment. Additional challenges may arise from data entry, especially if individual sites enter their own data for transmittal to the coordinating center. In these situations, explicit protocols for quality control (e.g., double entry of data, and scannable forms) should be considered in the design and implementation stage. The organizational and administrative burdens are increased even further when there are multiple levels of data collection (such as telephone interviews, mail-out questionnaires, consent forms to access medical records, and collection of biological samples) at multiple time periods (especially when active follow-up is needed). Cohort study research protocols may require elaborate data-management systems to monitor the status of the various components of data collection. Such management systems support individuals in the field who are charged with the multifaceted components, as well as study managers and investigators who monitor overall progress. Management of data from cohort studies can be incredibly challenging and should be considered when staffing needs are being defined. Challenges arise from data collected from multiple sources, merging of files, and "cleaning" of data files. Cleaning is necessary in the case of missing values, out-of-range entries, and inconsistencies (e.g., someone responds that they never smoke but subsequently report a habit of 2 packs per day). These issues are not peculiar to cohort studies, as cross-sectional surveys and case-control studies can be quite large, too. However, the relative inefficiency of cohort studies for investigation of rare diseases means that they are typically larger than other designs.

Follow-up Issues

The value of cohort studies can be realized only if an effective system can be implemented to follow the cohort for subsequent occurrence of disease or other outcomes. It may be helpful at this time to distinguish between *active* versus *passive follow-up*.

Active follow-up denotes the situation in which the investigator, through direct contact with the cohort, must obtain data on subsequent incidence of the outcome (disease, change in risk factor, change in biological marker). Such contact may be accomplished through follow-up mailings, phone calls, or written invitations to return to study sites/centers for subsequent medical evaluation and, in some cases, biospecimen collection. Follow-up requires a substantial amount of effort, especially for large cohorts. For instance, the Minnesota Breast Cancer Family Study[18] follows up on study participants with a mailed survey, a reminder postcard 30 days later, a second survey, and a telephone call to non-responders. In the present era of telephone technology—answering machines, caller identification (ID), and automated telemarketing solicitations—active follow-up is becoming increasingly labor intensive and oftentimes frustrating, especially in our mobile society where addresses change often. For some cohort studies, however, a persistent and labor-intensive effort is the only option for follow-up.

Contrast the foregoing scenario with *passive follow-up,* which does not require direct contact with cohort members. Passive follow-up is possible when databases containing the outcomes of interest are collected and maintained by organizations outside the investigative team. Epidemiologists sometimes are able to achieve record linkage between databases and the study cohort. An excellent example amenable to passive follow-up is cancer, for which the federal and many state governments mandate reporting. The Iowa Women's Health Study,[11] described earlier in Chapter 3, is able to conduct follow-up for cancer incidence within the state in this manner.

Passive follow-up is clearly not an option for many diseases. The only endpoint for which there is universal coverage is death; the National Center for Health Statistics collects mortality data, which are made available to the scientific community through the National Death Index (NDI). The success of linkage to the NDI depends upon the extent of demographic information collected on participants. Social Security numbers are the most effective data element for linkage. If Social Security numbers are unavailable, record linkage sometimes is possible for persons who have uncommon last names.

Sufficiency of Scientific Justification

The preceding sections emphasized that the establishment of a cohort study requires major investments in resources (time, money, and energy). Thus, there should be considerable scientific rationale for a cohort study. This rationale should be grounded on prior research from various perspectives: study designs other than cohort studies; several different investigators; and several different study populations. Additional justification for cohort studies may come from laboratory experiments or animal studies. Furthermore, the situation in which investigators would like to explore more than one outcome from a particular exposure provides one of the greatest justifications for a cohort study. Because of the nature of case-control studies, only a single outcome can be investigated at a time. Cohort studies are the only observational study design that permits examination of multiple outcomes at the level of the individual within a single study. Consider as an example the complex issue of hormone replacement therapy (HRT). Numerous epidemiologic studies have noted that HRT is associated with a slight, but detectable, increased risk of breast cancer. In fact, recommendations have been published in leading medical journals for the avoidance of HRT among women at elevated risk of breast cancer because of a family history.[18] Complicating such a recommendation is the observation from other epidemiologic studies that have associated HRT with a number of health benefits, including lower risks of coronary heart disease,[19,20] osteoporosis,[21,22] and Alzheimer's disease.[23] However, a study published in mid-2003 reported increased rates of dementia among older women on combination hormone replacement therapy (see box). The pros and cons of HRT use can be examined within an appropriately designed cohort study[24] with measures of HRT collected at baseline and a follow-up protocol designed to collect data on the multiple outcomes of interest.

Late Breaker—Hormone Replacement Therapy

"Rates of Dementia Increase Among Older Women on Combination Hormone Therapy

Older women taking combination hormone therapy had twice the rate of dementia, including Alzheimer's disease (AD), compared with women who did not take the medication, according to new findings from a memory substudy of the Women's Health Initiative (WHI). The research, part of the Women's Health Initiative Memory study (WHIMS) and reported in the May 28, 2003, *Journal of the American Medical Association (JAMA),* found the heightened risk of developing dementia in a study of women 65 and older taking Prempro™, a particular form of estrogen plus progestin hormone therapy.

The study also found that the combination therapy did not protect against the development of Mild Cognitive Impairment, or MCI, a form of cognitive decline less severe than dementia.

continues

'Because of possible harm in some areas and lack of a demonstrated benefit in others, we have concluded that combination hormone therapy should not be prescribed at this time for older, postmenopausal women to maintain or improve cognitive function,' says . . . [a government official affiliated with the National Institutes of Health]." ■

Source: Reprinted from National Institutes of Health, National Institute on Aging. *NIH News,* May 27, 2003. Available at: http://www.nih.gov/news/pr/may2003/nia-27.htm. Accessed June 12, 2003.

Measures of Interpretation and Examples

In the simplest case of two levels of exposure (yes/no), two incidence rates are calculated. The relative risk is defined as the ratio of the risk of disease or death among the exposed, to the risk among the unexposed.[1] Recall from Chapter 3 that risk is estimated in epidemiologic studies only by the cumulative incidence. When the relative risk is calculated with incidence rates or incidence density, then the term *rate ratio* is more precise.

$$\text{Relative risk} = \frac{\text{Incidence rate in the exposed}}{\text{Incidence rate in the nonexposed}}$$

Using the notation from the 2 by 2 table (Figure 6-1), the relative risk can be expressed as $[A/(A + B)] \div [C/(C + D)]$. A sample calculation is shown in Exhibit 7-2.

Some comments regarding interpretation of relative risk are in order. A relative risk of 1.0 implies that the risk (rate) of disease among the exposed is no different from the risk of disease among the nonexposed. A relative risk of 2.0 implies that risk is twice as high, whereas a relative risk of 0.5 indicates that the exposure of interest is associated with half the risk of disease.

Examples of Cohort Studies

Table 7-5 presents examples of major cohort studies, including when they were initiated, their main focus, study population, measurement of exposure at baseline and follow-up, and frequency of exposure follow-up. More detailed coverage of some of these studies is provided in this chapter and throughout the text. Exhibit 7-3 showcases four cohort studies that concern women's health.

EXHIBIT 7-2

Sample Problem: Relative Risk

The following is an example of how to use a fourfold table for calculation of relative risk. Deykin and Buka[25] studied suicide ideation and attempts in a population of chemically dependent adolescents believed by the researchers to be a group at high risk for self-destructive behavior. Boys who had been exposed to physical or sexual abuse and who stated that a report of abuse or neglect had been filed with authorities were more likely than boys who were absent such exposures to have made a suicide attempt. The data for history of sexual abuse among the boys are charted below:

History of sexual abuse	Suicide attempt	No suicide attempt	Totals
Yes	A = 14	B = 9	A + B = 23
No	C = 49	D = 149	C + D = 198

Relative risk = (14/23)/(49/198) = 0.609/0.247 = 2.46

Source: Data from EY Deykin and SL Buka. Suicidal ideation and attempts among chemically dependent adolescents. *American Journal of Public Health.* vol 84, pp 634–639; American Public Health Association, © 1994. The fourfold table was constructed by the authors from these data and from the percentage of suicide attempts reported for boys with a positive history and boys with a negative history of sexual abuse. Deykin and Buka reported 60.9% and 24.8% attempting suicide, respectively, and a relative risk of 2.4.

The remainder of this section provides examples of cohort studies built upon a common research theme: physical activity and CHD. The idea that physical activity is beneficial to humans is certainly not a new one. In *The Dialogues,* Timeus tells Socrates that "Moderate exercise reduces to order, according to their affinities, the particles and affections which are wandering about the body."[26(p405)] Two thousand years later the experts still are unable to agree on how much or how often exercise is needed or whether habitual physical activity (as opposed to exercise) is sufficient to maintain one's health. The rediscovery of the potential importance of physical activity was spurred by a landmark study of British transportation workers by Morris and colleagues in 1953.[27] Hoping to uncover "social factors which may be favourable or unfavourable to its occurrence,"[27(p1053)] the investigators conducted a study of roughly 31,000 men aged 35 to 64. Rates of angina pectoris, coronary

Table 7-5 Examples of Major Cohort Studies

Study [Year Begun]	Main Focus	Study Population [Sample Size]	Baseline Exposure Instruments*	Follow-Up Exposure Instruments*	Frequency of Exposure Follow-up
The Framingham Heart Study [1948]	Risk factors for cardiovascular disease	Residents of Framingham, MA, ages 28–62 years [*n* = 5,209]	Interview, clinic examination (PE, lab, tests)	Interview, clinic examination (PE, lab, tests)	Every 2 years
Colorado Plateau Uranium Miners Study [1950]	Occupational risk factors for cancer	White, male underground uranium miners, Colorado Plateau [*n* = 3,415]	Clinic examination (PE), questionnaire, environmental measures (airborne radiation)	Questionnaire (in-person or mailed), environmental measures (airborne radiation)	Triennial
American Cancer Society: Cancer Prevention Study 1 [1959]	Cigarette smoking and cancer mortality	U.S. men and women aged 30 years and older [*n* = 1,045,087]	Self-administered questionnaire delivered by volunteers	Self-administered questionnaire	Every 2 years
The Alameda County Study [1965]	Factors associated with health and mortality	Residents of Alameda County, CA, ages 16–94 years [*n* = 6,928]	Mailed questionnaire; telephone interview or home interview of nonrespondents	Mailed questionnaire; telephone interview or home interview of nonrespondents	At years 9, 18, and 29
Honolulu Heart Program 12 [1965]	Coronary heart disease and stroke in men of Japanese ancestry	Men of Japanese ancestry living on Oahu, HI, ages 45–65 years [*n* = 8,006]	Mailed questionnaire, interview, clinic examination (PE, lab, tests)		
The Oral Contraception Study of the Royal College of General Practitioners [1968]	Oral contraceptive use and cancer	Married premenopausal British women [*n* = 47,000]	Medical form completed by physician based on patient interview or medical record	Same	Every 6 months
Nurses' Health Study [1976]	Originally oral contraceptive use and cancer, expanded to women's health	Married female U.S. registered nurses ages 30–55 years [*n* = 121,700]	Mailed questionnaire	Mailed questionnaire Lab (toenail sample) Lab (home blood draw)	Every 2 years At year 6 At year 13

continues

Table 7-5 *continued*

Study [Year Begun]	Main Focus	Study Population [Sample Size]	Baseline Exposure Instruments*	Follow-Up Exposure Instruments*	Frequency of Exposure Follow-up
Port Pirie Cohort Study [1979]	Lead exposure and child development	Infants born in Port Pirie, South Australia, 1979–1982 [n = 723]	Lab (blood samples from pregnant mother and umbilical cord at birth)	Lab (blood samples)	At 6,15, and 24 months, annually up to 7 years, and at 11–13 years
Multicenter AIDS Cohort Study [1984]	Risk factors for HIV in gay men	U.S. homosexual men ages 18–70 years [n = 4,954]	Clinic examination (PE, lab), self-administered questionnaire, interview	Clinic examination (PE, lab), self-administered questionnaire, interview	Every 6 months
Coronary Artery Risk Development in Young Adults (CARDIA) [1985]	Risk factors for coronary heart disease in young adults	Black and white U.S. men and women ages 18–30 years [n = 5,115]	Telephone interview, clinic examination (PE, lab, tests), self-administered questionnaire, interview	Clinic examination (PE, lab, tests), self-administered questionnaire, interview	At years 2, 5, and 7
New York University Women's Health Study [1985]	Endogenous hormones and risk of breast cancer	New York women ages 35–65 years [n = 14,291]	Lab, self-administered questionnaire	Lab	Annual
Iowa Women's [Health] Study [1986]	Cancer in women	Iowa women ages 55–69 years [n = 41,837]	Mailed questionnaire with self body girth measures	None	
Study of Osteoporotic Fractures [1986]	Risk factors for fractures	Nonblack U.S. women aged 65 years and older [n = 9,704]	Questionnaire, clinic examination (PE, tests), abstraction (medication labels)	Questionnaire Clinic examination (PE, tests)	Year 1 Year 2
Cardiovascular Health Study (CHS) [1989]	Risk factors for cardiovascular disease in older adults	U.S. men and women aged 65 years and older [n = 5,201]	Home interview, clinic examination (PE, lab, tests), questionnaire, abstraction (medication labels)	Clinic examination (PE, tests), questionnaire, abstraction (medication labels) Clinic examination (lab) and all of above	Annual Triennial

continues

Table 7-5 *continued*

Study [Year Begun]	Main Focus	Study Population [Sample Size]	Baseline Exposure Instruments*	Follow-Up Exposure Instruments*	Frequency of Exposure Follow-up
Women's Health Initiative (WHI) Observational Study [1994]	Women's health	U.S. women, ages 50–79 years [$n = 100,000$]	Telephone interview, clinic examination (PE, lab, tests), interview, self-administered questionnaire, abstraction (medication labels)	Mailed questionnaire Clinic examination (PE, lab, tests), abstraction (medication labels), self-administered questionnaire	Annual At year 3

*Exposure instruments definitions: PE, physical examination or physical measures, such as anthropometrics, strength, etc.; lab, measures in blood and other specimens; tests, medical tests, such as electrocardiography, treadmill, bone mineral density, etc.; abstraction, abstraction of medication information from medication labels, medical record abstraction; environmental measures, measures in the environment (air or water); questionnaire, either self-administered or interviewer-administered (not explicitly stated); and interview, interviewer-administered questionnaire.

Source: Adapted with permission from E White, JR Hunt, and D Casso, Exposure measurement in cohort studies: the challenges of prospective data collection. *Epidemiologic Reviews*, vol 20. No 1, pp 44–45, 1998.

Four Cohort Studies that Investigate Women's Health

Nurses' Health Study: Affiliated investigators, housed at Brigham and Women's Hospital in Boston, mailed questionnaires beginning in 1976 to 170,000 nurses who resided in the 11 most populous U.S. states. Nurses (approximately $n = 122,000$ responding) were selected because they were knowledgeable about the technically worded questionnaire items and motivated to remain over the long term in the cohort study. The aim of Frank Speizer, the study's originator, was to examine the long-term potential consequences of use of oral contraceptives. Mailed every two years, the original questionnaire searched for the occurrence of various diseases and also probed health-related topics, such as smoking, hormone use, and menopausal issues. A later phase of the project initiated in 1980 was expanded to include diet and quality of life topics. A subset of the cohort submitted toenail samples (used for mineral analyses) and blood samples, employed in studies of biomarkers. In 1989, Dr. Walter Willett started the Nurses' Health Study II, which focused on oral contraceptive use, diet, and lifestyle risk factors in a population younger that the original Nurses' Health Study cohort. The Nurses' Health Study has generated an impressive list of scientific publications and many fundamental contributions to the store of health knowledge.[1]

Women's Health Initiative (WHI): The WHI, begun in 1991, concentrates on the major causes of death, disability, and frailty among postmenopausal women: coronary heart disease, breast and colorectal cancer, and osteoporotic fractures. Two major goals of the WHI are to provide estimates of the extent to which known risk factors predict heart disease, cancers, and fractures and to identify new risk factors for these and other diseases in women. One of the largest preventive studies of its kind in the United States, the WHI will have a projected 15-year duration. The WHI encompasses three major components: a randomized clinical trial for disease prevention, a study of community approaches to developing healthful behaviors, and an observational study (OS). The OS follows more than 93,000 postmenopausal women between the ages of 50 to 79 over an average of nine years. The respondents complete periodic health forms and visit a clinic three years after enrollment.[2]

continues

EXHIBIT 7-3 *continued*

> **Study of Osteoporotic Fractures:** From September 1986 to October 1987, this prospective cohort study enrolled 9,704 women aged 65 years of age and older. Subjects were selected from the rosters of four clinical centers: The Kaiser-Permanente Center for Health Research, Portland, OR; the University of Minnesota, Minneapolis; the University of Maryland, Baltimore; and the University of Pittsburgh. The University of California, San Francisco, acted as the research coordinating center. Investigators administered questionnaires, interviews, and examinations to obtain information on anthropometric characteristics, estrogen use and medical history. Follow-up measures included the incidence of fractures, validated by radiographic reports.[3]
>
> **Iowa Women's Health Study:** See Chapter 3, Exhibit 3-2. ■

Source: Adapted from [1]http://www.channing.Harvard.edu/nhs/ Accessed March 16, 2003; [2]http://www.nhlbi.nih.gov/whi/. Accessed March 16, 2003; [3]Sellmeyer DE, Stone KL, Sebastian A, et al. A high ratio of dietary animal to vegetable protein increases the rate of bone loss and the risk of fracture in postmenopausal women. *American Journal of Clinical Nutrition* 2001;73:118–122.

thrombosis, and sudden death were obtained for drivers, conductors, and underground railway workers. Conductors, whose job was physically more demanding than that of the other two groups, had significantly lower rates of CHD. The proposition that physical activity might be protective generated tremendous interest and spurred numerous investigations to confirm and refine the hypothesis.

The first example is a retrospective cohort study of railroad workers.[28] The cohort included 191,609 railroad industry employees in the United States between the ages of 40 and 64.[28] The "exposure" was work-related physical activity. Based on job descriptions, three groups were formed: clerks, switchmen, and section men, with activity levels of low, moderate, and heavy, respectively. With any cohort study that entails long periods of follow-up, a legitimate concern is whether exposures at the baseline period change over time, resulting in exposure misclassification. One advantage of using the railroad industry for this study was that the labor contracts between management and the brotherhoods contained seniority provisions that prevented a man from carrying his seniority from one job to another job controlled by a separate brotherhood. Because seniority brings benefits in terms of privileges and income, job changes associated with a switch to a different labor contract were uncommon. Follow-up for CHD end points was accomplished through the Railroad Retirement Board, which maintained an account for each man employed by any interstate railroad in the United States. Because the retirement and disability benefits to members were greater than those received from Social Security, follow-up rates were high. The number of deaths among members that were not detected by the board occurred almost exclusively among men who left the industry completely; the investigators estimated that this number was only 11 to 12 per 1,000 workers.

Average annual age-adjusted mortality rates of CHD per 1,000 men were calculated among men who had accumulated 10 years of service by the end of 1951 and were employed in 1954. Mortality rates per 1,000 were 5.7, 3.9, and 2.8 for clerks, switchmen, and section men, respectively. If one considers the rates among the sedentary clerks as the reference, then the relative risk of CHD death for the moderately active switchmen was 0.68, and 0.49 for the very active section men.

Although the study findings supported the hypothesis that physical activity is protective for CHD, there were some limitations inherent in the historical exposure data. In this particular situation, few data were available on other risk factors that might underlie the observed association. For example, no information was available about smoking, body mass index, blood pressure, family history of CHD, and hypertension. Therefore, additional studies were warranted.

The second example is of an ambispective, or historical prospective, cohort study. Reported by Paffenbarger and colleagues in 1984,[13] the study examined a history of athleticism and CHD in a cohort of male Harvard alumni from 1916 to 1950 ($N = 16,936$). Exposure assessments occurred at two time periods: a historical measure of physical activity based on college archives of student health and athletics, and a questionnaire mailed in 1962 or 1966 for which the response rate was 70%. The alumni questionnaire assessed post-college physical exercise, other elements of lifestyle, health status, and histories of parental disease. The assessment of physical activity included the number of stairs climbed per day, the number of city blocks or equivalent walked each day, and sports actively played (in hours per week). Responses were used to estimate kilocalories of energy expenditure per week. Follow-up of the cohort was achieved through questionnaires mailed in 1972 by the alumni office. The first questionnaire ascertained self-reports of physician-diagnosed CHD events. The second questionnaire, mailed in the same year to the survivors of the deceased cohort members, ascertained dates of death. Weekly updates of death lists by the alumni office provided the means to obtain death certificates for causes. To account for the varying amount of follow-up, person-years of observation were calculated. Heart attack rates were computed according to activity level as a student and as an alumnus. Men who participated in fewer than five hours per week of intramural sports as a student and fewer than 500 kilocalories per week of leisure time activity as an alumnus were designated as the reference group (85.5 per 10,000 person-years). Men who were college varsity athletes but became sedentary as adults had the same rate of first CHD attacks (relative risk, 1.0) as the reference group. In contrast, men who were active as adults (2,000+ kilocalories per week) had a much-reduced risk of CHD, regardless of whether they had been sedentary or active as students.

The third and final example of a cohort study is purely prospective in nature. Peters et al.[29] designed a study to address one of the major concerns of the previous body of literature on the subject of physical activity (occupational or leisure): Most occupational physical activity is not of sufficient intensity or duration to affect cardiorespiratory fitness. Exercise physiologists argued that physical fitness, not physical activity, was the appropriate and relevant exposure. A cohort of 2,779 firefighters and police officers in Los Angeles County between the ages of 35 and 55 was established. In contrast to the two previous studies, which based exposure levels on job title or questionnaires, level of physical work capacity was determined by use of a bicycle ergometer. The cohort was divided into two exposure categories based on a median split (the 50% point in a distribution). Measurements were taken also on a number of other risk factors, including blood pressure, relative weight, family history, cholesterol, and skinfolds. Follow-up for heart attacks was accomplished using county workers' compensation files, death certificates, and medical records; person-years of observation were tabulated. Because heart attacks and an expensive hospital stay were fully reimbursable by insurance, coverage was thought to be complete. Analyses were performed to control for smoking, obesity, blood pressure, cholesterol, family history, relative weight, and physical activity. Results suggested that the least physically fit had more than a twofold greater risk of heart attacks than the most physically fit. Risk was especially prominent (relative risk, 6.6) for those who had at least two additional risk factors (smoking, high serum cholesterol, or high blood pressure).

Nested Case-Control Studies

Although this section would seem to be more logically placed with Chapter 6 (case-control studies), an understanding of nested case-control studies requires an understanding of cohort studies. A **nested case-control study** is defined as a type of case-control study ". . . in which cases and controls are drawn from the population in a cohort study."[1] For example, suppose we have data from an ongoing cohort study of the relationship between use of birth control pills and breast cancer. The population of the cohort study would comprise both exposed and nonexposed persons; the former and latter would consist of women who take and do not take birth control pills, respectively. To perform a nested case-control study, the investigator would select a subset of the population from the cohort study; this subset would comprise the controls. The cases of breast cancer identified from the cohort study would comprise the cases in the case-control study. Figure 7-7 contrasts a cohort study with a nested case-control study.

What are the advantages of a nested case-control study? This design provides a degree of control over confounding factors, because exposure information and other data have been collected during the course of the cohort study. Another

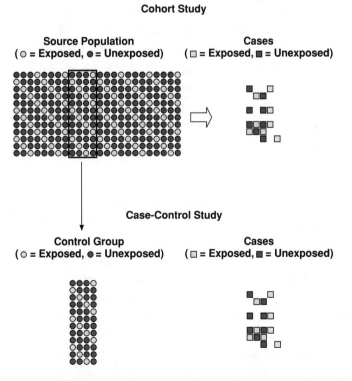

FIGURE 7-7 Illustration of cohort and nested case-control studies.
Source: Reprinted with permission from Rothman KJ. *Epidemiology: An Introduction.* New York, NY: Oxford University Press; 2002, p 74.

advantage relates to the reduced cost of collecting detailed exposure information from a subset of the cohort only; this procedure obviously would be less costly than obtaining information from every single person in the cohort.

An example of a nested case-control study is an investigation of suicide among electric utility workers. The study examined the association between exposure to extremely low-frequency magnetic fields and suicide.[30] Cases (536 deaths from suicide) and controls ($n = 5,248$) were selected from a cohort of 138,905 male utility workers. Findings supported an association between occupational exposure to electromagnetic fields and suicide.

A second example comes from Dearden et al.,[31] who conducted a case-control study that aimed to identify factors associated with teen fatherhood. Data came from the National Child Development Study, a longitudinal investigation of all children born in Great Britain between March 3 and March 9, 1958. This type of design, in which a subset of members from a larger cohort study is selected for analysis, was a nested case-control study. Data were collected at birth and at 7, 11, 16, and 23 years of age[32]; information about fatherhood status was available on 5,997 males. Cases were defined as teens who had fathered a child before their 20th birthday (n = 209). Controls, selected from the same follow-up group, were divided into two groups: 844 nonteen fathers (those who became fathers between the ages of 20 and 23), and 798 nonfathers (those who had no children by age 23). Teen fathers were found to be three times as likely as nonfathers to engage in lawbreaking behavior and to be absent from school, three to four times as likely to show signs of aggression, and eight times as likely to leave school at age 16.

Summary of Cohort Studies

Cohort studies have several clearly identified strengths. The cohort study is the first observational study design covered that permits direct determination of risk. Because one starts with disease-free subjects, this design provides stronger evidence of an exposure-disease association than the case-control scheme. In addition, cohort studies provide evidence about lag time between exposure and disease. In comparison to case-control studies, which have a greater potential for error, cohort studies facilitate generalization of findings. A tremendous advantage of cohort studies is that, if properly designed and executed, they allow examination of multiple outcomes. While case-control studies may not be efficient for exposures that are rare in the population, cohort studies are able to increase the efficiency for rare exposures by selecting cohorts with known exposures (such as certain occupational groups).

The main limitation of cohort studies, at least for those that are purely prospective, is that they take considerable effort to conduct. Because they are almost always larger than case-control studies, more time is required to collect the exposure information. Additional time passes while one waits for the outcomes to occur. The amount of time required to accumulate sufficient end points for meaningful analysis can be reduced by increasing the size of the cohort, but this increase has to be balanced against the longer time to assemble and measure the cohort as well as the increased financial costs. Given the large size of cohort studies and the need for multiple observation points, they are more difficult to implement and carry out than other observational designs, especially for rare diseases. Loss to follow-up can be a significant problem, limiting the sample size for analysis and raising questions about the results if loss is too high. With long-term follow-up, some exposures may change over time. This misclassification of exposure would attenuate the estimates of the relative risk. It is even conceivable that participation in the study itself may lead to changes in exposure. For example, suppose the investigator recruits a cohort to study the association of dietary fat and disease. As a result of participation, subjects' motivation to learn more about the hypothesis may subsequently lead to adoption of a low-fat diet. Ethical issues arise if good data already indicate that a particular exposure is harmful and one does nothing to intervene with at-risk subjects. Despite these limitations, the cohort study design is an important and valuable tool. For an in-depth coverage of cohort studies, refer to Samet and Munoz.[33]

Comparisons of Observational Designs

Chapters 6 and 7 have covered all of the major types of observational study designs used in public health practice. Table 7-6 summarizes these designs by giving a comparison of their characteristics, advantages, and disadvantages.

Conclusion

Chapter 7 has covered the cohort study, one of the most powerful epidemiologic study designs. We noted that cohort studies overcome many of the problems associated with temporality of data collection and rare exposures. Both the term cohort and the method of cohort analysis were defined. We provided several examples of cohort analyses, including Frost's tabular data on tuberculosis mortality. Related to cohort analyses are life tables and survival curves, which, respectively, estimate and graphically portray survival (often of patients in clinical trials) over time.

Table 7-6 Comparisons of Observational Study Designs

Study Attribute	Ecologic	Cross-Sectional	Name of Study Design Case-Control	Cohort
Type of Study	Descriptive and analytic	Descriptive	Analytic	Analytic
Number of Observations	Single point of observation (ecologic comparison study)	Single point of observation. Collect exposure and disease histories simultaneously.	Single point of observation.	Outcome determined prospectively. Exposure determined at baseline.
Information on Directionality of Exposure	Usually unknown	Unknown whether disease or exposure came first.	Exposure information collected retrospectively.	Exposure information collected at baseline. Outcome information collected prospectively.
Data Sources/Collection Methods	Existing data, such as mortality rates.	Data from sample surveys. May also use secondary data, i.e., school records, national surveys.	Primary data from surveys of patients. Secondary data, e.g., from disease registries, medical records.	Primary data for exposure and outcome. Some cohort designs use secondary data.
Unit of Observation	The group	The individual	The individual	The individual
Measures used	Correlation, chi-square	Prevalence estimates	Odds ratio	Relative risk
Advantages	Quick and easy to conduct. Inexpensive.	Can be completed within a short time frame. Inexpensive.	Often smaller in size than prospective studies. Quick and easy to complete. Cost effective. Useful for studying rare diseases.	Permit direct determination of risk. Provide stronger evidence of exposure-disease associations than other observational designs. Useful for studying rare exposures.

continues

Table 7-6 *continued*

Study Attribute	Name of Study Design			
	Ecologic	Cross-Sectional	Case-Control	Cohort
Disadvantages	Ecologic fallacy. Imprecise measurement of exposure-disease relationships.	Should not be used for studying disease etiology. Not useful for diseases of low frequency. Exposure-disease temporality not ascertained.	Uncertainty of the exposure-disease relationship. Inability to provide direct estimate of risk. Not useful for rare exposures. Recall bias.	Lengthy to conduct. Attrition. Difficult to carry out. Selection bias. Difficult to use with rare diseases.
Applications	Test specific etiologic hypotheses. Develop new etiologic hypotheses. Suggest mechanisms of causation. Identify new methods for disease prevention.	Depict mortality and morbidity from specific diseases. Generate hypotheses. Plan interventions. Describe the magnitude and distribution of a health problem. Assist in planning health services.	Infectious disease outbreak investigation. Chronic disease investigation when etiology unknown. Hypothesis testing.	Studies of chronic disease etiology Risk estimation. Hypothesis testing.
Examples	Association between breast cancer mortality and dietary fats. Air pollution and mortality by cities.	Prevalence of smokeless tobacco use among school-children. Number of vasectomies. Prevalence of congenital malformations.	Association between chili pepper consumption and gastric cancer risk. Anesthesia and neural tube defects. Smoking and cervical cancer.	Physical activity and coronary heart disease mortality. Child abuse and suicide. Exposure to toxic materials and mortality among workers.

The remainder of the chapter focused on methods associated with cohort studies. Population-based cohort studies were distinguished from exposure-based cohort studies. We also presented methods for the selection of comparison groups in cohort studies. Other issues included types of outcome measures, temporal differences in designs, and practical considerations in the operation of cohort studies. Relative risk, a measure of interpretation, was defined and illustrated. Finally, the chapter concluded with many examples of cohort studies, a review of the related topic of nested case-control studies, and a comparison of observational study designs.

Study Questions and Exercises

1. Define in your own words the following terms:
   a. Cohort
   b. Cohort effect
   c. Population-based cohort
   d. Exposure-based cohort
   e. Comparison groups in cohort studies
   f. Prospective cohort study
   g. Retrospective cohort study
   h. Ambispective cohort study

2. What are secular trends and cohort effects? Explain the relationship between these two terms.

3. Explain what is meant by the term relative risk and explain how it is used in cohort studies.

4. Describe the essential differences between life tables and survival curves.

5. A cohort study was conducted to study the association of coffee drinking and anxiety in a population-based sample of adults. Among 10,000 coffee drinkers, 500 developed anxiety. Among the 20,000 non-coffee drinkers, 200 cases of anxiety were observed. What is the relative risk of anxiety associated with coffee use?

6. How is a case-control study different from a retrospective cohort study? List the key criteria that, in general, would influence you to select one approach over the other.

7. Are relative risks of 2.0 and 0.5 the same or different in strength of association?

8. Cohort studies have some advantages over case-control studies in terms of the confidence with which their results are viewed. Suppose there have

been four case-control studies of an exposure-disease association and that the range of the odds ratios is from 28.0 to 49.0. Would you advocate a cohort study? Justify your answer.

9. Cohort studies allow the investigator to examine multiple outcomes and multiple exposures. Consider the following three exposures: smoking, low vitamin D intake, and severe cold weather. How many different outcomes could you examine in a cohort study that measured all three exposures at baseline?

10. High rates of follow-up are essential to the validity of cohort studies. What are some approaches that can be employed to ensure compliance when linkage to a central disease registry is not an option?

11. Summarize the strengths and weaknesses and advantages and disadvantages of the various types of observational study designs: ecologic, cross-sectional, case-control, and cohort.

12. Describe how you would conduct a nested case-control study of low socioeconomic status as a risk factor for teenage pregnancy.

13. Explain what is meant by the statement that cohort studies overcome the problem of temporality, which is not addressed by other types of observational study designs.

14. What are some of the practical issues that influence the design of a cohort study?

15. Discuss some of the possible outcomes for cohort studies, distinguishing between discrete events and disease markers.

References

1. Last JM. *A Dictionary of Epidemiology,* 4th ed. New York, NY: Oxford University Press; 2001.

2. Comstock GW. Cohort analysis: W.H. Frost's contributions to the epidemiology of tuberculosis and chronic disease. *Soz Präventivmed.* 2001;46:7–12.

3. Tolley HD, Crane L, Shipley N. Smoking prevalence and lung cancer death rates. In: *Strategies To Control Tobacco Use in the United States: A Blueprint for Public Health Action in the 1990s.* Bethesda, MD: National Institutes of Health; 1991.

4. National Center for Health Statistics. Mortality from diseases associated with smoking, United States, 1950–64. *Mon Vital Stat Rep.* 1966;20.

5. National Cancer Institute. *Risks Associated With Smoking Cigarettes With Low Machine-Measured Yields of Tar and Nicotine.* Smoking and Tobacco Control Monograph No. 13. NIH Pub. No. 02-5074. Bethesda, MD: U.S. Department of Health and Human Services, National Institutes of Health, National Cancer Institute; October 2001.

6. Chernick MR, Friis RH. *Introductory Biostatistics for the Health Sciences: Modern Applications Including Bootstrap.* Hoboken, NJ: John Wiley & Sons, Inc.; 2003.

7. Arias E. United States Life Tables, 2000. *National Vital Statistics Reports.* Hyattsville, MD: National Center for Health Statistics, 2002:51, No. 3.

8. Motulsky H. *Intuitive Biostatistics.* New York, NY: Oxford University Press; 1995. Available at: http://www.graphpad.com/www/book/survive.htm. Accessed March 17, 2003.

9. Dawber TR, Meadors GF, Moore FE. Epidemiological approaches to heart disease: the Framingham Study. *Am J Public Health.* 1951;41:279–286.

10. Francis T Jr, Epstein FH. Survey methods in general populations: Tecumseh, Michigan. In: Acheson RM, ed. *Comparability in International Epidemiology.* Princeton, NJ: Milbank Memorial Fund; 1965:333–342.

11. Bisgard KM, Folsom AR, Hong C-P, Sellers TA. Mortality and cancer rates in nonresponders to a prospective study in older women: 5-year follow-up. *Am J Epidemiol.* 1994;139:990–1000.

12. Robison LL, Mertens AC, Boice JD, et al. Study design and cohort characteristics of the Childhood Cancer Survivor Study: a multi-institutional collaborative project. *Med Pediatr Oncol.* 2002;38:229–239.

13. Paffenbarger RS, Hyde RT, Wing AL, Steinmetz CH. A natural history of athleticism and cardiovascular health. *JAMA.* 1984;252:491–495.

14. Tager IB. Outcomes in cohort studies. *Epidemiol Rev.* 1998;20:15–28.

15. Sellers TA, King RA, Cerhan JR, et al. Fifty-year follow-up of cancer incidence in a historical cohort of Minnesota Breast Cancer Families. *Cancer Epidemiol Biomarkers Prev.* 1999;12:1051–1057.

16. Hartmann LC, Schaid DJ, Woods JE, et al. Efficacy of bilateral prophylactic mastectomy in women with a family history of breast cancer. *N Engl J Med.* 1999;340:77–84.

17. Zheng W. Cancer risk reduction and diet: A cohort study of women. Grant No.: 2R01CA070867-07. Available at: http://crisp.cit.nih.gov. Accessed June 12, 2003.

18. Hoskins KF, Stopfer JE, Calzone KA, et al. Assessment and counseling for women with a family history of breast cancer. A guide for clinicians. *JAMA.* 1995;273:577–585.

19. Hu FB, Grodstein F. Postmenopausal hormone therapy and the risk of cardiovascular disease: The epidemiologic evidence. *Am J Cardiol.* 2002;90(suppl):26F–29F.

20. Psaty BM, Heckbert SR, Atkins D, et al. A review of the association of estrogens and progestins with cardiovascular disease in postmenopausal women. *Arch Intern Med.* 1993;153:1421–1427.

21. Nelson HD, Humphrey LL, Nygren P, et al. Postmenopausal hormone replacement therapy: scientific review. *JAMA.* 2002;288:872–881.

22. Lobo RA. Benefits and risks of estrogen replacement therapy. *Am J Obstet Gynecol* 1995;173:782–789.

23. Kawas C, Resnick S, Morrison A, et al. A prospective study of estrogen replacement therapy and the risk of developing Alzheimer's disease: the Baltimore Longitudinal Study of Aging. *Neurology.* 1997;48:1517–1521.

24. Sellers TA, Mink PJ, Anderson KE, et al. The role of hormone replacement therapy in the risk for breast cancer and total mortality in women with a family history of breast cancer. *Ann Intern Med.* 1997;127:973–980.

25. Deykin EY, Buka SL. Suicidal ideation and attempts among chemically dependent adolescents. *Am J Public Health.* 1994;84:634–639.

26. Fox SM III, Naughton JP, Haskell WL. Physical activity and the prevention of coronary heart disease. *Ann Clin Res.* 1971;3:404–432.

27. Morris JN, Heady JA, Raffle PAB, et al. Coronary heart disease and physical activity of work. *Lancet.* 1953;2:1053–1120.

28. Taylor HL, Klepetar E, Keys A, et al. Death rates among physically active and sedentary employees of the railroad industry. *Am J Public Health.* 1962;10:1697–1707.

29. Peters RK, Cady LD Jr, Bischoff DP, et al. Physical fitness and subsequent myocardial infarction in healthy workers. *JAMA.* 1983;249:3052–3056.

30. van Wijngaarden E, Savitz DA, Kleckner RC, et al. Exposure to electromagnetic fields and suicide among electric utility workers: A nested case-control study. *West J Med.* 2000;173:94–100

31. Dearden KA, Hale CB, Woolley T. The antecedents of teen fatherhood: a retrospective case-control study of Great Britain youth. *Am J Public Health.* 1995;85:551–554.

32. Shepherd PM. *The National Child Development Study: An Introduction to the Background to the Study and the Methods of Data Collection* (Working Paper I, National Child Development Study User Support Group). London, England: City University, Social Statistics Unit; 1985.

33. Samet JM, Munoz A, eds.. Cohort studies. *Epidemiol. Rev.* 1998;20(1).

Experimental Study Designs

LEARNING OBJECTIVES

By the end of this chapter the reader will be able to:

- state how study designs compare with respect to validity of causal inference
- distinguish between a controlled experiment and a quasi-experiment
- describe the scope of intervention studies
- define the term *controlled clinical trials* and give examples
- explain the phases in testing a new drug
- discuss *blinding* and *crossover* in clinical trials
- define what is meant by *community trials*
- discuss ethical aspects of experimentation with human subjects

CHAPTER OUTLINE

Introduction

In Chapters 6 and 7, we covered observational study designs. Chapter 8 focuses on experimental and quasi-experimental designs. We will examine how these study designs differ from observational studies as well as their unique advantages and disadvantages.

Modern epidemiologists often equate experimental epidemiology with randomized controlled clinical trials.[1] In the field of epidemiology, experimental designs are typically implemented as intervention studies, either controlled experiments or quasi-experiments. We will begin by taking an in-depth look at the two categories of intervention studies, which include clinical trials and community trials. The authors will provide examples of each type as well as a discussion of ethical aspects of human experimentation. A related topic will be special considerations in the design of clinical trials, such as sample selection and crossover designs. The chapter will conclude with a discussion of methods for evaluating the outcomes of community interventions.

Hierarchy of Study Designs

Chapters 6 and 7 identified strengths and weaknesses of observational studies for descriptive and analytic epidemiology, especially with respect to our confidence in inferring causation of disease. These assertions are summarized in Exhibit 8-1, which ranks study designs according to their validity.

Exhibit 8-1 also includes experimental designs (i.e., randomized clinical trials, which are covered in the present chapter). As Exhibit 8-1 indicates, all of the study designs from case studies to prospective cohort studies may be considered less powerful for etiologic inference than randomized clinical trials. The latter are generally regarded as the most scientifically rigorous method of hypothesis testing available in epidemiology. The emphasis is on rigor and not feasibility, for as we shall learn subsequently, not all research situations permit the use of this design.

Experimental designs, including clinical trials, enable us to overcome some of the deficiencies inherent in observational designs. The use of experimentation to derive knowledge about the causes of disease has intuitive appeal. In a controlled clinical trial, by exercising control over who will receive the exposure as well as the level of the exposure, the investigator more confidently may attribute cause and effect to associations than in nonexperimental designs.

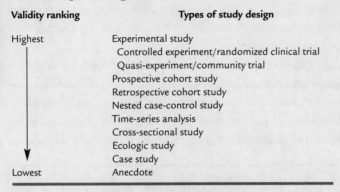

EXHIBIT 8-1

Validity for Etiologic Inference According to Study Designs

Validity ranking	Types of study design
Highest	Experimental study
	Controlled experiment/randomized clinical trial
	Quasi-experiment/community trial
	Prospective cohort study
	Retrospective cohort study
	Nested case-control study
	Time-series analysis
	Cross-sectional study
	Ecologic study
	Case study
Lowest	Anecdote

Source: Adapted from N Künzli and IB Tager. The semi-individual study in air pollution epidemiology: a valid design as compared to ecologic studies, *Environmental Health Perspectives,* vol 105, No 10, p 1079, 1997, National Institute of Environmental Health Sciences, U.S. Department of Health and Human Services.

Ranked immediately below controlled experiments are quasi-experiments.[2] As noted in Chapter 6, the investigator is unable to randomly allocate subjects to the conditions (intervention or control) of a quasi-experimental study. As a result, there may be contamination across the conditions of the study. It becomes more difficult to differentiate between the effects of the intervention and the control conditions than in a controlled experiment. (Of course, it also is possible for contamination to occur in a clinical trial.)

The reader should not conclude that experimental designs (such as randomized controlled trials) are always the most appropriate design for investigating the causes of disease. Experimental designs are not necessarily appropriate for testing all conceivable hypotheses, such as those in the fields of occupational and environmental health. To give an example, an epidemiologist might want to examine the relative contributions of smoking and radon exposure to lung cancer among uranium miners. For ethical reasons, this investigation could not be conducted as an experimental study because it would involve deliberate exposure of subjects to agents suspected of being harmful. An observational study design is the only realistic approach in this scenario. In the following sections, we will explore in greater detail the designs that we introduced previously.

Intervention Studies

Intervention studies are employed to test the efficacy of a preventive or therapeutic measure. This objective differs from the intent of observational studies, which is to generate enough knowledge about the etiology and natural history of a disease to formulate strategies for prevention.

Recall the two basic facets of research designs: manipulation of the study factor and randomization of study subjects (see Table 6-1). Controlled experimental studies involve randomization of subjects to exposures under the control of the investigator, whereas quasi-experimental studies involve external control of exposure without randomization. Both strategies are employed in intervention studies.

Intervention Designs Include:

- Controlled clinical trials (focus on the individual)
- Community interventions (focus on the group or community)

Note: Controlled clinical trials may be conducted both at the individual and community levels (for narrowly defined outcomes).

Broadly defined, there are two types of intervention designs: clinical trials and community trials. The key difference between the two types of intervention is that in clinical trials the focus is individuals, whereas the focus of community trials is groups or community outcomes. This difference in focus limits the types of interventions that are possible under each approach. Clinical trials are usually tightly controlled in terms of eligibility, delivery of the intervention, and monitoring of outcomes. The duration of clinical trials ranges from days to years. Participation is generally restricted to a highly selected group of individuals: commonly volunteers who have been diagnosed with a disease; volunteers who are screened subjects at high risk for disease; or other types of volunteers who may be interested in participating in the clinical trial and are deemed eligible for such participation. The randomized controlled trial is most appropriate for testing narrow hypotheses, such as tests of vaccines, treatments, or individuals' behavior change.[2] An example of behavior change is elimination of tobacco use among smokers. A clinical trial is not the most applicable design for complex interventions.

Usually, community trials cannot exert rigid control over members of the group or community, are typically delivered to all members rather than narrowly defined subsets, tend to be of longer duration, and usually involve primary prevention efforts. Thus, randomized controlled trials at the community level can be used only in special situations when there is a simple intervention, such as a response to a vaccine, and there is a sufficient number of communities to involve in the experiment.[2]

Clinical Trials

The concepts of clinical trials have a venerable history that spans a time period from early biblical and Greek references to increasing activity during the eighteenth and nineteenth centuries to present methodologic sophistication.[3] The first efforts were not formal clinical trials, as we know them today; however, the attempts at experimentation led the way to contemporary methods. For example, in 1537 Ambroise Paré applied an experimental treatment for battlefield wounds that used what he called a "digestive" made from turpentine, rose oil, and egg yolks. He observed that this concoction was more effective in treating wounds than application of boiling oil—the standard of the day. Later, in 1600, the East India Shipping Company found that lemon juice protected sailors from scurvy by comparing sailors on a ship supplied with lemon juice with sailors on ships that were not supplied. James Lind, in 1747, was credited with designing one of the first experiments that used a concurrently treated control group.[3] His experiment involved feeding 12 sailors who were suffering from scurvy six different types of diets; he noted that sailors who received citrus fruits had the best recovery from their malady. Other pioneering landmarks in the development of clinical trials include Jenner's efforts to develop a smallpox vaccine in the late eighteenth century and experiments with anesthetics, such as ether and chloroform, in the mid-nineteenth century. While the earliest planned experiments were carried out without the benefit of a control or comparison, subsequent research contributed to the development of control treatments and randomization. More recent historical developments have included the use of multicenter trials in which the results from several researchers are pooled. Multicenter trials have been instrumental in the development of treatments for infectious diseases (e.g., polio) and recently in chronic diseases that are of noninfectious origin (Exhibit 8-2).

"A clinical trial is a planned experiment designed to assess the efficacy of a treatment in man by comparing the outcomes in a group of patients treated with the test treatment with those observed in a comparable group of patients receiving a control treatment, where patients in both groups are enrolled, treated, and followed over the same time period."[3(p3)] Therefore, one starts by determining

EXHIBIT 8-2

The Why, What, When, and Where of Clinical Trials

We've all taken medication. It may have been in the form of over-the-counter cough medicine, or prescription pills to treat chronic conditions such as diabetes. But how did researchers discover if the medicine is effective, if it's safe, and if there are any potential side effects?

Testing and evaluating drugs is serious business, and clinical trials are right at the center of the process, according to Dorothy Cirelli, chief of the Patient Recruitment and Referral Center at the National Institutes of Health (NIH), U.S. Department of Health and Human Services (HHS). "Medical advances would not occur without clinical trials," she said.

Well known as a world leader in medical research, NIH developed the first treatment for the human immunodeficiency virus (HIV), as well as innovative therapies for breast cancer, leukemia, and lymphoma. For over a century, the agency has conducted clinical studies that explore the nature of illnesses. Clinical studies are currently under way for nearly every kind of cancer, HIV, cardiovascular disease, diabetes, obesity, and many other conditions—common and rare.

There are several types of clinical trials. By far the largest number are those that test new drugs. Prevention studies look at drugs or lifestyle changes that may help prevent disease. Diagnostic studies look at ways of detecting or finding out more about disease. Treatment studies may monitor new drugs or evaluate new combinations of established treatments.

The Food and Drug Administration (FDA), another HHS agency, is responsible for reviewing the scientific work of drug developers and implementing a rigorous drug approval process. The FDA, which some have called the world's largest consumer protection agency, works to protect the public by ensuring that products are safe, effective, and labeled for their intended use.

From Animals to Humans: Every year, hundreds of clinical trials are conducted at medical centers across the country. Drugs must be studied in properly controlled trials in order to determine if they work for a specific purpose. Drugs that have not been previously used in humans must

continues

EXHIBIT 8-2 *continued*

undergo preclinical test-tube analysis and/or animal studies involving at least two mammals to determine toxicity.

The toxicity information is then used to make risk/benefit assessments, and determine if the drug is acceptable for testing in humans.

NIH or the company developing the drug must conduct studies to show any interaction between the body and the drug. In addition, researchers must provide the FDA with information on chemistry, manufacturing, and controls. This ensures the identity, purity, quality, and strength of both the active ingredient and the finished dosage form.

The sponsor of the proposed new drug then develops a plan for testing the drug in humans. The plan is submitted to the FDA with information on animal testing data, the composition of the drug, manufacturing data, qualifications of its study investigators, and safety of the people who will participate in the trial. This information forms what is known as the Investigational New Drug Application (IND).

The entire drug development process is lengthy and expensive. On average it takes about 10 years to complete. But it is an effective system that generally protects the public from dangerous and ineffective drugs. ■

Source: Reprinted from J Brooks. Clinical trials: how they work, why we need them. In: *Closing the Gap,* December 1997/January 1998, pp 1-2. Washington, DC: Office of Minority Health, Public Health Service, U.S. Department of Health and Human Services.

eligibility of potential subjects. Eligibility rules must be carefully defined and rigidly enforced. Criteria for inclusion will vary by the type and nature of the intervention proposed. Once eligible subjects agree to participate, they are then randomly assigned to one of the study groups. Figure 8-1 illustrates a single intervention and single control (or placebo) arm of a trial, yet more than one experimental intervention can be run in parallel.

Prophylactic and Therapeutic Trials

A prophylactic trial is designed to evaluate the effectiveness of a substance that is used to prevent disease, such as a vaccine against measles or polio, or a prevention program, such as vitamin supplementation or patient education. A therapeutic trial involves the study of curative drugs or a new surgical procedure to evaluate how well they bring about an improvement in the patient's health.

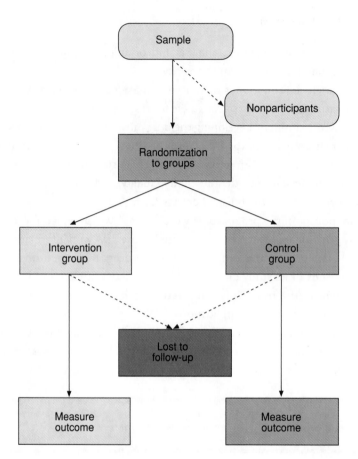

FIGURE 8-1 Schematic diagram of a clinical trial

One group is designated as the control arm of the trial; these subjects would receive the standard of care (for a surgery or drug trial), a placebo (for a vitamin trial), or no intervention (for the patient education trial).

Outcomes of Clinical Trials

Outcomes, or results of a clinical trial, are referred to as clinical end points. To assess the results, investigators compare rates of disease, death, recovery, or other appropriate outcome. The outcome of interest is measured in the intervention and control arms of the trial to evaluate efficacy. We have previously noted that the outcome of a clinical trial must be measured in a comparable manner in both the intervention and control conditions.

For some drugs, such as antihypertensive agents, it may not be feasible to conduct randomized large clinical trials that evaluate major clinical end points, such as strokes or myocardial infarctions.[4] As an alternative, surrogate end points may be used in small short-term trials. A surrogate end point for drug therapy in hypertension would be measures of subclinical disease or physical measures, including reduction of blood pressure.

Examples of Clinical Trials

The first example of a clinical trial is the double-blind Medical Research Council Vitamin Study.[5] Neural tube defects (NTDs) (e.g., anencephaly, spina bifida, or encephalocele) are among the most severe congenital malformations. The possibility that folic acid (a B vitamin) might be involved was raised as early as 1964.[6] Preliminary interventions had been promising but not conclusive. Therefore, a randomized trial was conducted at 33 centers in seven countries. The trial examined whether vitamin supplementation around the time of conception could prevent NTDs. The supplements used were folic acid or a mixture of seven other vitamins (A, D, B_1, B_2, B_6, C, and nicotinamide). Eligible subjects included women who were planning a pregnancy, had had a previous child with an NTD, and were not already taking vitamin supplements. A total of 1,817 women were randomized into one of four groups: folic acid, other vitamins, both, or neither. Subjects did not know to which group they were assigned. To monitor possible toxicity associated with the supplementation, forms were provided to all subjects. Of those randomized, 1,195 gave birth to a child with a known outcome. Whenever an NTD was reported, independent corroboration was sought. Classification was made without knowing to which group the mother had been randomized.

The rate of NTDs among women receiving folic acid (alone or in combination with other vitamins) was 1.0% (5 out of 514). The rate among those allocated to the other groups (other vitamins or nothing) was 3.5%, yielding a relative risk of 0.28 (95% confidence interval [CI], 0.12 to 0.71). The rate among women in the other vitamin-only group was only slightly lower than the rate among the women receiving nothing (relative risk, 0.80; 95% CI, 0.32 to 1.72). The trial results were regularly monitored. By April 12, 1991, the difference between the folic acid-supplemented group and the others was firmly established by case 27. The data-monitoring committee recommended that the trial be stopped; the steering committee agreed. The authors of the report concluded that folic acid supplementation could now be recommended for all women who had a previously affected pregnancy. Furthermore, they suggested that public health measures should be taken to ensure that all women of childbearing age receive adequate dietary folic acid and that consideration should be given to fortification of staple foods with it.

Another application of clinical trials is to evaluate the effectiveness of education efforts to prevent the spread of sexually transmitted diseases (STDs). The factors that contribute to an increased risk of STDs are multiple and complex and include social, behavioral, and environmental influences. Efforts to reduce the incidence of STDs among inner-city residents are especially difficult, given the fact that most education efforts are relegated to public clinics. Because the clinics often have limited resources, educational programs must be delivered by staff who may be inadequately trained in prevention and unprepared to provide information and skills to culturally diverse populations. O'Donnell and colleagues[7] conducted a clinical trial of video-based educational interventions on condom acquisition among men and women seeking services at a large STD clinic in South Bronx, New York. A total of 3,348 African-American and Hispanic male and female patients were assigned to one of three arms: video only, video plus interactive session, or control. The videos were 20 minutes in length, culturally appropriate, and designed to model appropriate strategies for overcoming barriers to consistent condom use. A proxy measure of condom use was employed. After clinic services and participation in the assigned treatment group, subjects were given coupons for free condoms at a nearby pharmacy. The rate of redemption of coupons for condoms was 21.2% among patients who received no intervention, 27.6% among patients who received video alone, and 36.9% among patients who received video plus interactive group sessions. The study's authors pointed out that because of the high prevalence of STDs in the population served by public clinics, the observed increases in the number of people practicing safer sex could have a significant impact on public health.

Blinding (Masking)

Objectivity of the data is a major source of concern about clinical trials. For example, some clinical trials make use of volunteers who are extremely grateful for the opportunity to participate. At the same time, the investigator may assess the trial's outcome by determining the participants' subjective impressions, for example, by means of a self-report questionnaire. This evaluation method may tend to overstate the intervention's clinical responses and benefits. Furthermore, subjects who learn that they had been randomized to the placebo arm of the trial may not wish to continue participation. For these reasons, a commonly used approach is a single-blind design. (A synonym for the term blinding is masking.) In this design the subject is unaware of group assignment. Informed consent is obtained before assignment, and the experimenter must treat and monitor all groups in a similar manner. Another concern and potential for problems lies in how the experimenter assesses the trial's outcome. This concern is especially warranted if the trial evaluates a new drug, the drug's manufacturer is financing the trial, and/or those performing the evaluations stand to benefit if the new drug is shown to be more effective than existing medications. To reduce the likelihood of biased assessment, an approach called a double-blind design is used; neither the subject nor the experimenter is aware of group assignment. For example, in a clinical trial of a new drug, one way to implement such a procedure is to have the placebo or treatment agents come in a preassigned container, the contents of which are unknown to the investigator and subjects at the time of the trial. All subjects are then treated and monitored in a similar manner.

Phases of Clinical Trials

Phases in a clinical trial refer to the stages that must occur in the development of a vaccine, drug, or treatment before it can be licensed for general use. A long and arduous process is required to bring a vaccine from the laboratory setting to eventual licensing,[8] and the same may be said for licensing of new drugs. The process of bringing a new vaccine to market requires the balance between protecting the public from a potentially deleterious vaccine and satisfying urgent needs for new vaccines. To illustrate, while researchers have devoted a great deal of attention to producing a vaccine for HIV, the problems in perfecting such a vaccine have been daunting. Generally, licensing of the product requires a phase I, phase II, and phase III evaluation. A description of these steps for the development of a new vaccine is in Exhibit 8-3.

In the evaluation of vaccines, phase I trials involve testing the new vaccine in adult volunteers, typically fewer than 100. Upon successful demonstration of a response in a small-scale study among the volunteers (e.g., antibody formation in response to a vaccine), the testing proceeds to phase II. This phase expands the testing to a group of approximately 100 to 200 subjects who are selected from the target population for the vaccine. Antibody responses and clinical reactions to the vaccine are examined. There may be a double-blind design with random allocation to study or placebo conditions. The third phase, which is used to assess protective efficacy in the target population, is the main test of the vaccine. Vaccine efficacy refers to the reduction in the incidence rate of a disease in a

EXHIBIT 8-3

Stages in the Development of a Vaccination Program

Pre-licensing evaluation of vaccine

- Phase I trials: Safety in adult volunteers
- Phase II trials: Immunogenicity and reactogenicity in the target population
- Phase III trials: Protective efficacy

Postlicensing evaluation

- Safety and efficacy of vaccine
- Disease surveillance
- Serologic surveillance
- Measurement of vaccine coverage

Source: Reprinted from N Begg and E Miller. Role of Epidemiology in Vaccine Policy. In *Vaccine,* vol 8, p 180. ©1990, with permission from Elsevier.

vaccinated population compared to an unvaccinated population.[8] After phase III testing has been completed, a license to manufacture the vaccine may be granted. Postlicensing evaluations of the vaccine need to continue to monitor its safety and efficacy.

The phases for testing an anticancer drug follow a similar pattern (Table 8-1). Laboratory studies in vitro and in vivo among animals may have suggested a new agent that has promising antitumor action. Phase I consists of testing the agent among human subjects. Phase II is concerned with testing the efficacy of the drug with various tumor types. At the conclusion of phase III trials, much information has been gathered about the agent.[9]

The lengthy process that is required to bring a new drug, vaccine, or treatment to the health care marketplace not only helps to protect the consumer, but also results in delay in bringing needed pharmaceutical agents to critically ill patients. Because of demands that advocacy groups have made on government agencies, proposals have been made to shorten the lead time to make new drugs more rapidly available. These legislative and policy modifications are intended to bring more speedy relief to patients who are afflicted with conditions such as acquired immune deficiency syndrome (AIDS) and cancer.

Table 8-1 A Description of Clinical Trials for a Cancer Drug

Phase	Goals	Objectives
I	Initial testing in humans following animal studies. Organized as escalating dose trials in which subjects are entered into a series of progressively higher dosage levels until life-threatening, irreversible, or fatal toxicity is experienced.	Identify dose-limiting toxicities. Establish maximally tolerated dose; optimal dosage range. Describe pharmacology of agent (e.g., metabolism, distribution, excretion).
II	Testing in selected tumor types ranging from highly chemosensitive to chemo-resistant.	Determine activity and therapeutic efficacy in a range of tumor types. Validate toxicity and dosage data.
III	Randomized trial comparing new therapy with existing therapies in terms of duration and quality of survival. Trial may have multiple study arms and involve sample stratification.	Determine value of new therapy in relation to existing therapies. Generate and publish recommendations for the medical community.

Source: Adapted with permission from C Engelking. Clinical trials: impact evaluation and implementation consideration. *Seminars in Oncology Nursing,* vol 8, No 2, p 149. © 1992, WB Saunders Company.

Randomization

The method of choice for assigning subjects to the treatment or control conditions of a clinical trial is randomization. Researchers must be very concerned about the error that might be introduced when some other method of subject assignment is used. In nonrandom assignment, any observed differences between study arms might simply reflect differences observed among participants of the trial. There are two general methods for randomization of subjects to the conditions of the trial, known as fixed and adaptive randomization.[3] Fixed randomization is easier to perform than adaptive randomization. However, a full discussion of them is beyond the scope of this text. The general concept of fixed randomization is that once subjects have been selected, pass the eligibility determination, and agree to participate they have an equal probability of being assigned to the intervention or control arm. The simplest form of randomization is the "flip of a coin," but more elaborate protocols that employ random numbers tables or computer algorithms are typically used. As part of randomization in some trials, subjects are stratified in order to improve comparability among conditions. For example, in order to control for sex and age differences, equal proportions of gender and age groups are included in the treatment and control groups. For randomization to be fully effective, a reasonably large number of subjects must be enrolled. For the sake of illustration, a study with only two men and two women could be randomized and result in each study arm having the same gender.

Crossover Designs

A treatment crossover refers to "Any change of *treatment* for a *patient* in a *clinical trial* involving a switch of *study treatments*."[3(p306)] These crossovers may be planned or unplanned. To illustrate, the protocol may specify in advance that a patient or group of subjects may be switched from one treatment condition to another treatment condition during the course of the trial and after a predetermined period of follow-up. Sometimes, in such crossovers, the patient is said to serve as his or her own control. An unplanned crossover refers to a switch of patients to different treatment conditions for various reasons. For example, patients in a coronary bypass treatment may have misgivings about this invasive surgical procedure, or patients in a medical care group may require surgical treatment because of deterioration in their condition.[10]

Ethical Aspects of Experimentation with Human Subjects

Miké and Schottenfeld[11] identified some of the ethical issues surrounding experimentation with human subjects, particularly with respect to clinical trials. Some of these issues include informed consent, withholding treatment known to be effective, protecting the interests of the individual patient, monitoring for toxicity and side effects, and deciding when to withdraw a patient from the study.

The ethical aspects of experimentation with human subjects are capable of generating much heated debate and strong emotional responses. It is generally agreed that the benefits of participation in an experimental study must clearly outweigh any possible risks to the subject. One side of the issue is that human experimentation, especially with drugs, may bring about certain iatrogenic reactions (adverse effects caused by the medications) that could have been avoided had the subject not participated in the experiment. The other viewpoint is that an experimental design (i.e., being in a control condition) requires that medication be withheld from people who might benefit from it. The problem of iatrogenic reactions may be circumvented through experimental studies with animals, although animal models may not apply directly to human beings.

In order to address both of these issues—the withholding of needed medication and the possibility of adverse effects from the medication—experimental drug trials use what is known as a sequential design. Let us consider a clinical trial to evaluate a new drug. In contrast with a sequential design, many drug trials use a preestablished number of subjects who are assigned a priori to the study and control conditions. The results of the trial are evaluated after all subjects have been assigned to the conditions of the trial, usually after an extended period of time. In a sequential design, investigators continuously monitor results and add subjects, i.e., there is no preestablished number of subjects. The trial is interrupted as soon as the results are statistically significant and either confirm or reject a positive outcome for the drug being tested. If the drug produces improvement in the patients' conditions, it then becomes available for use by members of the control group as well (or the drug is discontinued if it is found to produce adverse effects). In addition, in some clinical trials, experimental therapies are evaluated only on patients for whom all other treatments have failed.

There has been increasing interest in developing rigorous evaluations of psychological therapy interventions.[12] Selection of appropriate control subjects in such evaluations poses ethical concerns for subjects in placebo or no-treatment conditions. One concern relates to withholding benefits that might accrue from a psychosocial intervention. This concern is similar to the ethical issue of withholding an effective drug from a needy control patient. Another issue is finding a control group that is sufficiently comparable to the study group for which the intervention is being evaluated.

The National Institutes of Health have instituted a policy ". . . that requires oversight and monitoring of all intervention studies to ensure the safety of participants and the validity and integrity of the data."[13] This goal is accomplished through the use of a data and safety monitoring board (DSMB), comprised of an independent group of experts who advise investigators and funding agencies. For example, in the case of the Division of Microbiology and Infectious Diseases (DMID), "The primary responsibilities of the DSMB are to 1) periodically review and evaluate the accumulated study data for participant safety, study conduct and progress, and, when appropriate, efficacy, and 2) make recommendations to DMID concerning the continuation, modification, or termination of the trial."[14] Although phase III clinical trials are required to have a DSMB, phase I and phase II trials, in certain circumstances, also may require them.

Reporting of the Results of Clinical Trials

The results of a randomized controlled trial (RCT) may impact patient care greatly.[15] Readers of the results of a RCT need to comprehend key aspects of the trial—design, conduct, and analysis—as well as to determine the generalizability of its findings. To meet that need, a panel of experts developed the CONSORT statement.[16] The acronym CONSORT stands for Consolidated Standards of Reporting Trials. The current revision guides the reporting of randomized trials by providing a 22-item checklist and a flow chart, to be used by those who review, write, and assess the findings from a RCT. One of the main aims of CONSORT is to help authors optimize the quality of their reports of simple RCTs. Refer to Figure 8-2 for a CONSORT flow chart, which describes the flow of subjects through the phases of a RCT.

Summary of Clinical Trials

This brief overview of clinical trials reveals a number of their strengths. As opposed to the several varieties of observational studies, clinical trials provide the greatest control over the study situation. The investigator has the ability to control

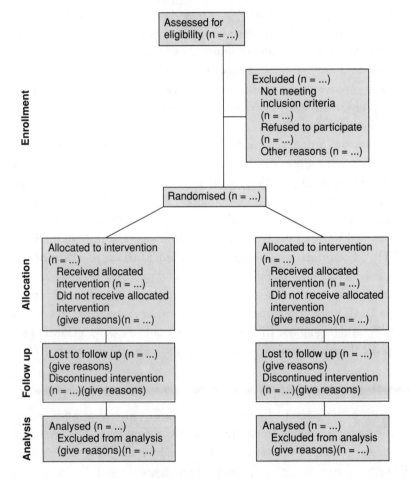

FIGURE 8-2 Flow diagram of the progress through the phases of a randomized trial. *Source:* Reprinted with permission from Moher D, Schultz KF, Altman DG. The CONSORT statement: revised recommendations for improving the quality of reports of parallel-group randomized trials. *Lancet.* 2001;357:1193

the amount of exposure (e.g., drug dosage), the timing and frequency of the exposure, and the period of observation for end points. For large trials, the ability to randomize subjects to study assignments reduces the likelihood that the groups will differ significantly with respect to the distribution of risk factors that might influence the outcome.

Clinical trials have several limitations. In particular, one of these is the very thing that was cited as an advantage: The setting for delivery and evaluation of the treatment tends to be artificial, so that the experimenter may find it difficult to determine whether the treatment would work well in the larger community or for unselected patient populations. Obviously, there is necessarily less control over all factors in a community setting than in a clinical trial. A second disadvantage is that adherence to protocols may be difficult to enforce, especially if the treatment produces undesirable side effects and presents a significant burden to the subjects. By the time a clinical trial is conducted, fairly good evidence usually exists in support of the exposure-disease association; withholding a potentially beneficial treatment from the control arm presents an ethical dilemma.

Community Trials

Although clinical trials play an important role in efforts to improve health and the delivery of medical care, they are limited in terms of the scope of their potential impact. Because they require such great control over subjects, they are not typically employed to evaluate the potential efficacy of large-scale public health interventions. Rather, intervention trials at the level of entire communities are needed to determine the potential benefit of new policies and programs. According to Rossi and Freeman, an intervention is "Any program or other planned effort designed to produce changes in a target population."[17(p15)] Note that the word *community* as used here is not meant to be taken literally. A community may well be some other defined unit, such as a county, state, or school district.

Like clinical trials, community trials start by determining eligible communities and their willingness to participate. Permission to enroll the community is typically given by someone capable of providing consent, such as a mayor, governor, or school board. To be able to evaluate the impact of a program properly, it is desirable to have some baseline measures of the problem to be addressed in the intervention and control communities. Such measures may include, for example, disease prevalence or incidence; knowledge, attitudes, and practice; or purchase of lean relative to fatty cuts of meat. After the relevant baseline measures have been taken, communities are randomized to receive or not receive the intervention. Both study assignments are followed for a period of time, and the outcomes of interest are measured (Fig. 8-3).

Years of etiologic research on atherosclerotic disease have contributed greatly to our understanding of risk factors for the disease. Many of these risk factors, such as elevated levels of serum cholesterol and low-density lipoprotein, can be reduced by lowering intake of dietary fat and cholesterol; cigarette smokers can quit; and hypertensive individuals can lower their body weight, exercise more, or

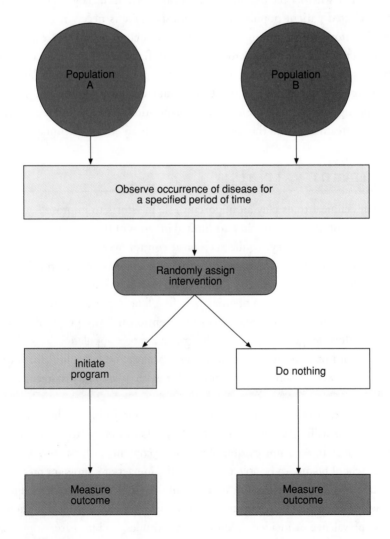

FIGURE 8-3 Schematic diagram of a community trial

use appropriate medication. By the 1970s, enough was known about these risk factors and their potential for modification that a number of community interventions were tested; a few of these interventions include the North Karelia Project, the Minnesota Heart Health Program, and the Stanford Five-City Project (Exhibit 8-4 and Fig. 8-4).

EXHIBIT 8-4

Stanford Five-City Project
Design, Methods, and Results

The Stanford Five-City Project was a major community trial designed to lower risk of cardiovascular diseases. Two treatment cities (Monterey and Salinas) and two control cities (Modesto and San Luis Obispo), located in northern California and ranging in size from 35,000 to 145,000 residents, were selected for study (the fifth city, Santa Maria, was included only for morbidity and mortality surveillance). Random assignment of cities to treatment and control conditions was precluded by constraints on community selection, particularly concerning independent media markets (Fig. 8-4).

The intervention was a six-year, integrated, comprehensive, community-wide multifactor risk reduction education program. The interventions had multiple target audiences and used multiple communication channels and settings. Before the intervention began, data from a baseline population survey were used to develop an overview of knowledge, attitudes, and behavior in treatment communities. The audience was segmented by age, ethnicity, socioeconomic status, overall cardiovascular risk, media use, organizational membership, and motivation to change behavior. Formative evaluation with these audience subgroups was used to refine educational strategies, programs, and materials. [Formative evaluation is defined later in this chapter.] Social learning theory guided the development of educational materials.

To evaluate the effect of the intervention on cardiovascular risk factors, four independent cross-sectional surveys of randomly selected households and four repeated surveys of a cohort were conducted. All persons from households randomly chosen from commercial directories, age 12 to 74 years, were eligible for recruitment into the survey. Eligible persons were

continues

EXHIBIT 8-4 *continued*

contacted by mail, telephone, and in person, and they were invited to attend survey centers located in the four cities. Trained health professionals interviewed participants about their demographic background, health knowledge, cardiovascular risk-related attitudes and behavior, including a 24-hour diet recall, and medical history. Weight was measured using a balance beam, and blood pressure was measured using a semiautomated cuff, after which venous blood samples were drawn for determination of total and high-density lipoprotein cholesterol concentrations. Prior fasting was not required. Cigarette smoking status was confirmed with biochemical testing.

Morbidity and mortality rate data are still being collected and have yet to be analyzed. However, changes in risk factors have been reported. These risk factor results . . .[showed]. . . changes during the six-year educational intervention in the individuals surveyed in the treatment towns compared with the control towns. With the exception of obesity, as measured by body mass index, risk factor changes were in healthful directions in both treatment and control towns, the changes in treatment towns exceeded those in control towns, and there was general consistency of these treatment-control differences across risk factors and in both the cohort and serial cross-sectional surveys. ■

Source: Reprinted with permission from SP Fortmann, JA Flora, MA Winkleby, et al. Community intervention trials: reflections on the Stanford Five-City Project experience. *American Journal of Epidemiology,* vol 142, No 6, pp 579–580, © 1995, The Johns Hopkins University School of Hygiene and Public Health.

As another example of a community trial, the design and methods of the Pawtucket Heart Health Program are described.[18] Nine cities in Rhode Island that met certain size and population stability criteria were identified. Pawtucket was randomly selected for the intervention, and an unnamed city with similar sociodemographic characteristics was chosen as the comparison city. The focus of the intervention was to help individuals adopt new, healthy behaviors and to create a supportive physical and behavioral environment. The program targeted three dimensions of activities: risk factors (e.g., elevated blood cholesterol, elevated blood pressure, and smoking), behavioral change (e.g., training, aid in development of social support, and maintenance strategies), and community activation (achieving goals while working through community groups and

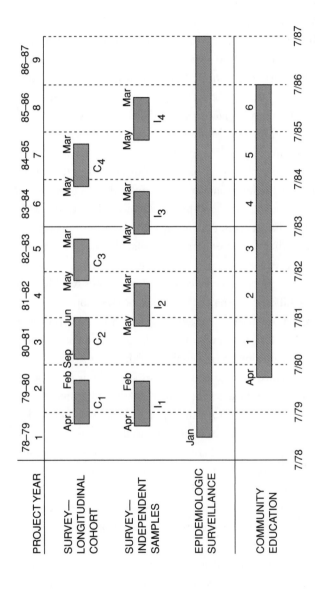

FIGURE 8-4 Design of the nine-year Stanford Five-City Project, encompassing the initial surveys and the intervention. The project was subsequently extended to 18 years, including four years of education maintenance activity (to 1990) and six additional years of surveillance (through 1992.) C_1–C_4, cohorts 1–4; I_1–I_4, independent samples 1–4. *Source:* Reprinted with permission from SP Fortmann et al, Community intervention trials: reflections on the Stanford Five-City Project experience, *American Journal of Epidemiology*, vol 142, No 6, p 579, © 1995, The Johns Hopkins University School of Hygiene and Public Health.

organizations). During a seven-year intervention period, "over 500 community organizations were involved at some level. These included all 27 public and private schools, most religious and social organizations and larger work sites, all supermarkets and many smaller grocery stores, 19 restaurants, and most departments of city government. In addition, a total of 3,664 individuals volunteered to assist in program delivery."[19(p778)] Efforts to create a supportive environment included identification of low-fat foods in grocery stores, installation of an exercise course, nutrition programs at the public library, and highlights of heart-healthy selections on restaurant menus. Efforts to permeate the community, its organizations, and social groupings placed particular emphasis on behavior change, low cost, ease of adoption, and visibility.

Evaluation of the community intervention included cross-sectional surveys in the intervention and control communities at baseline, four times over the course of the intervention, and after the intervention was completed. There was some evidence of lower mean cholesterol and blood pressure levels in Pawtucket, with significantly lower projected disease rates. According to the authors of the report, however, "The hypothesis that projected cardiovascular disease risk can be altered by community-based education gains limited support from these data. Achieving cardiovascular risk reduction at the community level was feasible, but maintaining statistically significant differences between cities was not."[19(p777)]

The Community Intervention Trial for Smoking Cessation (COMMIT) was conducted as a multicenter project beginning in 1989. The project sought to reach cigarette smokers and bring about long-term cessation of the habit.[20] This intervention trial involved 11 matched pairs of communities throughout the United States and Canada and was believed to affect more than 200,000 adult smokers.

The Community Clinical Oncology Program, begun in 1983, is sponsored by the National Cancer Institute.[21] As part of a larger clinical trials network, it is designed to evaluate the efficacy of new chemopreventive agents for cancer. In 1987, cooperative groups were formed that consisted of an administrative core, statistical center, member institutions, and affiliated physicians. These cooperative groups and the clinical trials network have been involved in such cancer prevention and control research activities as the implementation of the Tamoxifen and Finasteride Prevention Trials.

The authors point out that there are many other examples of community trials. In recent times, community-based interventions have been conducted for the purpose of HIV prevention. Many of these interventions may be characterized as rigorous and theory based with multi-arms, multi-sites, or using multiple outcome measures. An illustration of a multi-site study was a randomized controlled community trial that evaluated the impact of an HIV/AIDS prevention program in Tanzania.[22] Prevention programs were adopted in Arusha and Kilimanjaro, neighboring areas in Tanzania. The target study sites were all public primary schools, which were stratified for random assignment to intervention or comparison conditions. Investigators reported that intervention groups showed a significant increase in knowledge of AIDS information and had significantly more positive attitudes toward people with AIDS relative to the comparison groups. Another example of an AIDS-related community trial is shown in Exhibit 8-5.

Summary of Community Trials

Community trials are crucial because they represent the only way to estimate directly the realistic impact of a change in behavior or some other modifiable exposure on the incidence of disease. They are inferior to clinical trials with respect to the ability to control entrance into the study, delivery of the intervention, and

---

EXHIBIT 8-5

Project RESPECT

Project RESPECT is an example of a randomized controlled trial for prevention of HIV and other sexually transmitted diseases (STDs).[23] The trial sought to establish the efficacy of several counseling methods for reducing high-risk sexual behaviors. This effort involved collaboration among a clinic in Long Beach, California, as well as four other inner-city clinics across the United States.

The project had four interventions. In a study that has several different interventions, each type is called an arm. The four arms of project RESPECT were enhanced counseling (arm 1), brief counseling (arm 2), and didactic messages (arms 3 and 4). Arms 1 through 3 were followed up actively after enrollment with periodic questionnaires and STD tests for one year. Outcome measures were use of condoms and new occurrence of STDs.

The study sample comprised a total of 5,758 HIV-negative heterosexual patients (14 years of age and older) who presented at the five STD clinics for examinations. Project investigators randomly assigned subjects to one of the four arms of the trial (with approximately equal numbers of subjects in each arm). The results of this study demonstrated that brief counseling sessions for risk reduction (as opposed to didactic sessions) are effective in increasing condom use and preventing the occurrence of new STDs. ∎

monitoring of outcomes. With clinical trials one can potentially randomize a large enough number of subjects to ensure that the study groups are comparable with respect to both measured and unmeasured variables. This statement is less true of community trials; fewer study units (e.g., communities or subjects) are capable of being randomized. Accordingly, the likelihood remains that the intervention and control communities may differ with respect to racial composition, education level, age distribution, or some other unmeasured variable. In a dynamic population, residents who received the intervention may move away, and people may move into the community after the intervention has begun; such shifting in the composition of the study population may lead to loss of effect. If there are significant secular trends with respect to the prevalence of the exposure being modified, then it may be extremely difficult to demonstrate an effect of the intervention. For example, the prevalence of cigarette smoking among U.S. adults is decreasing irrespective of specific interventions in a given community. A related phenomenon is that of nonintervention influences. Continuing with the example of cigarette smoking, suppose the American Cancer Society decides to implement a national stop-smoking campaign characterized by television, radio, and newspaper messages. Its ability to succeed can affect both control and treatment communities involved in an intervention.

Evaluation of Community Interventions

The benefit of an intervention should never be assumed. Rather, it is important for the investigator to quantify and properly evaluate whether a program has achieved its intended results. Evaluations may be undertaken for a variety of reasons, and the form of the evaluation must obviously follow the function. A thorough coverage of evaluation is beyond the scope of this book. The reader is referred to the text by Rossi and Freeman[17] for greater detail. It is our intent to provide an overview as well as some of the specifics germane to assessment. The present authors note that evaluation is, ideally, a continuing activity that comprises four stages following in sequence: formative, process, impact, and outcome (Exhibit 8-6). The examples that we have provided in this chapter apply mostly to impact evaluation.

Posttest

One approach to evaluation is simply for the researcher to make observations only after the program has been delivered. The U.S. educational system typically follows the pattern for evaluation of classroom instruction. Students enter a class, endure lectures and presentations from the instructor, and then complete examinations to demonstrate that they have acquired knowledge. The advantage of

EXHIBIT 8-6

The Four Stages of Evaluation

Formative Evaluation: "a way of making sure program, plans, procedures, activities, materials, and modifications will work as planned. Begin formative evaluation as soon as the idea for a program is conceived."

Process Evaluation: Its purpose "is to learn whether the program is serving the target population as planned and whether the number of people being served is more or less than expected. Begin process evaluation as soon as the program goes into operation."

Impact Evaluation: Measures "whatever changes the program creates in the target population's knowledge, attitudes, beliefs, or behaviors." Requires collection of baseline information before the program starts and subsequent data after first encounter with the target group. Informs program planners whether they are making progress toward goals.

Outcome Evaluation: "For ongoing programs . . . , conduct outcome evaluations at specified intervals. . . . For one-time programs conduct outcome evaluation after the program is finished. The purpose is to learn how well the program has accomplished its ultimate goal." ■

Source: Adapted from NJ Thompson and HO McClintock. *Demonstrating Your Program's Worth: A Primer on Evaluation for Programs To Prevent Unintentional Injury.*1998, pp 21-22. Atlanta, GA: National Center for Injury Prevention and Control, Centers for Disease Control and Prevention.

this evaluation method is that it makes explanation of results easy. The obvious limitation is that there is usually no measure for baseline comparison. Perhaps the students who score highest on examinations came into the class with greater prior knowledge of the subject. In a similar vein, an evaluation of the effectiveness of a community program to increase consumption of fresh fruits and vegetables (a posttest-only design) would be unable to determine whether eating habits had actually changed.

Pretest/Posttest

In view of the criticisms leveled at the posttest-only design, one way to improve the evaluation is simply to add a baseline period of observation. The intervention and posttest observations would still be done. By making observations before and after the program is put into effect, one can measure change relative to baseline.

Pretest/Posttest/Control

Although the pretest/posttest design is better than the posttest-only design, the limitation of the former is that there is no measure of external influences that might induce changes in both study groups. One approach to address this deficiency is to add a control group that does not receive the intervention. Observations are made in both intervention and control groups before and after the program. Thus, the effect of any external influences can be estimated by any measured changes that occur in the nonintervention group. The "true" effect of the intervention therefore would be the "observed effect" in the intervention group minus the "nonintervention effect" from external factors as measured in the control group.

Solomon Four-Group Assignment

As alluded to earlier in the chapter, the mere fact that individuals are observed may result in behavior change. In a famous experiment designed to determine the effects of varying light intensity on the productivity of women assembling small electronic parts,[24] it was observed that a change, whether positive or negative, in the intensity of illumination produced an increase in worker productivity. The investigators reasoned that the workers took the fact that they had been singled out as an experimental group and given a great deal of attention as evidence that the firm was interested in their personal welfare. Termed the *Hawthorne effect* (after the site where the experiment was conducted), the phenomenon is not specific to social experiments but applies to any circumstance that involves human subjects. This is the basis for the placebo control in clinical trials of pharmacologic agents.

One possible solution to the problem of the Hawthorne effect is to design a study that includes four equivalent groups: two intervention and two control groups. Two are observed before and after the program, and the other two are observed only after the program. Thus, one has the pretest/posttest/control design with two additional arms, neither of which had a pretest observation. This design allows one to determine the effect of both the treatment and the observations. Although the Solomon four-group assignment has been used extensively in social science and educational research, epidemiologists seldom employ it. An obvious reason for its limited use is the increased cost inherent in adding two additional study arms. Furthermore, a reanalysis of the Hawthorne experiment cast considerable doubt on whether the work actually demonstrated any observation effect at all[25]; some researchers believe that such an effect is probably rare.[17]

Miscellaneous Issues

Several other issues apply to the design of experiments: external validity, statistical power, and noncompliance. We have already considered external validity in Chapter 5. This term refers to the ability to generalize the results of the clinical or community trial to a target population beyond the subjects of the study. External validity is very much connected with the manner in which the study subjects have been selected (e.g., white, middle-class men only or a more diverse sample). Findings from a controlled clinical trial of a new medication using a sample that has limited demographic composition, such as all white men, can only be generalized to a similarly narrow target population. As a result, the research community is required to increase the diversity of human subjects who participate in epidemiologic studies.

The issue of statistical power is linked to the size of the samples selected for the various conditions of the intervention. It refers to the ability of the study design to detect the hypothesized outcomes of the study. Studies that have larger samples in comparison to smaller samples have greater statistical power and reduced measurement error; of course, larger samples are more costly to collect than smaller samples.

Finally, noncompliance is a factor in experimental study design that has the potential to vitiate or nullify the effects of the intervention. For example, if the subjects in a randomized controlled clinical trial do not take a prescribed medication, the outcome of the trial may be reduced or may not be detectable. For a summary of intervention studies (comparisons of clinical trials and community trials), refer to Table 8-2.

Conclusion

This chapter has provided an overview and description of experimental study designs, both controlled experiments and quasi-experiments, which usually take the form of interventions in the field of epidemiology. Examples of intervention studies covered were clinical trials and community trials. The distinction between the two is that clinical trials focus upon individuals and community trials upon the group. While both clinical trials and community trials can take the form of controlled experiments, community trials, because of their complexity, are often conducted as quasi-experimental designs. Related to the types of study designs is their hierarchy with respect to ability to generate causal inferences. Other issues covered in this chapter were the applications and phasing of clinical trials as well as randomization and crossover designs.

Table 8-2 Summary of Intervention Studies (Clinical Trials versus Community Trials)

Clinical Trials	Community Trials
Prospective study that often uses a true experimental design.	Prospective study that often uses a quasi-experimental design.
Used for testing new medications, procedures (therapeutic trials), and substances to prevent disease (prophylactic trials).	Designed to produce changes (especially health-related) in a target population.
Focused on the individual	Focused on the community, school district, county or state
Randomization of subjects to the exposure (treatment or control conditions), in order to promote comparability of subjects with respect to measured and unmeasured variables	Fewer study units can be randomized to the study conditions. Intervention and control communities may differ with respect to race, education, age, and other unmeasured variables.
Manipulation (external control of exposure) is possible.	Manipulation (external control of exposure) is possible.
Duration ranges from days to years (in the case of some trials).	Generally longer time duration than clinical trials.
Strict human subject protocol to regulate eligibility of subjects; informed consent to participate required.	Informed consent of participating subjects required for collection of baseline, outcome, and other information.
Participation restricted to a highly selected group of individuals with disease, at high risk for disease, or volunteers.	Participation involves all members of a targeted community; intervention is applied more generally than in a clinical trial.
Tightly controlled in terms of eligibility, delivery of intervention (treatment), and monitoring of outcome.	Less rigid control over intervention in comparison to clinical trials.
Appropriate for testing narrow hypotheses, such as those related to vaccine treatment testing and evaluating new drugs.	Appropriate for determining the potential benefit of new policies and programs, such as those related to health.
Usually two groups (experimental and control) are compared in terms of an outcome.	Baseline measures taken in the intervention and control communities with follow-up at the end of the intervention.
Outcomes of clinical trials (clinical end points): compare rate of disease, death, recovery; outcome of interest is measured in the intervention and control arms of the trial to evaluate efficacy.	Outcomes of community trials: programs may be evaluated according to the four stages of evaluation—formative, process, impact, and outcome. Pre- and post-test measures compared.
Advantages: provide general control over the study situation with respect to amount of exposure, timing, frequency, and period of observation.	Advantages: estimate realistically the impact of behavior change or other modifiable exposure in the incidence of disease.
Disadvantages: Artificial setting of the treatment delivery and evaluation result in lack of generalizability (external validity). Difficulty of adherence to a protocol when trial produces side effects or preliminary results show it to be efficacious.	Disadvantages: loss of effect may occur due to the shifting in the study population composition. Secular trends in respect to prevalence of the exposure being modified make it difficult to determine the effect of the intervention.

continues

Table 8-2 *continued*

Clinical Trials	Community Trials
Blinding and double blinding are used to promote objectivity.	Blinding and double blinding not generally used.
Variations: crossover design, a change of treatments for the study patients that involves a switch of study treatments.	Variations: posttest only, pretest/posttest, and the Solomon four-group assignment
Examples: the folic acid randomized clinical trial; effectiveness of education efforts to reduce STDs. Refer to text.	Examples: the Pawtucket Heart Healthy Program; Project Respect. Refer to text.

Study Questions and Exercises

1. Define the following terms:
   a. Experimental study
   b. Quasi-experimental study
   c. Intervention study
   d. Controlled clinical trial
2. Compare and contrast the two categories of intervention studies (controlled clinical trials vs. community interventions) discussed in this chapter. What are some advantages and disadvantages of controlled experimental designs in comparison to quasi-experimental designs?
3. Explain the purposes of *blinding* and *randomization* in clinical trials.
4. Describe the phases of a clinical trial to license a vaccine or new medicine.
5. What is meant by a *crossover design?* Distinguish between a planned and unplanned crossover.
6. Can you foresee ethical problems that might arise in the development of new pharmaceutical agents for HIV?
7. What are some of the design strategies that are used to improve the validity of community trials?

Questions 8 and 9 pertain to Chapters 6, 7, and 8.

8. Epidemiologic studies of the role of a suspected factor in the etiology of a disease may be observational or experimental. The essential difference between experimental and observational studies is that in experimental studies:

    a. The study and control groups are equal in size.

    b. The study is prospective.

    c. The study and control groups are always comparable with respect to all factors other than the exposure.

    d. The investigator determines who shall be exposed to the suspected factor and who shall not.

    e. Controls are used.

9. From the descriptions provided, identify the type of study design that is being described:

    a. Smoking histories are obtained from all patients entering a hospital who have lip cancer and are compared with smoking histories of patients with cold sores who enter the same hospital.

    b. The entire population of a given community is examined, and all who are judged free of bowel cancer are questioned extensively about their diet. These people are then followed for several years to see whether their eating habits will predict their risk of developing bowel cancer.

    c. To test the efficacy of vitamin C in preventing colds, army recruits are randomly assigned to two groups: one given 500 mg of vitamin C daily, and one given a placebo. Both groups are followed to determine the number and severity of subsequent colds.

    d. The physical examination records of the incoming first-year class of 1935 at the University of Minnesota are examined in 1980 to see whether the freshmen's recorded height and weight at the time of admission to the university were related to their chance of developing coronary heart disease by 1981.

    e. Fifteen hundred adult men who worked for Lockheed Aircraft were initially examined in 1951 and were classified by diagnosis criteria for coronary artery disease. Every three years they have been examined for new cases of the disease; attack rates in different subgroups have been computed annually.

    f. A random sample of middle-aged sedentary women was selected from four census tracts, and each subject was examined for evidence of osteoporosis. Those found to have the disease were excluded. All others were randomly assigned to either an exercise group, which followed a two-year program of systematic exercise, or a control group, which had no exercise program. Both groups were observed semiannually for incidence of osteoporosis.

g. Questionnaires were mailed to every 10th person listed in the city telephone directory. Each person was asked to provide his or her age, sex, and smoking habits and to describe the presence of any respiratory symptoms during the preceding seven days.

References

1. Last JM, ed. *A Dictionary of Epidemiology,* 3rd ed. New York, NY: Oxford University Press; 1995.
2. Susser M. Some principles of study design for preventing HIV transmission: rigor or reality. *Am J Public Health.* 1996;86:1713–1716.
3. Meinert CL. *Clinical Trials: Design, Conduct, and Analysis.* New York, NY: Oxford University Press; 1986.
4. Psaty BM, Siscovick DS, Weiss NS, et al. Hypertension and outcomes research: from clinical trials to clinical epidemiology. *Am J Hypertens.* 1995;9:178–183.
5. Medical Research Council Vitamin Study Research Group. Prevention of neural tube defects: results of the Medical Research Council Vitamin Study. *Lancet.* 1991;338:131–137.
6. Hibbard BM. The role of folic acid in pregnancy with particular reference to anaemia, abruption, and abortion. *J Obstet Gynaecol Br Commonw.* 1964;71:529–542.
7. O'Donnell LN, San Doval A, Duran R, O'Donnell C. Video-based sexually transmitted disease patient education: its impact on condom acquisition. *Am J Public Health.* 1995;85:817–822.
8. Begg N, Miller E. Role of epidemiology in vaccine policy. *Vaccine.* 1990;8:180–189.
9. Engelking C. Clinical trials: impact evaluation and implementation considerations. *Semin Oncol Nurs.* 1992;8:148–155.
10. Gordis L. *Epidemiology.* Philadelphia, PA: Saunders; 1996.
11. Miké V, Schottenfeld D. Observations on the clinical trial. *Clin Bull.* 1972;2:130–135.
12. Schwartz CE, Chesney MA, Irvine MJ, Keefe FJ. The control group dilemma in clinical research: applications for psychosocial and behavioral medicine trials. *Psychosom Med.* 1997;59:362–371.
13. NIH. Further guidance on a data and safety monitoring for phase I and phase II trials. Notice: OD-00-038, June 5, 2000. Available at: http://grants.nih.gov/grants/guide/notice-files. Accessed: June 12, 2003.
14. NIAID. Clinical Research. Data and Safety Monitoring Board (DSMB) guidelines. Available at: http://www.niaid.nih.gov/dmid/clinresearch/dsm.htm. Accessed: April 17, 2003.
15. Begg C, Cho M, Eastwood S, et al. Improving the quality of reporting of randomized controlled trials: the CONSORT statement. *JAMA.* 1996;276: 637–639.
16. Moher D, Schultz KF, Altman DG. The CONSORT statement: Revised recommendations for improving the quality of reports of parallel-group randomized trials. *Lancet.* 2001;357:1191–1194.
17. Rossi PH, Freeman HE. *Evaluation: A Systematic Approach,* 4th ed. Newbury Park, CA: Sage; 1989.

18. Carleton RA, Lasater TM, Assaf A, Lefebvre RC, McKinlay SM. The Pawtucket Heart Health Program, I: an experiment in population-based disease prevention. *RI Med J.* 1987;70:533–538.

19. Carleton RA, Lasater TM, Assaf AR, et al. The Pawtucket Heart Health Program: community changes in cardiovascular risk factors and projected disease risk. *Am J Public Health.* 1995;85:777–785.

20. COMMIT Research Group. Community Intervention Trial for Smoking Cessation (COMMIT): summary of design and intervention. *J Natl Cancer Inst.* 1991;83:1620–1628.

21. Kaluzny AD, Warnecke RB, Lacey LM, et al. Cancer prevention and control within the National Cancer Institute's clinical trials network: lessons from the Community Clinical Oncology Program. *J Natl Cancer Inst.* 1993;85:1807–1811.

22. Klepp K, Ndeki SS, Leshabari MT, Hannan PJ, Lyimo BA. AIDS education in Tanzania: Promoting risk reduction among primary school children. *Am J Public Health.* 1997;87:1931–1936.

23. Kamb ML, Fishbein M, Douglas JM, et al. Efficacy of a risk-reduction counseling to prevent human immunodeficiency virus and sexually transmitted diseases: a randomized controlled trial. *JAMA.* 1998;280:1161–1167.

24. Roethlisberger FJ, Dickson W. *Management and the Worker.* Cambridge, MA: Harvard University Press; 1939.

25. Franke RH, Kaul JD. The Hawthorne experiments: first statistical interpretation. *Am Sociol Rev.* 1978;43:623–642.

CHAPTER 9

Measures of Effect

LEARNING OBJECTIVES

By the end of this chapter the reader will be able to:

- explain the meaning of absolute and relative effects
- calculate and interpret the following measures: risk difference, population risk difference, etiologic fraction, and population etiologic fraction
- define the role of statistical tests in epidemiologic research
- apply five criteria for evaluation of epidemiologic associations

CHAPTER OUTLINE

Introduction

One of the major challenges to an epidemiologist is presentation of research findings in a meaningful and interpretable manner. Much of the basic vocabulary ("epi-speak") for presentation of data and results was defined in Chapter 3. As part of the presentation on study designs in Chapters 6 and 7, the terms *odds ratios* (OR) and *relative risk* (RR) were defined and illustrated. The purpose of this chapter is to extend the discussion begun in Chapter 6 by introducing several additional measures that are useful when one is attempting to evaluate the potential implications of an exposure-disease association. For the science of public health, the ability to extrapolate the health ramifications for the larger population from the findings of individual studies is critical to the planning of programs and delivery of resources. A knowledge of the measures presented in this chapter will facilitate planning and evaluation of proposed interventions. We also demonstrate that the exposure-disease association can have quite different implications for risk to the individual and impact upon the population.

Absolute Effects

One of the simplest ways to compare the disease burden in two groups is to calculate the absolute difference in disease frequency. This type of comparison also is referred to as a difference measure of association, or attributable risk.[1] An absolute effect may be based on differences in incidence rates, cumulative incidence, prevalence,[2] or mortality.[3] An attributable risk is also known as a rate difference or risk difference.[2,4]

Risk Difference

I_e = Incidence rate of disease in exposed group
I_{ne} = Incidence rate of disease in nonexposed group

Recall from Chapter 2 the discussion about causality in epidemiology. Rothman's comments are particularly relevant:

> A *cause* is an act or event or a state of nature which initiates or permits, alone or in conjunction with other causes, a sequence of events resulting in an *effect*. A cause which inevitably produces the effect is *sufficient*. The inevitability of disease after a sufficient cause calls for qualification: disease usually requires time to become

manifest, and during this gestation, while disease may no longer be preventable, it might be fortuitously cured, or death might intervene. . . . Most causes that are of interest in the health field are components of sufficient causes but are not sufficient in themselves. . . . Causal research focuses on components of sufficient causes, whether necessary or not.[5(p588)]

Along the lines of these statements by Rothman, it is asserted elsewhere in this book that many chronic diseases, for example, coronary heart disease (CHD), result not from a single exposure but rather from the combined influences of several exposures, such as environmental and lifestyle factors, that operate over a long time period. Therefore, removal of only one of the exposures (e.g., high serum cholesterol) that leads to a chronic disease, such as CHD, would not result in complete elimination of the disease; other risk factors would still be operative and contribute to the rate of disease. One approach to estimate the realistic potential impact of removing an exposure from the population is to calculate the risk difference in disease frequency (i.e., incidence rates) between the exposed and the nonexposed groups. According to Rothman, a risk difference "represents the incidence rate of disease with the exposure as a component cause."[2(p35)]

> *Risk difference:* The difference between the incidence rate of disease in the exposed group (I_e) and the incidence rate of disease in the nonexposed group (I_{ne}); risk difference = $I_e - I_{ne}$.[4]

As mentioned above, the measure of disease frequency used in the determination of absolute effects may be incidence density, cumulative incidence, prevalence, or mortality. Thus, to be perfectly accurate, when the measure of disease frequency is cumulative incidence, the term *risk difference* could be used. When incidence density measures are used as the measure of disease frequency, the term *rate difference* is most appropriate. For prevalence and mortality, the most precise terms would be *prevalence difference* and *mortality difference,* respectively. Regardless of the measure of disease frequency used, the basic concept of absolute effects is the same: The measure of disease frequency among the nonexposed group is subtracted from the measure of disease frequency among the exposed group.

As an example, hip fractures pose a significant public health burden for the aged population. In 1990, there were an estimated 1.7 million hip fractures worldwide and more than 240,000 in the United States alone.[6] Investigators at the Mayo Clinic in Rochester, Minnesota, examined seasonal variations in fracture rates, comparing the rates during winter with those during summer.[7] For women younger than age 75, the incidence I_e of fractures per 100,000 person-days was highest in the winter (0.41), and the incidence I_{ne} was lowest in the summer (0.29). The risk difference between the two seasons ($I_e - I_{ne}$) was 0.41 − 0.29, or 0.12 per 100,000 person-days. *[handwritten: lea ps. 95]*

Population Risk Difference

I_p = Overall incidence rate of disease in a population
P_e = Proportion of the population exposed
P_{ne} = Proportion of the population not exposed

Population risk difference is defined as a measure of the benefit to the population derived by modifying a risk factor. That is, this measure addresses the question of how many cases in the whole population can be attributed to a particular expo- sure. To understand fully the concept of population risk difference, consider that the incidence rate (risk) of disease in the population (denoted by the symbol I_p), for the simplest case of a dichotomous exposure (exposed or nonexposed), is made up of four components: the incidence rate (risk) of disease in the exposed group, I_e; the incidence rate (risk) of disease in the nonexposed group, I_{ne}; the proportion of the population exposed, P_e; and the proportion of the population not exposed, P_{ne}. The nonexposed group is sometimes called the reference group. The relation- ship among the four components may be expressed by the following formula:

[handwritten: lp = exposed: ne]
$$I_p = (I_e)(P_e) + (I_{ne})(P_{ne})$$

Ignore, for the moment, the proportion exposed (P_e) and the proportion not exposed (P_{ne}). If one were to remove the effects of exposure associated with higher rates of disease, the overall rate of disease in the population then would be expected to decrease to the rate observed among the nonexposed, or reference, group. Thus, subtraction of the rate (risk) of disease among the nonexposed (I_{ne}) from the rate of disease among the population (I_p) provides an indication of the potential impact of a public health intervention designed to eliminate the harmful exposure.

Population risk difference: The difference between the rate (risk) of disease in the nonexposed segment of the population (I_{ne}) and the overall rate (I_p).

Just as for the risk difference, the measures of disease frequency used to calculate population risk differences may be generalized to include the cumulative incidence (risk), incidence density (rates), prevalence, or mortality. Remember: Risk difference is the risk in the exposed minus the risk in the nonexposed; population risk difference is the risk in the population minus the risk in the nonexposed subset of the population.

As another example, nonsteroidal anti-inflammatory drugs (NSAIDs) are among the most frequently used drugs in the United States. It has been estimated that 75 million prescriptions are dispensed annually at a cost of about $2.5 billion.[8] To examine the association of NSAID usage and peptic ulcer disease among elderly persons, Smalley et al.[9] determined the incidence rate of serious ulcer disease among users and nonusers of NSAIDs. The study was based on 103,954 elderly Tennessee Medicaid recipients followed from 1984 to 1986. A total of 1,371 patients were hospitalized with peptic ulcer disease after 209,068 person-years of follow-up. The incidence (density) rate of peptic ulcer disease in the study population (I_p) was calculated to be 6.6 per 1,000 person-years [$(1{,}371/209{,}068) \times 1{,}000$]. The rate ($I_{ne}$) among nonusers of NSAIDs was only 4.2 per 1,000 person-years. The population risk difference ($I_p - I_{ne}$) was 6.6 − 4.2, or 2.4 per 1,000 person-years. The risk difference may be computed also: It was known that the observed incidence rate (I_e) of peptic ulcer disease among users of NSAIDs was 16.7 per 1,000 person-years. Therefore, the risk difference ($I_e - I_{ne}$) was 16.7 − 4.2, or 12.5 per 1,000 person-years.

Relative Effects

Interpretation of the absolute measures of effect can sometimes be enhanced when expressed relative to a baseline rate. For example, RR (discussed in Chapter 7) provides an estimate of the magnitude of an association between exposure and disease.[4] Such a ratio also can be described as a relative effect. Note that all relative effects contain an absolute effect in the numerator.

Previously, we defined RR as the ratio of the cumulative incidence rate in the exposed (I_e) to the cumulative incidence rate in the nonexposed (I_{ne}), or I_e/I_{ne}. This is actually a simplification of the true formula for RR, in which the numerator is $I_e - I_{ne}$ (the risk difference). If one divides both terms in the numerator by I_{ne}, one is left with the formula (I_e/I_{ne}) − (I_{ne}/I_{ne}). The first term, I_e/I_{ne}, was previously defined as the RR. Because any number (or variable) divided by itself is 1, the second term becomes 1, and the expression becomes RR − 1. Typically the − 1 is ignored. Occasionally, however, one may encounter statements such as

"30% greater risk among the exposed"; this statement implies that the RR ratio of I_e/I_{ne} is 1.3 but that the 1 has been subtracted. The interpretation is exactly the same. RRs between 1.0 and 2.0 sound bigger when stated as a percentage, however (e.g., 1.3 vs. 30%).

Etiologic Fraction

One of the conceptual difficulties with RR is that the rate of disease in the referent (nonexposed) group is not necessarily 0. In fact, for a common disease that is theorized to have multiple contributing causes, the rate may still be quite high in the referent group as a result of other causes in addition to the exposure of interest. One implication of multiple contributing causes is that, even in the absence of exposure to the single factor of interest, a number of cases still would have developed among the nonexposed population. An approach to estimating the effects due to the single exposure factor is to compute the etiologic fraction. It is defined as the proportion of the rate in the exposed group that is due to the exposure. Also termed attributable proportion or attributable fraction, it can be estimated by two formulas. To estimate the number of cases among the exposed that are attributable to the exposure, one must subtract from the exposed group those cases that would have occurred irrespective of membership in the exposed population.

$$\text{Etiologic fraction} = \frac{I_e - I_{ne}}{I_e} \qquad \text{(Eq. 1)}$$

Note that the difference between Equation 1 and RR is the rate in the denominator, I_e instead of I_{ne}. The numerator represents an acknowledgment that not all the cases among the exposed group can be fairly ascribed to the exposure; some fraction would have occurred anyway, and this fraction is estimated by the rate in the nonexposed. This formula can be applied to data from cohort or cross-sectional studies. The appropriate measures of disease frequency must be utilized: cumulative incidence, incidence density, or mortality from cohort studies or prevalence of disease from cross-sectional studies.

With a little arithmetic, it is possible to express Equation 1, the formula for etiologic fraction, in another convenient form. If one considers Equation 1 as two separate fractions, one obtains $1 - (I_{ne}/I_e)$. Note that (I_{ne}/I_e) is merely the reciprocal of the original definition of RR. Thus, one is left with $1 - (1/\text{RR})$. If one expresses the 1 as RR/RR, the formula requires only an estimate of RR, obviously beneficial for those situations in which the actual incidence rates are unknown (Equation 2). Thus, this formula may be applied when the data at hand, whether from a report or a published article, include only the summary measures. More important, because the OR provides an estimate of RR, this formula is applicable to data from case-control studies.

$$\text{Etiologic fraction} = \frac{RR - 1}{RR} \qquad \text{(Eq. 2)}$$

For example, what fraction of peptic ulcer disease in elderly persons is attributable to NSAIDs? Recall from the previous example that I_{ne} was 4.2 and I_e was 16.7 per 1,000 person-years.[9] The risk difference was computed to be $16.7 - 4.2$, or 12.5 per 1,000 person-years. The etiologic fraction from Equation 1 is $12.5 \div 16.7$, or 74.9%. Thus, roughly three-fourths of the cases of peptic ulcer disease that occurred among NSAID users were attributed to that exposure.

To demonstrate that both formulas are equivalent, one may compute the etiologic fraction using Equation 2. To do this, one must first compute the RR. In this example the answer is $16.7 \div 4.2$, or 3.98. The etiologic fraction is therefore 2.98 divided by 3.98. Both formulas should yield the same answer, an outcome that the reader may wish to verify.

In general, low RRs equate to a low etiologic fraction, and high RRs equate to a high etiologic fraction. A reasonable question to ask at this point is what risk difference reveals beyond what one could already infer from the RR? Perhaps this question is best answered with an illustration. Take the case of two diseases, A and B, and two exposure factors, X and Y. The rate of disease A is 2 per 100,000 per year among individuals exposed to factor X and 1 per 100,000 per year among those not exposed to factor X. The rate of disease B is 400 per 100,000 per year among individuals exposed to factor Y and 200 per 100,000 per year among those not exposed to factor Y. Therefore, for either disease the RR associated with the relevant exposure is 2.0 (i.e., $2 \div 1$ or $400 \div 200$). Exposure factors X and Y both appear to pose a significant health hazard, a doubling of risk of disease. Consider what is obtained by examining the risk difference: For disease A the risk difference is $2 - 1$ or 1 per 100,000 per year, and for disease B the risk difference is $400 - 200$ or 200 per 100,000 per year. Although the RRs for factor X and factor Y are the same, the risk differences for the two factors are quite disparate. If one were to design an intervention to improve public health, the RRs for factors X and Y would not be terribly informative. The risk difference calculations would suggest, however, that control of exposure Y might pay greater dividends than control of exposure X (ignoring, for the moment, critical issues such as cost and feasibility).

Population Etiologic Fraction

As we have seen, from the perspective of those with a disease the etiologic fraction gives an indication of the potential benefit of removing a particular exposure to a putative disease factor. That is, does a particular exposure account for 5% of the etiology of the disease or 95%? An alternative perspective to consider is that of the population. The population etiologic fraction provides an indication of the effect of removing a particular exposure on the burden of disease in the population. A possible scenario is one in which a dichotomous (present or absent) exposure factor is associated with risk of disease and 25% of the population is exposed to the factor. As was pointed out earlier, the total rate of disease in the population may be thought of as a weighted average of the rate of disease among the 25% of the population exposed and the rate of disease among the 75% of the population not exposed (the concept of weighted average was applied, in Chapter 3, to the direct method of age adjustment). If the offending exposure is reduced, the lower limit of disease rate that can be achieved is the background rate observed among the nonexposed segment of the population. Again, two formulas for the population etiologic fraction will be presented.

The population etiologic fraction represented by Equation 3 is the proportion of the rate of disease in the population that is due to the exposure (also termed the attributable fraction in the population). It is calculated as the population risk difference divided by the rate of disease in the population.

$$\text{Population etiologic fraction} = \frac{I_p - I_{ne}}{I_p} \qquad \text{(Eq. 3)}$$

As an example, consider again the study of NSAIDs and peptic ulcer disease among elderly persons.[9] I_{ne} was 4.2, I_p was 6.6 per 1,000 person-years, and the population risk difference was computed to be $6.6 - 4.2$, or 2.4 per 1,000 person-years. For this example, the population etiologic fraction is $(2.4/6.6) \times 100 = 36.4\%$. Therefore, if everyone in the population stopped taking NSAIDs, the rate of peptic ulcer disease would decrease by more than one-third. Notice that compared to the perspective of those with the disease, this figure of 36.4% is far less than the etiologic fraction of 74.9%.

When the incidence rate in the population is unknown, an alternative formula (Equation 4) may be applied. This formula requires information about two components: the RR of disease associated with the exposure of interest, and the prevalence of the exposure in the population (P_e).

$$\text{Population etiologic fraction} = \frac{P_e(RR - 1)}{P_e(RR - 1) + 1} \times 100 \qquad \text{(Eq. 4)}$$

Case-control studies do not allow estimation of disease rates in the total population or in the nonexposed population; therefore, Equation 3 population etiologic fraction cannot be used. Equation 4, however, lends itself to interpretation of data from case-control studies because the OR can be substituted for RR. The missing piece of information is the prevalence of the exposure in the population. Recall from Chapter 6 (selection of controls in a case-control study) that the purpose of a control group is to provide an estimate of the expected frequency of the exposure of interest. With certain assumptions, the frequency of exposure among the control group can be used to approximate the overall frequency of exposure in the population.

Example 1: Given that the prevalence (P_e) of current NSAID use in the study by Smalley et al.[9] was 0.13, compute the population etiologic fraction using Equation 4. The RR had been previously determined to be 3.98. Plugging the values for RR and P_e into Equation 4, one obtains:

$$\frac{0.13(3.98 - 1)}{0.13(3.98 - 1) + 1} \times 100 = \frac{0.387}{1.387} \times 100 = 27.9\%$$

This answer is slightly lower than the results obtained by using Equation 3 for population etiologic fraction because the prevalence figure P_e did not include former or indeterminate users of NSAIDs. Mathematically the two formulas yield the same result, however.

Example 2: Suppose you are dealing with an exposure that confers a high RR for disease (e.g., RR = 20), but the prevalence (P_e) of the exposure in the population is low (e.g., 1 per 100,000). Compare the etiologic fraction with the population etiologic fraction using these data. Compute the etiologic fraction using Equation 2. We obtain:

$$\frac{20 - 1}{20} \times 100 = 95\%$$

From Equation 4, we obtain:

$$\frac{(0.00001)(20 - 1)}{(0.00001)(20 - 1) + 1} \times 100 = 0.019\%$$

Thus, 95% of the cases that occurred among the exposed were attributable to the exposure. Because the exposure was rare in the population, however, it contributed little to the total disease rate.

These two examples illustrate that the impact of an exposure on a population depends upon:

- the strength of the association between exposure and resulting disease
- the overall incidence rate of disease in the population
- the prevalence of the exposure in the population

One may also infer that exposures of high prevalence and low RR can have a major impact on public health. Chapter 2 provided an example of an individual's slight risk of cardiovascular disease mortality associated with a high serum cholesterol level; that is, the etiologic fraction was low. Because a substantial proportion of the population has high cholesterol, however (i.e., has a high prevalence of hypercholesterolemia), the benefit to the population from reducing cholesterol could be substantial. In contrast, the foregoing example of a rare exposure with a high RR for disease demonstrates that a single exposure factor can account for the vast majority of cases of disease among the exposed but that removal of that particular exposure from the population will have little impact on the overall incidence of disease.

Statistical Measures of Effect

In addition to the preceding methods of expressing epidemiologic study results (absolute and relative effects), epidemiologists frequently employ and rely on statistical tests to help interpret observed associations. An illustration of statistical tests arises from a study of the effects of passive smoking (by parents) on the prevalence of wheezing respiratory illness among their children.[10] The results indicate that mothers who smoked at the time of the survey were 1.4 times more likely to report wheezing respiratory illness among their children than mothers who did not smoke. The reasons for this outcome may be as follows:

1. Passive smoking by a parent does, in fact, increase children's risk of wheezing respiratory illness.
2. Some additional exposure has not been properly allowed for in the analysis.
3. The results represent nothing more than a chance (random) finding.

Only after options 2 and 3 have been ruled out can one reasonably conclude that passive smoking increases children's risk of wheezing respiratory illness.

Significance Tests

Underlying all statistical tests is a null hypothesis, usually stated as, "There is no difference in population parameters among the groups being compared." The parameters may consist of the prevalence or incidence of disease in the population. For example, the prevalence or incidence might represent an actual count of cases of disease or could arise from positive serologic evidence of infection with a disease agent, such as positive antibody titers (discussed in Chapt. 12) to the tick-borne illness Lyme disease. A discussion of the particular statistical test to be employed, the choice of which is determined by a number of considerations, is beyond the scope of this book. Suffice it to say that, in deciding whether to fail to reject or to reject the null hypothesis, a test statistic is computed and compared with a critical value obtained from a set of statistical tables. The significance level is the chance of rejecting the null hypothesis when, in fact, it is true.

The P Value

The P value indicates the probability that the findings observed could have occurred by chance alone. The converse is not true: A nonsignificant difference is not necessarily attributable to chance alone. For studies with a small sample size, the sampling error is likely to be large, which may lead to a nonsignificant test even when the observed difference is caused by a real effect.

Confidence Interval

A confidence interval (CI) is a statistical measure that is considered by many epidemiologists to be more meaningful than a point estimate; the latter is a single number—for example, a sample mean, an incidence rate, or a relative risk—that is used to estimate a population parameter. A CI is expressed as a computed interval of values that, with a given probability, contains the true value of the population parameter.[11] The degree of confidence is usually stated as a percentage; the 95% CI is commonly used. Although it is beyond the scope of this book to demonstrate how to construct CIs, it is important, nonetheless, to know how to interpret them. A CI can be interpreted as a measure of uncertainty about a parameter estimate (e.g., a mean, OR, RR, or incidence rate).

- In terms of utility, a 95% CI contains the "true" population estimate 95% of the time.

- Thus, if one samples a population 100 times, the 95% CI will contain the true estimate (i.e., the population parameter) 95 times. Alternatively, if one were to repeat the study 100 times, one would observe the same outcome 5 times just by chance.
- CIs are influenced by the variability of the data and the sample size.

The hypothetical example presented in Table 9-1 reports the OR for a case-control study with three different sample sizes. The exposure, disease, study population, and survey instrument are the same in all three cases. In fact, everything is identical except for the size of the study groups.

Perhaps the first sample size was obtained for a small-scale pilot study. Twenty cases and 20 controls are included. An OR of 2.0 is observed, but the 95% CI includes 1.0; the results are therefore consistent with no association. Suppose, alternatively, that one is able to study 50 per group instead of only 20. The same point estimate of association is observed, and the 95% CI also includes the null value of 1.0. The degree of precision of the magnitude of the OR is improved; the interval is narrower, but the results are still not statistically significant. In the final scenario there are unlimited resources, and one is able to study 500 individuals in each group. With this extra effort and expense, the same study results are obtained: an OR of 2.0. The larger sample size has allowed for a more precise estimate of the effect to be obtained (the 95% CI is narrower). The outcome is now statistically significant, as the null value of 1.0 is now excluded from the 95% CI for the OR. The point to be made is that the estimate of an effect from an epidemiologic study is not necessarily incorrect just because the sample size is small; a small sample size merely may not produce precise results (i.e., there is a wide CI around the estimate of effect).

Clinical Versus Statistical Significance

The preceding discussion of statistical significance should suggest to the reader that P values are only a part of the evaluation of the validity of epidemiologic data.

Table 9-1 ORs, P Values, and 95% CIs for a Case-Control Study with Three Different Sample Sizes

Parameter Computed	Sample Size		
	20	50	500
OR	2.0	2.0	2.0
P	0.50	0.20	0.001
95% CIs	0.5, 7.7	0.9, 4.7	1.5, 2.6

One also should be aware of an important caveat of large sample sizes: Small differences in disease frequency or low magnitudes of RR may be statistically significant. Such minimal effects may have no clinical significance, however. For example, suppose an investigator conducted a survey among pregnant women in urban and suburban populations to assess folic acid levels. Furthermore, suppose that there were 2,000 women in each group, that the average folic acid levels differed by 1.3%, and that this difference was statistically significant. In this example, the sample size was large enough to detect subtle differences in exposure; biologically and clinically, such small differences may be quite insignificant.

The converse of the large sample size issue is that, with small samples, large differences or measures of effect may be clinically important and worthy of additional study. Thus, mere inspection of statistical significance could cause oversight. The lack of statistical significance may simply be a reflection of insufficient statistical power to detect a meaningful association. Statistical power is defined as "The ability of a study to demonstrate an association if one exists. The power of a study is determined by several factors, including the frequency of the condition under study, the magnitude of the effect, the study design, and sample size."[11(p128)] One example of the magnitude of the effect is how large the relative risk is found, i.e., whether RR = 1.0, 5.0, or 10.0.

Another problem inherent in the use of statistical significance testing is that it may lead to mechanical thinking. In his Cassel Memorial Lecture to the Society for Epidemiologic Research Annual Meeting in June 1995, Rothman[12] noted that John Graunt's famous epidemiologic contributions were made in the absence of a knowledge of statistical significance testing.

Evaluating Epidemiologic Associations

The ability to evaluate critically epidemiologic associations reported in the literature is a realistic and attainable goal for the public health practitioner. Although the basic skills to perform such an evaluation are covered in this book, there is no substitute for practice. As an aid to the reader, five key questions that should be asked are presented below.

Could the Association Have Been Observed by Chance?

The major tools that are used to answer this question are statistical tests. Although any public health practitioner should have a basic understanding of biostatistics, he or she should not underestimate the value of a competent biostatistician as a source of help.

Could the Association Be Due to Bias?

The term *bias,* which refers to systematic errors, is discussed in detail in Chapter 10. At this point it is sufficient to say that one should critically evaluate how the study groups were selected, how the information about exposure and disease was collected, and how the data were analyzed. Errors at any of these stages may lead to results that are not valid.

Could Other Confounding Variables Have Accounted for the Observed Relationship?

Confounding refers to the masking of an association between an exposure and an outcome because of the influence of a third variable that was not considered in the design or analysis. The issue of confounding and how to control it is covered in Chapter 10. Based on one's understanding of the natural history and epidemiology of a disease, one needs to consider whether important known confounding factors have been omitted from the study.

To Whom Does This Association Apply?

Although population-based samples are important in epidemiologic research, and although these sampling procedures enhance the likelihood of generalizability of results, they do not guarantee such an outcome. Furthermore, in some situations a great deal can be learned from an unrepresentative study sample. If a study has been properly conducted among a certain stratum of the population, for example, white women between the ages of 55 and 69 who live in the state of Iowa, then one could certainly generalize to other white women who live in the Midwest. If the diets of the women in Iowa are indicative of the diets of American women of this age group, however, then any observed diet-disease associations may apply to a much broader population.

In addition to the representativeness of the sample, many investigators believe that participation rates are crucial to the validity of epidemiologic findings. Participation rates, the percentage of a sample that completes the data collection phase of a study, must be at a sufficiently high level. For example, some top tier public health journals may not publish a report in which the participation rate was less than 70%. Ironically, high participation rates do not necessarily ensure generalizability, and in certain circumstances generalizability may be high even if participation rates are low. Consider a study of a potential precursor of colorectal cancer: the rate of proliferation of cells in the rectal mucosa. Measurement of the proliferation rate of the rectal epithelium requires a punch biopsy, obtainable as part of a sigmoidoscopy or colonoscopy procedure. Suppose one conducts a case-control study of patients with adenomatous polyps (a known precursor of colorectal cancer) and controls free from colon polyps or cancer. Cases are found to have significantly higher rates of rectal cell proliferation than the controls. Because of the invasive nature of the procedure, however, the participation rates are only 10% among the eligible cases and 5% among eligible controls. Does this necessarily mean that the findings cannot be generalized? The key issue is whether the exposure of interest influenced the decision process of the eligible cases and controls to participate. In this example, it is difficult to imagine how an unmeasured characteristic, such as the rate of rectal cell proliferation, could possibly influence participation. Therefore, despite participation rates that usually would be regarded as unacceptable, one may still be able to generalize the findings, especially the underlying biology, to a broader population.

Does the Association Represent a Cause-and-Effect Relationship?

The answer to this question is determined by careful consideration of each of the criteria of causality that were identified and described in Chapter 2: strength of the association, temporality, dose-response, consistency, biologic plausibility, specificity, analogy, and coherence. Refer to Chapter 2 to review these concepts.

Conclusion

This chapter covered two new measures of effect, absolute and relative effects, that may be used as aids in the interpretation of epidemiologic studies. In addition, the chapter presented guidelines that should be taken into account when one is interpreting an epidemiologic finding. Absolute effects, the first variety of which is called risk differences, are determined by finding the difference in measures of disease frequency between exposed and nonexposed individuals. A second type of absolute effect, called population risk difference, is found by computing the difference in measures of disease frequency between the exposed segment of the population and the total population. Relative effects are characterized by the inclusion of an absolute effect in the numerator and a reference group in the denominator. One type of relative effect, the etiologic fraction, attempts to quantify the amount of a disease that is attributable to a given exposure. The second type of relative effect, the population etiologic fraction, provides an estimate of the possible impact on the population rates of disease that can be anticipated by removal of the offending exposure. With respect to interpretation of epidemiologic findings, one should be cognizant of the influence of sample size upon the statistical significance of the results. Large sample sizes may lead to clinically unimportant, yet statistically significant, results; small sample sizes may yield statistically nonsignificant results that are clinically important. Finally, the chapter closed with a series of five questions that should be asked when one attempts to interpret an epidemiologic observation.

Study Questions and Exercises

1. Calculate the etiologic fraction when the relative risk (RR) for disease associated with a given exposure is 1.2, 1.8, 3.0, and 15.0.
2. The impact of an exposure on a population does not depend upon:
   a. the strength of the association between exposure and disease
   b. the prevalence of the exposure
   c. the case fatality rate
   d. the overall incidence rate of disease in the population

The next seven questions (3 through 9) are based on the following data: The death rate per 100,000 for lung cancer is 7 among nonsmokers and 71 among smokers. The death rate per 100,000 for coronary thrombosis is 422 among nonsmokers and 599 among smokers. The prevalence of smoking in the population is 55%. (Refer to Chapt. 7 for formulas for RR.)

3. What is the RR of dying of lung cancer for smokers versus nonsmokers?
4. What is the RR of dying of coronary thrombosis for smokers versus nonsmokers?
5. What is the etiologic fraction of disease due to smoking among individuals with lung cancer?
6. What is the etiologic fraction of disease due to smoking among individuals with coronary thrombosis?
7. What is the population etiologic fraction of lung cancer due to smoking?
8. What is the population etiologic fraction of coronary thrombosis due to smoking?
9. On the basis of the RR and etiologic fractions associated with smoking from lung cancer and coronary thrombosis, which one of the following statements is most likely to be correct?
   a. Smoking seems much more likely to be causally related to coronary thrombosis than to lung cancer.

b. Smoking seems much more likely to be causally related to lung cancer than to coronary thrombosis.

c. Smoking seems to be equally causally related to both lung cancer and coronary thrombosis.

d. Smoking does not seem to be causally related to either lung cancer or coronary thrombosis.

e. No comparative statement is possible between smoking and lung cancer or coronary thrombosis.

10. A cohort study was conducted to investigate the association between coffee consumption and anxiety in a population-based sample of adults. The data are presented in Appendix 9.

a. What is the RR of anxiety associated with coffee use?

b. Calculate the risk (rate) difference.

c. What is the etiologic fraction?

d. Determine the population etiologic fraction.

References

1. Kelsey JL, Thompson WD, Evans AS. *Methods in Observational Epidemiology.* New York, NY: Oxford University Press; 1986.

2. Rothman KJ. *Modern Epidemiology.* Boston, MA: Little, Brown; 1986.

3. Kleinbaum DG, Kupper LL, Morgenstern H. *Epidemiologic Research: Principles and Quantitative Methods.* Belmont, CA: Lifetime Learning; 1982.

4. Hennekins CH, Buring JE. *Epidemiology in Medicine.* Boston, MA: Little, Brown; 1987.

5. Rothman KJ. Causes. *Am J Epidemiol.* 1976;104:587–592.

6. Cooper C, Campion G, Melton LJ III. Hip fractures in the elderly: a world-wide projection. *Osteoporosis Int.* 1992;2:285–289.

7. Jacobsen SJ, Sargent DJ, Atkinson EJ, O'Fallon WM, Melton LJ III. Population-based study of the contribution of weather to hip fracture seasonality. *Am J Epidemiol.* 1995;141:79–83.

8. Burke LB, Baum C, Jolson HM, et al. *Drug Utilization in the United States—1989, Eleventh Annual Review.* Dept of Health and Human Services publication PB91-198838. Washington, DC: Department of Health and Human Services; 1991.

9. Smalley WE, Ray WA, Daugherty JR, Griffin MR. Nonsteroidal anti-inflammatory drugs and the incidence of hospitalizations for peptic ulcer disease in elderly persons. *Am J Epidemiol.* 1995;141:539–545.

10. Stoddard JJ, Miller T. Impact of parental smoking on the prevalence of wheezing respiratory illness in children. *Am J Epidemiol.* 1995;141:96–102.

11. Last JM, ed. *A Dictionary of Epidemiology,* 3rd ed. New York, NY: Oxford University Press; 1995.

12. Rothman gives Cassel Memorial Lecture at SER. *Epidemiol Monit.* 1995;16:1.

APPENDIX
9

Cohort Study Data for Coffee Use and Anxiety

Table 9A-1

Coffee Use	Anxiety		Total
	Yes	No	
Yes	500	9,500	10,000
No	200	19,800	20,000

Data Interpretation Issues

LEARNING OBJECTIVES

By the end of this chapter the reader will be able to:

- distinguish between random and systematic errors
- state and describe the main sources of bias
- identify techniques to reduce bias at the design and analysis phases of a study
- define what is meant by the term *confounding* and provide three examples
- describe the methods that can be used to control confounding

CHAPTER OUTLINE

Introduction

As Exhibit 10-1 suggests, findings from epidemiologic studies are often quite newsworthy. One of the real dangers of obtaining epidemiologic information solely from media reports, however, is the selective nature of the coverage; the media may focus on the one positive result among a larger quantity of negative data. Another more troubling issue is whether the study being reported was even scientifically valid. One must not only understand the study's results and implications, but also be able to evaluate critically the study's design and methodology, a task that requires considerably greater knowledge and skills than merely assimilating the findings. Despite the peer review process adopted by scientific journals, methodologically flawed studies do appear in print and do attract media attention. One cannot assume that just because a study was published in a reputable journal the findings should not be questioned.

Where do possible deficiencies in media reports and published research leave the public health practitioner? To gain a more complete picture of any particular report, one really should retrieve and read the original article firsthand. More important, one should have the basic skills to evaluate critically the report as to selection of study subjects, measurement of exposure and outcome, analysis of data, and interpretation of results. This chapter provides a foundation for such skills.

Validity of Study Designs

The validity of a study is defined as "The degree to which the inference drawn from a study, especially generalizations extending beyond the study sample, are [sic] warranted when account is taken of the study methods, the representativeness of the study sample, and the nature of the population from which it is drawn."[1(p171)] Study validity embodies two components: internal and external validity.

Internal Validity

A study is said to have internal validity when there have been proper selection of study groups and a lack of error in measurement. The goal is to be able to ascribe any observed effect to the exposure under investigation. Thus, the manner of selection of cases and controls, or exposed and nonexposed groups, must be critically reviewed. Maintenance of internal validity also necessitates appropriate measurement of the following:

EXHIBIT 10-1

Press Coverage: Leaving Out the Big Picture

In the past two years, thorough readers of the *Los Angeles Times* would have learned about an extraordinary range of potential cancer causes. Among these putative hazards of modern life are hot dogs, breast implants, dioxin, stress, asbestos, allergy drugs, gas leaks, living in Orange County, tubal ligation, sunscreen, Asian food, pesticides, vasectomy, liquor, working in restaurants, Retin-A, vegetables, dietary fat, delayed child-bearing, impurities in meat, and lesbianism. This litany of fear was accompanied by a similar, although shorter, series of reports on dietary habits and lifestyles that may reduce cancer risk. Parallel coverage appeared in other newspapers and magazines and on television. To many scientists, though, the media would do well to curb its appetite for such news.

The problem, many researchers say, is that journalists often misunderstand the context of the research. Because of the limitations of risk factor epidemiology, most individual studies cannot produce authoritative findings. "Articles published in medical journals are often misconstrued by the lay press to be more definitive than they really are," says Larry Freedman, a biostatistician at the National Cancer Institute. "Broccoli prevents cancer, garlic prevents cancer—all these things do appear in the literature. But epidemiologists understand very well that these studies are far from definitive. It's only when a body of evidence exists over many, many studies that epidemiologists should really get serious about giving the public advice."

Instead of presenting surveys of the big, evolving picture, he and others say the media tend to report each new study in isolation, as a new breakthrough. Such reporting, some scientists say, is encouraged by press releases put out by journals and researchers' institutions. But whoever is to blame, says Noel Weiss, an epidemiologist at the University of Washington, Seattle, the result is "just too many false alarms. When we do have a serious message, I fear it won't be heeded because of the large number of false messages." ■

Source: Reprinted with permission from Charles C Mann. Press Coverage: Leaving Out the Big Picture, *Science,* vol 269, p 166. © 1995 American Association for the Advancement of Science.

- *Exposure.* Was characterization of exposure based on a questionnaire? If so, was the questionnaire administered in person or as a telephone survey, or was it mailed to the study subject for self-administration? To illustrate, the investigator may collect some types of data with reasonable accuracy by using mailed questionnaires, but careful probing that can be achieved only through in-person interviews may be required to collect other types of data. Were the instruments validated? It is important to know whether the questionnaires used actually measured what they purported to measure. Is the reliability known? If the instrument were administered to the same individual on separate occasions, would it provide the same response? Were biologic samples collected to quantify exposure? If so, were the procedures to collect the samples standardized according to timing of collection? For example, suppose you were interested in urinary hormone levels of pre-menopausal women. It would be important to know whether the samples were all collected during the same phase of the menstrual cycle. Were the laboratory assays used appropriate? Although it is not possible to cover all variations on the theme, this brief overview indicates some of the types of questions that should be pondered with respect to exposure assessment.

- *Outcome.* Whether the outcome of interest is a particular disease, behavior, or intermediate marker, the criteria used to define the outcome should be fully described. Was the outcome based solely on self-report, or was an examination performed by trained health professionals according to a standard protocol? How were the subjects with and without the outcome of interest identified? Were all eligible subjects successfully located? Did a high proportion participate? If the study was prospective in nature, were all end points identified? Was there loss to follow-up? Clearly, a number of important considerations pertain to assessment of the outcome and the formation of the study groups.

- *Association between exposure and disease.* The two preceding categories reflect aspects of measurement of exposure and outcome; this category relates to assessment of the association between them by raising the following questions: Were the data properly analyzed? Was adjustment made for extraneous factors that might influence the results? Some types of data analysis require certain assumptions about the nature (distribution) of the data. Were the assumptions tested? Do they appear reasonable given the context of the study? Are there crucial analyses that appear to have been omitted?

External Validity

The preceding section discussed internal validity, a requirement that must be satisfied for a study to have external validity. External validity is a more encompassing process than the ability to extrapolate from a sample population to a target population. External validity implies the ability to generalize beyond a set of observations to some universal statement. According to Last, "A study is externally valid or generalizable if it can produce unbiased inferences regarding a target population (beyond the subjects in the study). This aspect of validity is only meaningful with regard to a specified external target population."[1(p171)]

The basic process of generalizing study results is neither mechanical nor statistical, for one must understand which conditions are relevant or irrelevant to the generalization. Although representativeness of the sample is a condition of external validity, generalizability also is independent of how representative of the target population the study groups are; this statement applies particularly when one uses epidemiology to improve understanding about the biologic basis of a disease.

An example is a feeding study designed to evaluate the utility of plasma carotenoids (compounds found in plant foods thought to have anticarcinogenic properties) as a marker of vegetable intake.[2] Subjects (volunteers who agreed to participate) were randomized into a crossover feeding study of four experimental diets of nine days each. Thus, after spending nine days consuming a particular experimental diet, the subjects were "crossed over" to one of the other diets. It should be noted that volunteers for health studies tend to be more educated and health conscious than the general population. In this particular study, however, 11 exclusion criteria were applied to restrict the pool of volunteers. These included a medical history of gastrointestinal disorders, food allergies, weight loss or gain greater than 4.5 kg within the past year, major changes in eating habits within the past year, exercise regimens requiring significant short-term dietary changes, antibiotic use within the past three months, body weight greater than 130% of ideal, current treatment for a diagnosed disease, alcohol intake greater than two drinks per day, oral contraceptive use, and unwillingness to consume all foods provided in the study. Although these exclusion criteria greatly improved the internal validity of the study, they might have decreased the generalizability of the study if the subjects enrolled were physiologically atypical with respect to how their plasma carotenoid levels responded to a high-vegetable diet.

The preceding example reaffirms the notion that clinical trials are often initially based on a highly selected subgroup of patients. Nonetheless, the information gleaned from such trials often can be generalized to a much broader category of patients.

Sources of Error in Epidemiologic Research

In the context of epidemiologic research, one should consider two categories of error: random and systematic. Random errors reflect fluctuations around a true value of a parameter (such as a rate or a relative risk) because of sampling variability. They occur as a result of poor precision, sampling error, or variability in measurement.

Factors That Contribute to Random Error

Poor Precision

This type of random error occurs when a study factor is not measured sharply. Consider the analogy of aiming a rifle at a target that is not in focus. The target may correctly yield the proper direction in which one should be aiming, but the blurry picture makes it difficult to hit the bull's-eye, causing bullets to scatter all over the target. Increasing the sample size of a study or the number of measurements will yield greater precision. For example, in the Bogalusa Heart Study, a prospective study of the early natural history of cardiovascular disease in a small, rural Louisiana community, an average of six blood pressure readings was used to characterize an individual child's blood pressure.[3] Each child was randomly assigned to two of three trained observers who each made three independent blood pressure measurements. By taking the average of six readings, the random error was reduced, thereby improving precision.

Sampling Error

In the field of epidemiology, one wishes to make inferences about a target population without necessarily having to measure each member of the target population. The target population may be the general population of the entire United States or a specified subset, such as residents of California, children aged 5 to 9, African Americans, or Hmong residents of the Minneapolis-St Paul area of Minnesota. For this reason, one typically selects samples from the target population that are of a more manageable size for study than would occur if every member of the target population were examined.

Sampling error is relevant to all types of epidemiologic studies—cross-sectional, case-control, cohort, or intervention. For example, when one conducts a case-control study of colorectal cancer in the state of Utah, the study group of cases may be considered a sample of all cases of colorectal cancer in the United

States. When one draws a sample from a larger population, the possibility always exists that the sample selected is not representative of the target population. Nonrepresentative samples may occur without any intention or fault of the investigators even if subjects are randomly selected. To a certain extent, sampling error may be thought of as just plain bad luck of the draw, just as there can be an unusual run of cards in poker or run of colors in a roulette game. Although there is no way to prevent a nonrepresentative sample from occurring, increasing the size of the sample can reduce the likelihood of its happening.

Variability in Measurement

The validity of a study will be greatly enhanced if the data that are collected are objective, reliable, accurate, and reproducible. Even under the best of circumstances, however, errors in measurement can and do occur. For example, the Bogalusa Heart Study investigators were concerned about the stability of laboratory measures over long periods of time.[3] To determine consistency in measurement, a blind sample from randomly selected individuals was included when samples of blood were sent to the laboratory for analysis. In fact, perfect agreement was rarely achieved despite the fact that the same procedures were used and the samples were from the same individuals and collected at the same time. The lack of agreement in results from time to time reflects random error inherent in the type of measurement procedure employed.

Factors That Contribute to Systematic Errors

Bias (Systematic Errors)

Deviation of results or inferences from the truth, or processes leading to such deviation. Any trend in the collection, analysis, interpretation, publication, or review of data that can lead to conclusions that are systematically different from the truth.[1(p15)]

A much more serious problem for the validity of a study than random errors is systematic errors, or bias. As the definition of bias given above implies, systematic errors can be introduced at any point in an investigation. These errors can be conveniently grouped into three broad categories: selection bias, information bias, and confounding.

Selection Bias

Selection bias arises when the relation between exposure and disease is different for those who participate and those who would be theoretically eligible for study but do not participate.[4] Such bias may occur during the follow-up period of a study, during the period of recruitment for the study, or even before the study begins. For example, the healthy worker effect represents a source of bias that may occur when only employed individuals, such as an occupational cohort, are eligible for a study. Workers typically are relatively healthy people who have had the opportunity to find and maintain employment. Physically or mentally disabled individuals may not have enjoyed a similar opportunity and thus would not be represented in the study.

As another example, recall the Iowa Women's Health Study, described in Chapter 3. The target population consisted of women between the ages of 55 and 69. From the total eligible pool of licensed female drivers, a 50% random sample of women in this age range was selected.[5] Not all age-eligible subjects were identified using this method because only 94% of women in this age category actually had a valid Iowa driver's license and thus the potential to participate. Data were available on the self-reported height and weight of all participants and nonparticipants from the driver's license data tape provided by the state motor vehicle agency. These data from respondents and nonrespondents provided a rare opportunity to examine possible selection bias. It was found that respondents were on average three months younger and 0.38 kg/m^2 lighter than nonrespondents. Based on 1980 census data, respondents were slightly more likely than nonrespondents to live in rural, less affluent counties. One advantage of conducting the study in Iowa is that one's driver's license number is the same as one's Social Security number. This circumstance facilitated efficient record linkage with the State Health Registry for documentation of subsequent cancer occurrence. Bisgard et al.[6] compared the rates of cancer incidence and mortality between respondents and nonrespondents. Results suggested greater occurrence of smoking-associated diseases among the nonrespondents, a finding consistent with a lower response rate of smokers to a health survey.

Information Bias

Information bias can be introduced as a result of measurement error in assessment of both exposure and disease. One example of information bias is recall bias, which denotes a phenomenon whereby cases may be more likely to recall past exposures than controls. Suppose that in a study of childhood leukemia mothers are interviewed regarding drug use during pregnancy. Mothers of cases are likely to have spent considerable periods of time pondering their children's illness. Although the frequency of exposure may actually be equivalent in both study groups, better recall among the cases than among the controls would yield positive evidence of an association. A special case of recall bias is recollection of a family history of disease, labeled family recall bias.[7] Cases learn of a family history of a disease from relatives after the diagnosis is made. As a result of family recall bias, data on the occurrence of the same disease among family members is likely to be more complete among cases than among controls. Although the true prevalence of the disease among family members of cases and controls may be similar, this bias would give the appearance of a higher prevalence among cases.

Interviewer/abstractor bias can occur when well-intentioned interviewers probe more thoroughly for an exposure in a case than in a control. Similarly, an abstractor may pore over records more thoroughly to identify an exposure in a case than in a control.

Prevarication (lying) bias is a type of information bias that may occur when participants have ulterior motives for answering a question and thus may underestimate or exaggerate exposures. For example, questions asked of married, apparently heterosexual men with acquired immune deficiency syndrome may not necessarily reveal past homosexual behavior. Surveys of individuals who have drinking disorders or members of religious groups that disallow alcohol use may yield false responses.

Information bias may occur also in relation to ascertainment of health outcomes. Consider again the Iowa Women's Health Study cohort of postmenopausal women. One of the exposures of interest was a positive family history of selected cancers, especially breast cancer. The National Cancer Institute (NCI) recommends the use of screening mammography for the early detection of breast cancer; the NCI argues that although mammography is imperfect, it is the best available tool for breast cancer screening. Nevertheless, according to data from the 1993 National Health Information Survey, the frequency of receiving mammograms among women in the age category 55 to 69 is low. Fewer than 50% of women over age 50 reported having a mammogram in the previous year.[8] A positive family history of breast cancer is an established risk factor for the disease, however, and some data suggest that women with a known family history of the disease are more likely to be administered mammograms than women with a negative history of the disease.[9] Accordingly, a physician who knows of a patient's family history of breast cancer may refer the patient for a mammogram, increasing the likelihood of detecting a malignancy in the exposure group of interest.

Confounding

Confounding is the term used to describe distortion of the estimate of the effect of an exposure of interest because it is mixed with the effect of an extraneous factor. According to Susser, a confounding variable is "an independent variable that varies systematically with the hypothetical causal variable under study. When uncontrolled, the effects of a confounding variable cannot be distinguished from those of the study variable."[10(p95)] According to a good working definition, confounding occurs when the crude and adjusted measures of effect are not equal. Formal statistical tests can be performed to evaluate the statistical significance of a confounder. A reasonable rule of thumb is that a change in the estimate of effect by at least 10% when crude and adjusted measures of effect are compared suggests the influence of a confounder.

Although the categories of error (selection bias, information bias, and confounding) are not mutually exclusive, only confounding, practically speaking, can be controlled in the data analysis. To be a confounder, the extraneous factor must satisfy the following three criteria:

1. be a risk factor for the disease (not necessarily causal, but at least a marker for the actual cause of the disease)
2. be associated with the exposure under study in the population from which the cases derive (e.g., smoking would not be a confounder in an occupational cohort study if unassociated with occupational exposure)
3. not be an intermediate step in the causal path between exposure and disease

An excellent illustration of confounding is known as Simpson's paradox.[11] A man enters a shop to buy a hat and sees two tables, each with 30 hats. At the first table he determines that 90% of the black hats fit but only 85% of the gray hats fit. Over at the second table he notices that, similar to the first table, a greater proportion of black hats than gray hats fits (15% vs. 10%). Unfortunately, the shop is closing and the man is forced to return the next day. Much to his chagrin, when he returns he sees that the store clerk has placed all 60 of the hats on a single table. Although on the previous day the greatest proportion of hats that fit at each table were black in color, he soon discovers that, now that all the hats have been mixed together on the same table, 60% (18 of 30) of the gray hats fit but only 40% (12 of 30) of the black hats fit (Table 10-1).

This intriguing example is neither obvious nor intuitive. Confounding can be equally vexing; sometimes associations can be so distorted that even the direction is reversed.[12] An example of confounding is the positive association between air pollution and bronchitis. Air pollution varies directly and systematically with

Table 10-1 An Analogy to Confounding: Simpson's Paradox

Table	Hat Color	Number	Number That Fit	Percentage That Fit
1	Black	10	9	90
	Gray	20	17	85
2	Black	20	3	15
	Gray	10	1	10

urban density and overcrowding, factors that may facilitate the spread of respiratory-associated diseases, such as bronchitis. In this situation, crowding represents a confounding variable.

Another example is the inverse relation between coronary heart disease (CHD) mortality and altitude described by Buechley et al.[13] Some investigators had reported that populations residing at high altitudes had lower heart disease mortality because of the protective effect of adaptation to reduced oxygen tension. A confounding variable that had not been previously accounted for was ethnicity: Hispanics in New Mexico tended to live at higher altitudes and to have lower CHD rates than other ethnic groups. Thus, there was an apparent association between altitude and CHD mortality because of unrecognized differences in ethnic composition of the regions being compared.

A more complicated example is obesity and lung cancer. Obesity has been associated with an increased risk of cancer at a number of sites. A notable exception appears to be lung cancer, for which several studies have suggested a modest inverse association.[14,15] Cigarette smoking is directly associated with lung cancer risk, however, and inversely associated with body mass index, which is a measure of obesity.[16] A careful analysis of the obesity-lung cancer association with proper control for the confounding effect of tobacco exposure suggested that the previous observations were spurious.[17] A pictorial representation of the model is presented in Figure 10-1.

Summary

To recapitulate, error can be introduced into an epidemiologic study at many stages. An overview of these sources of error is depicted in Figure 10-2.

Techniques to Reduce Bias

There is a variety of methods available to reduce or prevent the occurrence of bias in epidemiologic research. Some guidelines that may help prevent selection bias are as follows:

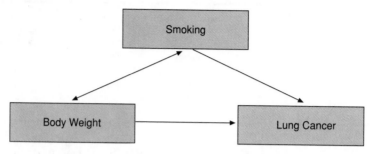

FIGURE 10-1 Graphic representation of how smoking confounds the body weight-lung cancer association

- Develop an explicit (objective) case definition.
- Enroll all cases in a defined time and region.
- Strive for high participation rates (incentives).
- Take precautions to ensure representativeness.
- For cases:
  1. Ensure that all medical facilities are thoroughly canvassed.
  2. Develop an effective system for case ascertainment.
  3. Consider whether all cases require medical attention; consider possible strategies to identify where else the cases might be ascertained.
- For controls:
  1. Try to compare the prevalence of the exposure with other sources to evaluate credibility.
  2. Attempt to draw controls from a variety of sources.

One way to prevent nonrepresentative sampling of eligible cases is to develop, before data collection, explicit definitions about what constitutes a case. Study personnel should be trained to follow the guidelines irrespective of the exposure status of the case. There can be no doubt about the representativeness of the cases if all cases in the target population are selected for study. Definition of the number of cases eligible by time period and geographic region, for example, a three-year period in a five-state area, gives precision to the denominator. An established case registry facilitates the identification of cases; if a registry is not available, a surveillance network of medical facilities where patients would be seen should be established, and all such facilities should be enrolled. Health conditions that do not universally motivate afflicted persons to seek medical attention raise a special concern for the investigator; those who present for medical care may represent only the most severe cases who are atypical with respect to their exposure patterns.

Low participation rates always raise concerns about the validity and generalizability of a study. One approach to enhance participation is to use incentives. These may take the form of T-shirts, key chains, buttons, stickers, coupons for discounts on healthful food choices, free medical evaluation, and even monetary compensation.

Techniques to reduce information bias include the following:

- Use memory aids and validate exposures.
- Blind interviewers as to subjects' study status.
- Provide standardized training sessions and protocols.

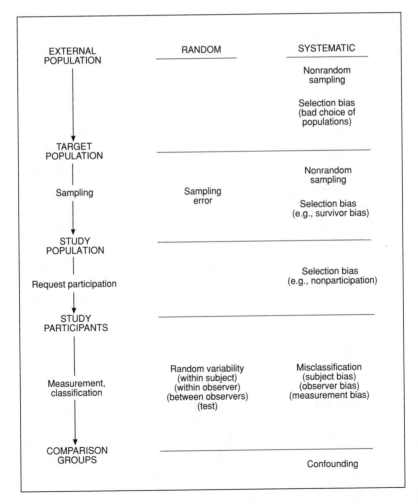

FIGURE 10-2 Sources of error and bias in epidemiologic studies

- Use standardized data collection forms.
- Blind participants as to study goals and participants' classification status.
- Try to ensure that questions are clearly understood through careful wording and pretesting.

The problem of recall bias can be reduced by using memory aids to prompt for responses. For example, when one is conducting an interview of subjects to determine foods eaten over the previous day (a 24-hour recall), it is helpful to structure the interview to refer to particular meals and snack times. The use of food models to indicate portion sizes can help quantify intakes, and posters of commonly eaten snack foods are useful reminders. Studies of oral contraceptive use have utilized pictures of the pill dispensers to help subjects identify brand names and formulations.

Although a study staff committed to the research is an asset, well-intentioned interviewers or abstractors may introduce bias in data collection. Whenever possible, staff should be blinded as to the status of the study subjects: case versus noncase, exposed versus nonexposed. In some situations it also may be desirable to blind the subjects themselves to the true goals of the study. This strategy can help reduce the likelihood of subjects providing responses to please the investigator, attempting to anticipate the "correct" answer to a given question, or producing what they consider socially desirable answers. Clearly, biases introduced by the study subjects are less of an issue when the exposure is a biologic factor that cannot be purposely changed by the subject. One situation in which biases from study subjects might be an issue, however, would be if the biases influenced their decision to participate. Although ethical conduct of research on humans dictates that subjects be informed of the reason for the study and the basis for their invitation to participate, the specific hypothesis to be tested need not be revealed. Development of standardized data collection forms and survey instruments helps ensure that complete data are collected on all subjects in a uniform manner.

Methods to Control Confounding

There are two general approaches to control for confounding. Prevention strategies represent an attempt to control confounding through the study design itself. Analysis strategies seek to control confounding through the use of statistical analysis methods.

Control of Confounding

Prevention strategies
- Randomization
- Restriction
- Matching

Analysis strategies
- Stratification
- Multivariate techniques

Three Prevention Strategies to Control Confounding

The first prevention strategy is randomization of study subjects. The intended net effect is to ensure equal distributions of the confounding variable in each exposure category. This strategy is an extremely efficient approach with a number of clearly defined advantages. Randomization of subjects, if the sample size is sufficiently large, provides control of all factors known and unknown. It is a fairly convenient method, is inexpensive, and permits straightforward data analysis. The primary disadvantages are that randomization can be applied only to intervention studies when investigators have control over the exposure and are able to assign subjects to study groups. Even then, randomization works well only for large sample sizes. If the number of subjects is small, a chance remains that the distribution of confounding variables will be dissimilar across study groups.

The second prevention strategy, restriction of admission criteria, may prohibit variation of the confounder in the study groups. For example, if age is thought to be a potential confounder, the study could simply be restricted to subjects within a narrow age category. Restriction is extremely effective in providing complete control of known confounding factors; it shares with randomization the virtues of being convenient and inexpensive and permitting relatively easy data analysis compared with some of the alternatives. The difficulties encountered with restriction include the distinct possibility that there may still be residual confounding if restrictions are not sufficiently narrow. Moreover, restriction will not address problems created by unknown confounding. From a practical standpoint, restriction may shrink the pool of available subjects to an unacceptably low level. Depending on the health problem studied, one may not be able to generalize the results beyond restricted categories.

Matching of subjects in the study groups according to the value of the suspected or known confounding variable to ensure equal distributions is the third prevention strategy; an example of a potential confounding variable that might be controlled using matching is age. Several types of matching are available. In frequency matching, the number of cases with the particular match characteristics is tabulated. For example, if one is matching on five-year age groups, a frequency distribution of the cases by age group would be generated. Each five-year age group is called an age stratum. Controls are then selected until the required number of controls for each stratum has been acquired. If the controls are to be studied concurrently with the cases, one can generate an expected frequency of cases for each matching stratum based on previously observed rates. Another type of matching is individual matching, the pairing of one or more controls to each case based on similarity of one or several variables, for example, sex or race.

The use of matching to control confounding has a number of clear advantages. In terms of sample size requirements for follow-up studies, matching is efficient in that fewer subjects are required than in unmatched studies of the same hypothesis.[11] Matching also may enhance the validity of a follow-up study. Despite these advantages, matching can be costly, often requiring extensive searching and recordkeeping to find matches. For example, Ross and colleagues[18] conducted a case-control study of renal cancer to evaluate the potential role of analgesics in carcinogenesis. A total of 314 cases of incident cancer of the renal pelvis were identified through the Cancer Surveillance Program. Of these, 61 died before contact, 20 refused to be interviewed, and another 30 were prohibited from participating by the attending physician, leaving 203 cases. Controls were matched to cases on birth date (± 5 years), race, sex, and neighborhood. A predetermined walking algorithm, starting with the residence of the case, was applied for the selection of controls. The procedure continued until a suitable control was found or until 40 houses had been approached. Successful matches were found for 187 (92%) of the cases, and an average of 22 household units were approached per case to find an appropriate control.

For case-control studies, matching may introduce confounding rather than control for it. Confounding typically occurs by matching subjects on factors associated with exposure but then ignoring the matching in the analysis stage. The result is often an estimate of effect that is biased toward the null value (i.e., an odds ratio of 1.0). When one matches subjects on a potential confounder, that particular exposure variable can no longer be evaluated with respect to its contribution to risk; the distribution of the exposure variable is constrained to be similar (perhaps even identical) in both groups. When one matches on several factors, such as age, sex, and neighborhood, there is a danger of making the study groups so similar that one has essentially matched oneself out of business. That is, the exposure that is associated with the outcome of interest (not the confounder) becomes equivalent in the two study groups, and no meaningful associations are identified. Depending on how imprecise the matching variables are, one also can have residual confounding. For example, in a nested case-control analysis of alcohol and lung cancer risk in the Iowa Women's Health Study cohort, cases and noncases were matched on pack-years of smoking.[19] Careful inspection of the data revealed that within strata of pack-years cases tended to have slightly higher mean exposure levels than noncases.

Two Analysis Strategies to Control Confounding

Although it can be somewhat more comforting to conduct a study in which the potential for known confounding can be addressed in the design phase, issues of cost and feasibility may make it necessary instead to address confounding in the analysis stage. Furthermore, attempts to minimize confounding in the design phase obviously can be done only for known confounders. Often the presence of a confounding factor is not observed or detected until analyses are under way, making analysis strategies for dealing with confounding important tools indeed.

The first analysis strategy, stratification, occurs when analyses are performed to evaluate the effect of an exposure within strata (levels) of the confounder. A general approach is to define homogeneous categories or narrow ranges of the confounding variable. One can then combine stratum-specific effects into an overall effect by standard statistical principles and methods (e.g., the Mantel-Haenszel procedure).[20] There are three advantages to this approach. First, performing analyses within strata is a direct and logical strategy. Second, there are minimum assumptions that must be satisfied for the analyses to be appropriate. Third, the computational procedure is quite straightforward.

The difficulties with stratification arise in several areas. The basic process of stratification of the data may result, unfortunately, in small numbers of observations in some strata. When dealing with a continuous variable or an ordinal variable with a relatively large number of categories, one is faced with a variety of ways to form strata. Knowing or deciding which cut points are most appropriate may be difficult. If several confounding factors must be evaluated, necessitating stratification across two or more variables, each of which may have multiple levels, one can easily run into difficulty in interpretation. Finally, from a statistical standpoint, categorization almost always results in loss of information.

The second analysis strategy involves multivariate techniques in which computers are used to construct mathematical models that describe simultaneously the influence of exposure and other factors that may be confounding the effect. This strategy tends to be more feasible with smaller numbers of study subjects than stratification, although multivariate techniques generally require large sample sizes. Another advantage of this tactic pertains to the use of continuous versus categoric variables in the analysis of confounding. When factors that must be controlled are entered into the models as continuous variables, the problem of creating categoric variables is obviated. Continuous variables may be converted to categoric variables by establishing cut points for categories. The epidemiologist may be faced with theoretical difficulties in knowing or deciding where to form such cut points. Another major advantage of multivariate modeling is that it allows for simultaneous control of several exposure variables in a single analysis.

The main disadvantage of multivariate techniques is their great potential for misuse. There are some restrictive assumptions about the distribution of the data that should be, but are not always, examined. The choice of the model may be difficult, especially when the investigator is faced with a large number and wide variety of variables that could be selected. The widespread availability and user-friendly nature of commercial computer software make the method accessible to some data analysts who may not have had adequate instruction in its appropriate applications. When they are misapplied, multivariate techniques have the potential to contribute to incorrect model development, misleading results, and inappropriate interpretation of the effects of hypothesized confounders.

Bias in Analysis and Publication

Although not a reflection of errors in selection, measurement, or analysis (confounding), it is important to consider another source of bias that can have a profound influence. This type of bias is presented in a separate section of the chapter because it is generally outside the control of individual investigators. Publication bias is a phenomenon that occurs because of the influence of study results on the chance of publication. In particular, studies with positive results are more likely to be published than studies with negative results,[21] and to be published more quickly.[22,23] The net effect is a preponderance of false-positive results in the literature. The bias is compounded when published studies on a topic are subjected to meta-analysis. These tend to give an even greater air of importance because of the intent to summarize and synthesize a large number of studies on a given topic. Moreover, meta-analyses of observational studies may be used as the rationale for large clinical trials. Recent comparisons of results from meta-analyses and subsequent randomized clinical trials confirm that results cannot be accurately predicted roughly 35% of the time.[24] This raises the question of whether meta-analyses should include unpublished data. Cook et al.[25] reviewed 150 published meta-analyses and found that only 30% included unpublished data in their primary analysis, although 78% of authors surveyed and 47% of journal editors felt that unpublished material definitely or probably should be included in scientific overviews.

Although each of us as public health professionals probably adheres to a professional code of conduct and integrity in the work that we do, we cannot control the actions of our peers. In these days of "publish or perish" pressures within academia, and the increasing collaboration of universities with private businesses in sponsored research, not all actions are above reproach and one must have a dose of skepticism about what appears in the literature. For example, although not necessarily fraudulent, it can be difficult to ascertain whether or not study results from an observational study were tests of a priori hypotheses or post hoc analyses masqueraded as such. This is particularly worrisome in these days of large data sets, powerful analysis packages, and high-speed computers. Readers of the literature may have difficulty telling whether or not reported results were merely the product of "data dredging" and actually only a chance observation that would be most difficult to replicate.

Further raising the cloud of suspicion is the habit of deleting certain study subjects because they are considered outliers, or when a number of cut points are considered in the analysis and only the ones that yield statistically significant results are presented. Unfortunately, although most scientific journals have a peer review process, such actions are exceedingly difficult to detect. Moreover, there are tendencies for editors to base their decisions on suitability for publication based on the direction or strength of the study findings.[26]

Conclusion

The ability to evaluate critically sources of error in epidemiologic research is necessary not only to interpret properly the plethora of media reports, but also to design and analyze studies. Two main types of research errors must be considered: random errors, which occur because of sampling error, lack of precision, and variability in measurement; and systematic errors (bias), which occur through selection of subjects, collection of information about exposure and disease, and confounding. This chapter presented a number of techniques to reduce bias and introduced some helpful methods to control confounding. Prevention strategies include randomization of subjects into exposure groups, restriction of admission criteria, and matching subjects on the potential confounder. Analysis strategies include stratification and multivariate modeling.

Study Questions and Exercises

1. In a study to determine the incidence of a chronic disease, 150 people were examined at the end of a three-year period. Twelve cases were found, giving an incidence rate of 8%. Fifty other members of the initial cohort could not be examined; 20 of these 50 could not be examined because they died. Does this loss of subjects to follow-up represent a source of bias that may have affected the study results?

2. A case-control study was carried out in which 120 of 200 cases of stomach cancer and 50 of 200 control subjects gave a history of exposure to radiation. In further analysis, however, the investigators noticed that 50% of the cases but only 25% of the controls were men. What would be a practical and efficient way to eliminate differences between cases and controls with respect to sex?

3. Two automated blood cell counters are tested twice using a prepared suspension of leukocytes containing 8,000 cells/mm^3. The cell counts by device A are 8,400 cells/mm^3 the first time and 8,350 cells/mm^3 the second. Device B's counts are 8,200 and 7,850 cells/mm^3, respectively. Which device (A or B) gives leukocyte counts with greater validity? Which device gives leukocyte counts with greater reliability?

4. You are planning a case-control study of lung cancer to test the hypothesis that vegetable consumption is protective against lung cancer. Would you match on smoking? Explain your answer.

5. A follow-up study was conducted of 3,000 military troops deployed at an atomic test site in Nevada to detect the occurrence of leukemia. A total of 1,870 persons were successfully traced by the investigators, and an additional 443 contacted the investigators on their own as a result of publicity about the study. Four cases of leukemia occurred among the 1,870 individuals traced by the investigators, and an additional four occurred among those individuals who contacted the investigators on their own. Could interpretation of the study results be subject to bias?

6. You are conducting a study of insulin resistance and its relationship to body weight. Using a weight scale as your instrument to measure body weight, you find the scale always reads 30 kg regardless of who is standing on it. Discuss the validity and reliability of the scale.

Questions 7 through 10 are multiple choice. Select the correct answer from the options that follow each question.

7. You are investigating the role of physical activity in heart disease, and your data suggest a protective effect. While presenting your findings, a colleague asks whether you have thought about confounders, such as factor X. Under which of the following conditions could this factor have confounded your interpretation of the data?
   a. It is a risk factor for some other disease, but not heart disease.
   b. It is a risk factor associated with the physical activity measure and heart disease.
   c. It is part of the causal pathway by which physical activity affects heart disease.
   d. It has caused a lack of follow-up of test subjects.
   e. It may have blinded your study.

8. Surgeons at hospital A report that the mortality rate at the end of a one-year follow-up after a new coronary bypass procedure is 15%. At hospital B, the surgeons report a one-year mortality rate of 8% after the same procedure. Before concluding that the surgeons at hospital B had vastly superior skill, which of the following possible confounding factors would you examine?
   a. the severity (stage) of disease of the patients at the two hospitals at baseline
   b. the start of the one-year follow-up at both hospitals (after operation vs. after discharge)
   c. differences in postoperative care at the two hospitals
   d. equality of follow-up for mortality
   e. all of the above

9. Which of the following is *not* a method to control for the effects of confounding?
   a. randomization
   b. stratification
   c. matching
   d. blinding

10. The strategy that will *not* help reduce selection bias is:
    a. development of an explicit case definition
    b. the use of incentives to encourage high participation
    c. a standardized protocol for structured interviews
    d. enrollment of all cases in a defined time and region

References

1. Last JM, ed. *A Dictionary of Epidemiology,* 3rd ed. New York, NY: Oxford University Press; 1995.
2. Martini MC, Campbell DR, Gross MD, Grandits GA, Potter JD, Slavin JL. Plasma carotenoids as biomarkers of vegetable intake: the University of Minnesota Cancer Prevention Research Unit Feeding Studies. *Cancer Epidemiol Biomark Prev.* 1995;4:491–496.
3. Berenson GS, McMahan CA, Voors AW, et al. *Cardiovascular Risk Factors in Children: The Early Natural History of Atherosclerosis and Essential Hypertension.* New York, NY: Oxford University Press; 1980.
4. Greenland S. Response and follow-up bias in cohort studies. *Am J Epidemiol.* 1977;106:184–187.
5. Folsom AR, Kaye SA, Potter JD, et al. Association of incident carcinoma of the endometrium with body weight and fat distribution in older women: early findings of the Iowa Women's Health Study. *Cancer Res.* 1989;49:6828–6831.
6. Bisgard KM, Folsom AR, Hong C-P, Sellers TA. Mortality and cancer rates in nonrespondents to a prospective study of older women: 5-year follow-up. *Am J Epidemiol.* 1994;139:990–1000.
7. Sackett DL. Bias in analytic research. *J Chronic Dis.* 1979;32:51–63.
8. National Cancer Institute. NCI promotes proven benefits of mammography. *News & Features.* Fall 1997. Available at: http://www.nih.gov/news/nf/womenshealth/2.html.
9. Vargas AM, Sellers TA, Kaye SA, et al. Mammography utilization patterns in older women. Unpublished manuscript.
10. Susser M. *Causal Thinking in the Health Sciences.* New York, NY: Oxford University Press; 1973.
11. Rothman KJ. *Modern Epidemiology.* Boston, MA: Little, Brown; 1986.
12. Rothman KJ. A pictorial representation of confounding in epidemiologic studies. *J Chronic Dis.* 1975;28:101–108.
13. Buechley R, Key C, Morris D, et al. Altitude and ischemic heart disease in tricultural New Mexico: an example of confounding. *Am J Epidemiol.* 1979;109:663–666.
14. Kabat GC, Wynder EJ. Body mass index and lung cancer risk. *Am J Epidemiol.* 1992;135:769–774.
15. Knekt P, Heliovaara M, Rissanen A, et al. Leanness and lung cancer risk. *Int J Cancer.* 1991;49:208–213.
16. Rigotti NA. Cigarette smoking and body weight. *N Engl J Med.* 1989;320:931–933.
17. Drinkard CR, Sellers TA, Potter JD, et al. Association of body mass index and body fat distribution with risk of lung cancer in older women. *Am J Epidemiol.* 1995;142:600–607.

18. Ross RK, Paganini-Hill A, Randolph J, Gerkins V, Henderson BE. Analgesics, cigarette smoking, and other risk factors for cancer of the renal pelvis and ureter. *Cancer Res.* 1989;49:1045–1048.

19. Potter JD, Sellers TA, Folsom AR, McGovern PG. Alcohol, beer and lung cancer in postmenopausal women: the Iowa Women's Health Study. *Ann Epidemiol.* 1992;2:587–595.

20. Mantel N, Haenszel W. Statistical aspects of the analysis of data from retrospective studies of disease. *J Natl Cancer Inst.* 1959;22:719–748.

21. Begg CB, Berlin JA. Publication bias and dissemination of clinical research. *J Natl Cancer Inst.* 1989;81:107–115.

22. Stern JM, Simes RJ. Publication bias: evidence of delayed publication in a cohort study of clinical research projects. *Br Med J.* 1997;315:640–645.

23. Ioannidis JP. Effect of the statistical significance of results on the time to completion and publication of randomized efficacy trials. *JAMA.* 1998;279:281–286.

24. LeLorier J, Gregoire G, Benhaddad A, Lapierre J, Derderian F. Discrepancies between meta-analyses and subsequent large randomized, controlled trials. *N Engl J Med.* 1997;337:536–542.

25. Cook DJ, Guyatt GH, Ryan G, et al. Should unpublished data be included in meta-analyses? Current convictions and controversies. *JAMA.* 1993;269:2749–2753.

26. Dickersin K. The existence of publication bias and risk factors for its occurrence. *JAMA.* 1990;263:1385–1389.

Screening for Disease in the Community

Introduction

The public health field has increasingly recognized the importance of screening programs for the secondary prevention of morbidity and mortality. The effort to control diseases by early detection through screening has led to a basic change in the nature of medical practice from an exclusive focus upon a small number of ill persons to a targeting of large numbers of asymptomatic persons.[1] Screening programs for coronary heart disease risk factors have elicited the public's awareness of hypertension control and dietary components of hypercholesterolemia. Breast cancer screening by mammography for early malignancies may contribute to the high five-year survival rates for this cancer site. According to research findings, breast cancer screening is efficacious for women 50 years of age and older. Exhibit 11-1 describes one opinion regarding the current debate over the effectiveness of screening women who are in the 40- to 49-year-old group. This chapter discusses screening for disease in the population, including reliability and validity of measures, concepts and terminology of screening, sensitivity and specificity, and positive and negative predictive values.

Screening for Disease

A tenet of public health is that primary prevention of disease is the best approach. If all cases of disease cannot be prevented, however, then the next best strategy is early detection of disease in asymptomatic, apparently healthy individuals. Screening can be defined as the presumptive identification of unrecognized disease or defects by the application of tests, examinations, or other procedures that can be applied rapidly. The qualifier *presumptive* is included in the definition to emphasize the preliminary nature; diagnostic confirmation is required, usually with the benefit of more thorough clinical examination and additional tests. Some

EXHIBIT 11-1

Should Women Aged 40 Through 49 Years Receive Routine Mammography Screening?

One of the more remarkable aspects of the efforts to promote breast cancer screening has been the influence of rigorously conducted research. From an epidemiologic standpoint, the sequence of events could not have been better orchestrated.

In the 1950s and early 1960s, mammography emerged as a procedure that could lead to the detection of breast cancer at an earlier stage of the disease than could be detected in general clinical practice. This raised the question of whether mammography could be an effective screening tool when applied in the population at large. . . .

The HIP trial (initiated in 1963 at the Health Insurance Plan of Greater New York with contract support from the National Cancer Institute) enrolled women aged 40 through 64 years for annual screening; the control group continued to receive usual care.[2]

Thirty years of randomized controlled trials, diverse in content and design, have been conducted in various parts of the world.[3] . . . Case-control and quasi-experimental studies have added to the information about the value of mammography. During the 1970s, the Breast Cancer Detection Demonstration Project in the United States demonstrated that mammography screening had increased the capability to detect breast cancer early among young and older women; additional improvements in mammography have occurred since then. . . .

. . . guidelines from the National Cancer Institute (NCI), American Cancer Society, and other organizations . . . specify mammography screening every year or two for women aged 40 through 49 years and every year for women aged 50 years and older, and clinical breast examinations every year for all women aged 40 and older. . . . The results of the randomized controlled trials suggest that the guidelines should be changed.

One might best summarize the current situation by using the data from randomized controlled trials presented at the International Workshop on Screening for Breast Cancer in February 1993.[4] The task force charged with drawing conclusions that might affect screening guidelines found as follows: . . . The benefits of mammography screening for women aged 40

continues

EXHIBIT 11-1 *continued*

through 49 years are uncertain; the evidence from trials is "consistent in showing no benefit 5–7 years after entry (to screening), an uncertain, and, if present, marginal benefit at 10 to 12 years." In short, the value of mass mammography screening at these ages is judged to be questionable on the basis of currently available information. . . .

The NCI statement that was released in early December 1993, "Updating the Guidelines for Breast Cancer Screening," calls attention to the controversy about routine screening mammography for women aged 40 through 49 and the lack of convincing evidence on any reduction of breast cancer mortality related to screening in this age group. . . . New guidelines would emphasize mammography screening at 1- to 2-year intervals for women aged 50 years and older; for asymptomatic women aged 40 through 49 years, the guidelines would emphasize that patients and health care professionals should together discuss the uncertainty of the benefits, along with the risk factors, of mammography screening.

There will be voices raised against a change that focuses routine mammography screening on women aged 50 and older, just as there are challenges (albeit less frequent) to screening at any age. But in making decisions on mammography screening for millions of women, we need to continue to rely on evidence from research, and the uncertainty of the available evidence for women aged 40 through 49 calls for a change in guidelines that excludes these women from programs for mass, routine screening with mammography. ■

Source: Reprinted from S Shapiro. The call for change in breast cancer screening guidelines. *American Journal of Public Health,* vol 84, No 1, pp 10–11, with permission of the American Public Health Association, © 1994.

screening programs are conducted on an ad hoc basis to screen interested and concerned individuals for specific health problems, such as hypertension, cervical cancer, or sickle-cell disease. An example of an ad hoc screening program would be administration of a free thyroid test (serum level of thyroxine) to passersby in a shopping center or members of a senior citizens center.[5] Other screening programs may be applied on a mass basis to almost all individuals in the population; an example is screening for phenylketonuria (PKU) among all neonates.

It should be noted that screening differs from diagnosis, which is the process of confirming an actual case of a disease.[6,7] As a result of diagnosis, medical intervention, if appropriate, is initiated. Diagnostic tests are used in follow-up of positive screening test results (e.g., phenylalanine loading test in children positive on PKU screening) or directly for screening (e.g., fetal karyotyping in prenatal screening for Down's syndrome). For example, if a thyroid test is administered to determine an exact cause of a patient's illness, it would then be a diagnostic test.[5] The thyroid test also could be a screening test, however, as will be demonstrated subsequently.

Multiphasic Screening

Although screening programs can be restricted to early detection of a single disease, a more cost-effective approach is to screen for more than one disease. Multiphasic screening is defined as the use of two or more screening tests together among large groups of people.[8] The multiphasic screening examination may be administered as a preemployment physical, and successfully passing the examination may be a necessary condition for employment in the organization. As a perquisite (benefit) of employment, some large companies repeat the screening examination on an annual basis and direct suggestive findings to the employee's own physician while maintaining confidentiality of the results. Typical multiphasic screening programs assess risk factor status as well as individual and family history of illness, and they also collect physiologic and health measurements. Multiphasic screening also is a cornerstone of health maintenance organizations, such as Kaiser Permanente and Group Health.

Mass Screening and Selective Screening

Mass screening (also known as population screening) refers to screening on a large scale of total population groups, regardless of any a priori information as to whether the individuals are members of a high-risk subset of the population. Selective screening, sometimes referred to as targeted screening, is applied to subsets of the population at high risk for disease or certain conditions as the result of family history, age, or environmental exposures. It is likely to result in the greatest yield of true cases and represents the most economical utilization of screening measures. For example, screening tests for Tay-Sachs disease might be applied to individuals of Jewish extraction whose ancestors originated in Eastern Europe because this group has a higher frequency of the genetic alteration.

Mass Health Examinations

There are several other activities that are somewhat similar to screening but differ in one or more critical areas. Population or epidemiologic surveys aim to elucidate the natural history, prevalence, incidence, and duration of health conditions in defined populations.[8] The purpose of such surveys is to gain new knowledge regarding the distribution and determinants of diseases in carefully selected populations. Thus, they are not considered screening because they imply no health benefits to the participants.[9]

Epidemiologic surveillance, defined in Chapter 1, aims at the protection of community health through case detection and intervention (e.g., tuberculosis control).[10] It refers to the continuous observation of the trends and distribution of disease incidence in a community or other population over time to prevent disease or injury.[11] Sources of data for surveillance may consist of morbidity and mortality reports, for example, those reported by the Centers for Disease Control and Prevention. Surveillance activities have detected an increase in tuberculosis in the United States as well as an increase in measles cases; the latter disease was brought under control by stepped-up immunization of children. Surveillance programs are used for detection and control of conditions ranging from infectious diseases to injuries to chronic diseases.

Case finding, also referred to as opportunistic screening, is the utilization of screening tests for detection of conditions unrelated to the patient's chief complaint.[5,12] An example would be administration of a screen for colon cancer to a patient who came to a physician complaining of pharyngitis.

Appropriate Situations for Screening Tests and Programs

A number of criteria must be considered carefully before a decision is made to implement a screening program.[8] Although the ideal situation is one in which all criteria are satisfied, numerous examples can be cited to illustrate how screening programs that violate one or more of these issues can still be extremely valuable (Exhibit 11-2).

Social

Of major importance is the magnitude of the health problem for which screening is being considered. Magnitude is relevant in a number of dimensions: to the community, in terms of economics, and medically. From the community perspective, the disease or outcome must be viewed as a major health problem. This means that there is general consensus that the health problem is of sufficiently high priority as to justify the commitment of resources to implement and carry out the program.

Appropriate Situations for Screening

Social: The health problem should be important for the individual and the community. Diagnostic follow-up and intervention should be available to all who require them. There should be a favorable cost-benefit ratio. Public acceptance must be high.

Scientific: The natural history of the condition should be adequately understood. Identification should occur during prepathogenesis with sufficient lead time (see text for definition of *lead time*). There is sound case definition in addition to a policy regarding whom to treat as patients. A knowledge base exists for the efficacy of prevention and the occurrence of side effects. The prevalence of the disease or condition is high.

Ethical: The provider initiates the service and, therefore, should have evidence that the program can alter the natural history of the condition in a significant proportion of those screened. Suitable, acceptable tests for screening and diagnosis of the condition as well as acceptable, effective methods of prevention are available. ■

Source: Data are from JMG Wilson and F Jungner. Principles and practice of screening for disease, *Public Health Papers,* No 34, World Health Organization, 1968; and from AL Cochrane and WW Holland. Validation of screening procedures. *British Medical Bulletin,* vol 27, pp 3–8, Churchill Livingstone, 1971.

Furthermore, acceptance of the program by the public must be high. For example, an effective screening test for a major health problem will not necessarily result in an effective screening program if the public refuses to participate.

Although it may be tempting to do so, one must not automatically assume that screening programs are beneficial. Early detection efforts, if they are to be successful over the long run, must be cost-effective. Thus, one must consider the costs of the test itself, the costs of follow-up examinations, and the costs of treatments avoided. The most clear-cut evidence of cost-effectiveness manifests itself when the cost of the program itself is more than offset by the savings of more expensive treatment that would have been necessary had the condition advanced to a more serious stage. Oftentimes this may not be the case, however, and one must consider as benefits improvements in quality of life and the value of years of life saved. Negative costs should be considered also: There are emotional costs to healthy individuals who are falsely labeled as ill by a screening test and emotional costs to individuals (and their loved ones) who are diagnosed early and yet die quickly anyway.

An obvious determinant of the cost-benefit ratio of a screening program is the current cost to the medical community in the absence of screening. How much money is being spent to treat individuals with the disease? How many hospital beds are being utilized? What is the number of health personnel expended on the problem? Diseases and conditions that are costly to treat may still be considered for early detection even if the scientific justification for screening is weaker than for a disease that represents less of a medical burden.

Scientific

Early detection efforts are most likely to be successful when the natural history of the disease is known. This knowledge permits identification of early stages of disease and appropriate biologic markers of progression. For example, it is known that individuals with high cholesterol and high blood pressure are at increased risk for coronary heart disease. Because these risk factors precede onset of an acute myocardial infarction, identification of such high-risk individuals may lead to medical intervention (changes in diet, exercise, weight loss, or use of drugs) to prevent the disease. This example illustrates that there also should be good tests (screening and diagnostic) to measure blood pressure and blood cholesterol and that effective treatment should be available.

Ethical

It is most desirable to implement screening programs for diseases that, when diagnosed early, have their natural history altered—that is, for which effective treatment is available. Note, however, that screening is sometimes done for diseases for which effective treatment is not available. For example, we are yet without a cure for acquired immune deficiency syndrome. Screening is nonetheless important to prevent spread of the disease from infected to uninfected individuals and to improve the prognosis of those who may be affected. For those diseases for which effective treatments are available, it is important to consider the capacity of the medical community to handle the increased number of individuals requiring definitive diagnoses. Suppose a volunteer organization decides to offer a free health screening for high cholesterol at the local community center and that 10,000 citizens attend. Suppose further that 1,000 citizens are found to have high cholesterol. These individuals are mailed a letter informing them of their results with the suggestion to see their physician for further evaluation. A number of ethical issues can be envisioned. What if physicians in the local medical community are unable to accommodate the sudden increased demand for their services? What if these individuals lack medical insurance and have no physician?

Characteristics of a Good Screening Test

There are five attributes of a good screening test: simple, rapid, inexpensive, safe, and acceptable[8,9,13]:

1. *Simple:* The test should be easy to learn and perform. One that can be administered by nonphysician medical personnel will necessarily cost less than one that requires years of medical training.
2. *Rapid:* The test should not take long to administer, and the results should be available soon. The amount of time required to screen an individual is directly related to the success of the program: If a screening test requires only five minutes out of a person's schedule, it is likely to be perceived as being more valuable than one that requires an hour or more. Furthermore, immediate feedback is better than a test in which results may not be available for weeks or months. Results of a blood pressure screening are usually known immediately; results of a screen for high cholesterol must await laboratory analysis.
3. *Inexpensive:* As discussed earlier, cost-benefit is an important criterion to consider in the evaluation of screening programs. The lower the cost of a screening test, the more likely it is that the overall program will be cost beneficial.
4. *Safe:* The screening test should not carry potential harm to screenees.
5. *Acceptable:* The test should be acceptable to the target group. An effective protocol has been developed to screen for testicular cancer, but acceptance rates among men have not been as high as for a similar procedure, mammography, among women.

Evaluation of Screening Tests

Recall that the purpose of a screening test is to classify individuals as to whether they are likely to have disease or be disease free. To do this, a measuring instrument or combination of instruments is required. Examples of such instruments are clinical laboratory tests, a fever thermometer, weighing scales, and standardized questionnaires. The preceding section made no mention of how well the screening test should actually work. That is not to imply that this is not an important issue. Rather, it is a more complex subject that first requires introduction of several new concepts. The first and second of these concepts are reliability and validity.

Reliability types:
- Repeated measurements
- Internal consistency
- Interjudge

Validity types:
- Content
- Criterion-referenced
  - Predictive
  - Concurrent
- Construct

Reliability

Reliability, also known as precision, is the ability of a measuring instrument to give consistent results on repeated trials. According to Morrison, reliability of a test refers to "its capacity to give the same result—positive or negative, whether correct or incorrect—on repeated application in a person with a given level of disease. Reliability depends on the variability in the manifestation on which the test is based (e.g., short-term fluctuation in blood pressure), and on the variability in the method of measurement and the skill with which it is made."[1(p10)]

Repeated measurement reliability refers to the degree of consistency between or among repeated measurements of the same individual on more than one occasion. For example, if one were to measure the height of an adult at different times, one would expect to observe similar results. That is because, in part, one's true value of height is relatively constant (although we are actually slightly shorter at the end of the day than we were at the beginning!). There also might be slight errors in measurement from one occasion to another, however—some overestimates and some underestimates. Although one might expect to measure height reliably, other measures, such as blood pressure, may be much more unreliable than height. Technicians' skills in the measurement of blood pressure, slight variations in the calibration of the manometer cuff, and variability in subjects' true blood pressure levels from one occasion to another would affect the reliability of blood pressure measurements.

Internal consistency reliability evaluates the degree of agreement or homogeneity within a questionnaire measure of an attitude, personal characteristic, or psychologic attribute. For example, a researcher may be interested in studying the relationship between general anxiety level and peptic ulcer. A multi-item paper-and-pencil measure for general anxiety may be utilized in the research. The Kuder-Richardson reliability coefficient measures the internal consistency reliability of this type of measure.[14] It is based on the average intercorrelation of a set of items in a multi-item index. Chronbach's α coefficient is used also to measure internal consistency reliability; an α value of 0.7 or greater is believed to indicate satisfactory reliability and suggests that a set of items is measuring a common dimension.[15] These two reliability measures are particularly applicable to epidemiologic research that uses survey measures, such as interviews or self-report questionnaires.

Interjudge reliability refers to reliability assessments derived from agreement among trained experts. The ratings of psychiatrists in psychiatric research, for example, may be used to measure an individual's degree of psychiatric impairment. To obtain an estimate of the reliability of the rating procedure, the average percentage of agreement of the judges who are rating an attribute may be calculated.

There are several ways to express the reliability (precision) of a set of measurements.[13] One is to obtain repeated measurements of an attribute for a single person and then obtain the standard deviation of the measurements, known as the standard error of measurement. A second is the reliability coefficient, which is an indicator of repeated measurement reliability. It is a correlation coefficient that quantifies the degree of agreement between measurements taken on two different occasions.

Validity

Also known as accuracy, validity is the ability of a measuring instrument to give a true measure (i.e., how well it measures what it purports to measure).[16] Validity can be evaluated only if there exists an accepted and independent method for confirming the test measurement. Validity is an important component of epidemiologic research, including areas outside screening. Variations on the theme of validity are presented in the next few sections. The issues discussed extend beyond the role of validity in screening for a disease. However, they may be applicable to screening for high-risk behaviors.

Content validity is often used to measure the validity of survey instruments or paper-and-pencil measures. Content validity "refers to the degree to which a measure covers the range of meanings included within the concept."[17(p133)] It concerns the extent to which the items in a questionnaire seem to be valid for measuring the domain of the phenomenon that they are supposed to measure; that is, the measurement includes and fully covers all the aspects of the dimension being measured. For example, the content validity of a test of mechanical aptitude would measure whether the test contains items that cover a full range of mechanical abilities. This type of validity also is referred to as rational or logical validity.[13]

Criterion-referenced validity generally refers to validity that is found by correlating a measure with an external criterion of the entity being assessed.[7] The two types of criterion-referenced validity are predictive validity and concurrent validity. Predictive validity denotes the ability of a measure to predict some attribute or characteristic in the future. To illustrate this type of validity, consider the association between type A behavior and coronary heart disease. Researchers attempted to demonstrate the validity of the type A measure through its positive correlations with future incidence of coronary heart disease. The future outcome that was being predicted is known as a validity criterion. Another term for this type of validity is *empirical* or *statistical validity*. Similar to predictive validity is concurrent validity, which refers to validity measurement by correlating a measure with an alternative measure of the same phenomenon taken at the same point in time; typically the concurrent validating criterion is more cumbersome than the new measure. Much work has been devoted to self-administered measures of mental health characteristics for use in epidemiologic studies. An example would be the validation of a self-administered depressive symptoms questionnaire against the criterion of psychiatric diagnosis.

Construct validity refers to the degree to which the measurement agrees with the theoretical concept being investigated.[7] Construct validity involves the confirmation of a theoretical construct, such as anxiety. In designing a paper-and-pencil test of anxiety, the investigator would first need to specify what types of behavior are associated with anxiety. Then the investigator would need to compose items that measure these behaviors and demonstrate that they are consistent with a theoretical conception of anxiety. Construct validity is concerned primarily with the meaning of the items in a measure[14] and whether the measure is associated logically with other variables specified in a theoretical framework.[17] Construct validity is important to epidemiologic measures, such as scales of depressive symptomatology.

Interrelationships Between Reliability and Validity

Figure 11-1 is designed to assist the reader in differentiating between reliability and validity and also in understanding how the two terms are interrelated. In part A, the periphery of the target shows a measure that is highly reliable but invalid. The bullets have hit the target in the same general area (i.e., have clustered around

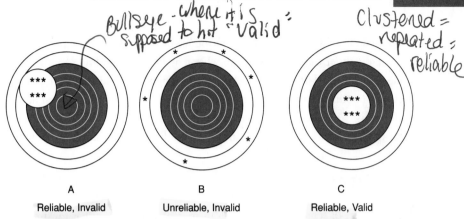

[handwritten annotations: "Bullseye - where it is supposed to hit = valid", "Clustered = repeated = reliable"]

A	B	C
Reliable, Invalid	Unreliable, Invalid	Reliable, Valid

FIGURE 11-1 Graphic representation of reliability and validity

the same general area) but have missed the bull's-eye of the target. Part B of the figure shows a measure that is neither reliable nor valid. The bullets have scattered randomly around the target and have not consistently hit the bull's-eye. Part C of the figure illustrates a measure that is both reliable and valid. The bullets have consistently hit the bull's-eye and also cluster in the same general area. Thus, it is possible for a measure to be highly reliable but invalid. Reliability means only that the same measurement results are being reproduced on repeated occasions. Conversely, however, it is not possible for a measure to be valid but unreliable. If the measure consistently hits the bull's-eye on repeated occasions, then the measure is, by definition, both reliable and valid.

Sources of Unreliability and Invalidity

[handwritten annotation: "halo effect = influenced by perception, previous ideas, traits, etc."]

Measurement bias refers to constant errors that are introduced by a faulty measuring device and tend to reduce the reliability of measurements. For example, a blood pressure manometer may be miscalibrated so that it consistently underestimates or overestimates true blood pressure values. Psychiatrists and clinicians also might introduce measurement biases in their judgments, which would be revealed if one rater had an average group of judgments that was higher than the mean ratings of other judges.

The halo effect is another kind of bias that affects the validity of questionnaire measurements. An illustration is completion of a checklist evaluation of an employee by a supervisor who has formed a general opinion about the employee. The supervisor might tend to evaluate all items of behavior in the same general direction without carefully rating specific aspects of the employee's behavior.

Social desirability effects are biases introduced when a respondent answers questions in a manner that corresponds to what may be the prevailing socially desired mode of behavior. For example, teenage boys might respond to an interviewer's questions about sexual behavior by exaggerating the frequency of sexual activity because this would be a socially desirable response among some peer groups. The factor of social desirability tends to affect the validity of questionnaire responses.

Measures of the Validity of Screening Tests

In the context of screening, there are four measures of validity that must be considered: sensitivity, specificity, predictive value (+), and predictive value (−). Figure 11-2 represents a sample of individuals who have been examined with both a screening test for disease (rows) and a definitive diagnostic test (columns). Thus, we are able to determine how well the screening test performed in identifying individuals with disease.

- *Sensitivity:* the ability of the test to identify correctly all screened individuals who actually have the disease. In Figure 11-2, a total of a + c individuals were determined to have the disease, according to some established gold standard, a definitive diagnosis that has been determined by biopsy, surgery, autopsy, or other method[5] and has been accepted as the standard. Sensitivity is defined as the number of true positives divided by the sum of true positives and false negatives. Suppose that in a sample of 1,000 individuals there were 120 who actually had the disease. If the screening test correctly identified all 120 cases, the sensitivity would be 100%. If the screening test was unable to identify all individuals who should be referred for definitive diagnoses, then sensitivity would be less than 100%.

- *Specificity:* the ability of the test to identify only nondiseased individuals who actually do not have the disease. It is defined as the number of true negatives divided by the sum of false positives and true negatives. If a test is not specific, then individuals who do not actually have the disease will be referred for additional diagnostic testing.

- *Predictive value (+):* the proportion of individuals screened positive by the test who actually have the disease. In Figure 11-2, a total of a + b individuals were screened positive by the test. Predictive value (+) is the proportion a/(a + b) who actually have the condition, according to the gold standard.

- *Predictive value (−):* an analogous measure for those screened negative by the test; it is designated by the formula d/(c + d).

FIGURE 11-2 Fourfold table for classification of screening test results. Definitions: True positives are individuals who both have been screened positive and truly have the condition; false positives are individuals who have been screened positive but do not have the condition; false negatives are individuals screened negative who truly have the condition; and true negatives are individuals who both have been screened negative and do not have the condition.

Note that the only time these measures can be estimated is when the same group of individuals has been examined using both the screening test and the gold standard. According to McCunney:

> False positive results are inherent in most laboratory reference limits, simply because of the manner by which those limits are established. People whose results are beyond 2 standard deviations from the mean are by definition "abnormal." In general, 1 out of 20 "well people" have an abnormal test result—without evidence of illness . . . the rates of false positive results reported from a variety of health fairs [range from approximately 3% for blood chemistry tests for iron to over 20% for triglycerides].[18(p299)]

The accuracy of a screening test is found by the following formula: $(a + d)/(a + b + c + d)$. Accuracy measures the degree of agreement between the screening test and the gold standard. A sample calculation for accuracy as well as sensitivity, specificity, and predictive value is shown in Exhibit 11-3.

Effects of Prevalence of Disease on Screening Test Results

Sensitivity and specificity are stable properties of screening tests and, as a result, are unaffected by the prevalence of a disease. Predictive value, however, is very much affected by the prevalence of the condition being screened. Many screening tests are validated upon groups that have a contrived prevalence of disease (e.g., approximately 50%). This prevalence would usually be higher than what is found in clinical practice.[5]

In Table 11-1, the cells of a 2 by 2 table have been arranged horizontally. Sensitivity and specificity are stable properties of screening tests that remain constant across groups that have different prevalences of disease. The data from Exhibit 11-3 have been transposed to row A. Sensitivity and specificity were previously calculated to be 94.1% and 89.8%, respectively. The prevalence of disease was 51.0%. In row B the prevalence of disease is 10.0%. The number of cases of disease $(a + c)$ in row B is found by multiplying $500 \times 0.10 = 50$. The number of true positives (a) is the number of cases of disease multiplied by the sensitivity of the test: $50 \times 0.94 = 47$. The number of true negatives (d) is the number of diagnosed negatives multiplied by the specificity of the test: $450 \times 0.90 = 405$. The numbers of false negatives (c) and false positives (b) are found by subtraction (3 and 45, respectively). For row B, the predictive value (+) is $[a/(a + b)] \times 100 = 51.1\%$, and the predictive value (−) is $[d/(c + d)] \times 100 = 99.3\%$. Thus, when the values for sensitivity and specificity found in row A are applied to the data in row B, among a group of people who have a 10% prevalence of disease,

EXHIBIT 11-3

Sample Calculation of Sensitivity, Specificity and Predictive Value

Suppose the following data are obtained from a screening test applied to 500 people:

Screening test result	Condition according to gold standard		
	Positive	**Negative**	**Total**
Positive	a = 240	b = 25	a + b = 265
Negative	c = 15	d = 220	c + d = 235
Total	a + c = 255	b + d = 245	a+b+c+d = 500

Sensitivity = a/(a + c) = (240/255) × 100 = 94.1%
Specificity = d/(b + d) = (220/245) × 100 = 89.8%
Predictive Value (+) = a/(a + b) = (240/265) × 100 = 90.6%
Predictive Value (−) = d/(c + d) = (220/235) × 100 = 93.6%
Prevalence = (a + c)/(a + b + c + d) = (255/500) × 100 = 51.0%
Accuracy = (a + d)/(a + b + c + d) = (460/500) × 100 = 92.0%

the predictive value (+) decreases to 51.1% and the predictive value (−) increases to about 99%.

When the prevalence of a disease falls, the predictive value (+) falls and the predictive value (−) rises. The clinical implications of low predictive value (+) are that any individual who has a positive screening test would have low probability of having the disease; an invasive diagnostic procedure would probably not be warranted for this patient. Table 11-1 demonstrates the effects of changing the prevalence of disease upon predictive values. When the prevalence of disease drops from about 51% to 10%, the predictive value (+) drops from about 91% to 51%, and the predictive value (−) increases from about 94% to 99%.

Table 11-1 Effects of Disease Prevalence on the Predictive Value of a Screening Test

	Cell Values				Total		No. of Cases of Disease	Predictive	Predictive
Row	a	b	c	d	(a+b+c+d)	Prevalence	(a+c)	Value (+)	Value (−)
A	240	25	15	220	500	51.0%	255	90.6%	93.6%
B	47	45	3	405	500	10.0%	50	51.1%	99.3%

Relationship Between Sensitivity and Specificity

Figure 11-3 illustrates the relationship between sensitivity and specificity. When the screening test result is a continuous or ordered variable with several levels, then the choice for a cut point that discriminates optimally between suspected diseased and normal individuals is a trade-off. Figure 11-3 demonstrates the effects of choosing various cut points. The figure shows a hypothetical distribution of trait values (e.g., fasting blood glucose, an indicator of diabetes) for normals and a distribution curve for the diseased population that overlaps the curve for the normal population. For example, fasting blood glucose levels may approximate the normal distribution with a mean of 100 mg/dL. A subject may have an elevated glucose level in the high range for a population (e.g., 120 mg/dL) and not be diabetic. Some diabetic individuals who are at the lower end of the curve for the diseased group also may have glucose levels in the high normal range. Thus, the two distributions may overlap: Some nondiseased individuals may have elevated glucose levels, and some diseased individuals may have glucose levels in the lower ranges for the abnormal group. The cut point may be set at B to maximize both sensitivity and specificity. If the cut point is moved to A by lowering the specific blood glucose level that is to be classified as abnormal, almost all the individuals who have the disease will be screened as positive, and sensitivity will approach 100%. Specificity will be lowered because more of the nondiseased individuals will be classified as diseased. By moving the cut point to C, which represents a higher blood glucose level than point A or B, specificity will be increased at the expense of sensitivity.

Another example of establishing a cut point to distinguish between diseased and nondiseased people is setting the referral criteria for screening for glaucoma.[19] By using the criterion of 15 mm Hg intraocular pressure, the sensitivity of the screening test would be high, and few persons with glaucoma would be missed. At the same time, many persons who did not have the disease would be incorrectly classified. If a high referral point were selected (e.g., 33 mm Hg), the majority of those without glaucoma would not be referred, but many with the disease would be missed by the screening test. Thus, this example demonstrates that sensitivity and specificity are complementary. "The key to a successful screening is to balance the referral criteria so that both the overreferrals and underreferrals are minimized."[19(p360)]

In summary, if one wishes to improve sensitivity, the cut point used to classify individuals as diseased should be moved farther in the range of the nondiseased.

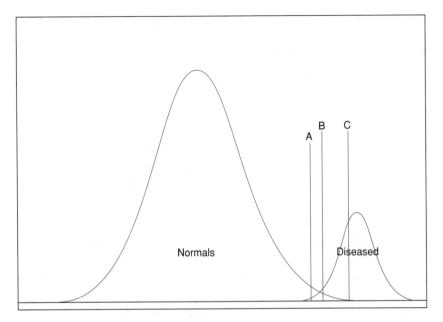

FIGURE 11-3 Interrelationship between sensitivity and specificity

To improve specificity, the cut point should be moved farther in the range typically associated with the disease. There are a number of additional procedures that can improve both sensitivity and specificity:

- *Retrain screeners:* If the test requires human assessment (e.g., blood pressure readings), then improving the precision of measurement through additional training sessions will reduce the amount of misclassification.
- *Recalibrate screening instrument:* For those tests that utilize technology (e.g., a weighing device or a densitometer), it may be possible to reduce the amount of imprecision through refinement of the methodology.
- *Utilize a different test:* In some situations there may be more than one way to measure the outcome of interest. Suppose there are two laboratory assays available to quantify serum cholesterol. If one assay performs poorly (low reliability and validity), it may be possible to replace it with a better assay.
- *Utilize more than one test:* Because of the variability in some measures, it is easy to misclassify an individual as high or low. By taking more than one measure of blood pressure and averaging the results, the ability to label an individual correctly as hypertensive will be improved, resulting in improved measures of sensitivity and specificity.

Evaluation of Screening Programs

Despite the intuitive appeal of screening programs, their utility should never be assumed. Rather, it is imperative that they be evaluated with the same rigor used to identify risk factors in the pathogenesis of disease. The ideal design is a randomized controlled trial. Under this approach, subjects are randomized either to receive the new screening test or program or to receive usual care. If the disease of interest is fatal, then the appropriate end point would be differences in mortality between the two groups. For nonfatal diseases, such as cataracts, differences in incidence between the screened and nonscreened populations should be estimated. Another approach, although less rigorous, is to conduct ecologic time trend studies in geographic areas with and without screening programs. Finally, the case-control method can be applied also: Cases are fatal (or likely to be fatal) cases of the disease, controls are nonfatal cases of the disease, and the exposure is participation in a screening program. Regardless of the approach that is taken, evaluation of screening programs is subject to several sources of bias that have not been described before. Figure 11-4 depicts the natural history of disease in relation to the time of diagnosis.

Suppose the disease begins at time A and results in death at time D. A case detected as the result of screening may be picked up at time B, whereas a case that is picked up as a result of clinical signs and symptoms may not be detected until time C.

- *Lead time bias:* the perception that the screen-detected case has a longer survival simply because the disease was identified earlier in the natural history of the disease. Thus, although these two individuals had identical dates of onset and death, there is an apparent increase in survival for the screen-detected case. The extent of this bias is estimated as the difference between time periods B and C.
- *Length bias:* used particularly with respect to certain cancer screening programs. In particular, tumors that are detected by a screening program tend to be slower growing and hence have an inherently better prognosis than tumors that are more rapidly growing and are detected as a result of clinical manifestation.
- *Selection bias:* Although this topic has been covered earlier, it is particularly relevant to the evaluation of screening programs. In particular, individuals who are motivated enough to participate in screening programs may have

FIGURE 11-4 Natural history of disease in relation to time of diagnosis. C to D, survival time for unscreened case; B to D, survival time for screened case; B to C, lead time.

a different probability of disease (as a result of other healthy behaviors) than individuals who refuse participation.

In conclusion, the foregoing section has discussed a number of factors that need to be taken into account in the evaluation of screening tests. Indeed, many of the issues remain controversial, as noted in Exhibit 11-4 for the prostate-specific antigen test.

Issues in the Classification of Morbidity and Mortality

The central theme of this chapter has been screening for disease in the community and the related topics of reliability and validity of measurement. Schemes for the nomenclature and classification of disease are central to the reliable measurement of the outcome variable in epidemiologic research. The terms *nomenclature* and *classification* are defined as follows: A nomenclature is a highly specific set of terms for describing and recording clinical or pathologic diagnoses to classify ill persons into groups. A system of nomenclature must be extensive so that all conditions encountered by the practitioner in a particular health discipline can be recorded. Classification, in contrast, lends itself to the statistical compilation of groups of cases of disease by arranging disease entities into categories that share similar features.[20]

EXHIBIT 11-4

Controversies in Screening

As an example of why it is important to evaluate the potential outcomes of new screening modalities, consider the case of prostate-specific antigen (PSA). As a marker, PSA is potentially useful for early detection of prostate cancer (as a form of adenocarcinoma). In venous blood samples, PSA levels greater than 10 ng/mL are associated with a positive predictive value of 66% for adenocarcinoma. For PSA levels between 4 and 10 ng/mL, the positive predictive value for adenocarcinoma declines to approximately 24%.[21] There is a complementary increment in false negative rates. Consequently, such high false negative rates tend to correspond with demands for biopsies as definitive diagnoses. The establishment of age-specific reference ranges[22] represents one approach to improve sensitivity while holding specificity constant, with a corresponding effect on positive and negative predictive values.

Prostate cancer is a disease for which incidence rates at autopsy are much higher than incidence rates based on clinical diagnoses. Anywhere from 40% to 80% of 90-year-old men will have pathologic evidence of prostate cancer at death, even if they had never been diagnosed with the disease.[23] Among elderly men all forms of cancer are much more prevalent than among younger men. Clinical medicine is unable to resolve the ethical issue of which type of cancer men should die with versus die from. The importance for the distinction arises from the risks for complications associated with surgical treatment of prostate cancer. These risks, for example, impotence and incontinence, have significant effects on quality of life. Thus, it is important to consider the negative effects of screening (unnecessary treatment) as well as the positive. Moreover, screening may incur significant financial burdens for patients; by some estimates, an ultrasound-guided biopsy and pathologic examination of the tissue cost approximately $1,000 during the 1990s.[24]

Unfortunately, to date, no available data demonstrate that the use of PSA as a screening marker is unequivocally associated with decreased mortality. In addition, the widespread adoption of PSA since its introduction in the 1980s makes conduct of a randomized controlled clinical trial extremely difficult. Although such trials are now under way, decades will probably elapse before definitive answers are at hand.

continues

EXHIBIT 11-4 *continued*

> The controversies surrounding PSA argue for the utility of careful observational research. For example, Jacobsen et al.[25] studied the incidence of prostate cancer in Olmsted County, Minnesota, and concluded that the recent increases in prostate cancer incidence are due to increased utilization of PSA, and that early detection efforts may be effective in identifying more early-stage cancers. Recent downward trends in prostate cancer mortality are the first suggestive evidence that PSA might be achieving the desired ends of any early detection program. ▪

The classification systems used are in some cases purely arbitrary because they are determined by the function that is to be served by classification; nevertheless, all practitioners in a discipline need to have at their disposal a standardized system for classification of diseases. Many classification systems for diseases are theoretically possible; they might be based upon age, circumstance of onset, geographic location, or some other factor connected with the purpose for which they are to be used. The categories of disease should be general so that there will be a limited number of categories that take into account all the diseases that might be encountered. The use of general categories facilitates the epidemiologic study of disease phenomena by giving rise to groups of interrelated morbid conditions. The classifications of disease must be distinct so that a disease falls into only one category of the classification system. Each category of the classification system must refer to diseases that are sufficiently frequent to permit several cases of disease to fall into the category. Otherwise, there would be an excessively detailed list of categories to contain the range of morbid conditions. Finally, a well-devised classification system permits standardization across different agencies and even countries so that comparisons in morbidity and mortality from disease can be made.

Two types of criteria are used for the classification of ill persons: causal and manifestational.[20] It is possible to classify cases of disease according to a causal basis (e.g., tuberculosis or syphilis) or according to manifestation (e.g., affected anatomic site—hepatitis or breast cancer). Epidemiologic research relies primarily on manifestational criteria for classification in the hope that there will be a strong enough connection with causal factors to make possible etiologic studies.[20]

One example of a classification system is the *Diagnostic and Statistical Manual of Mental Disorders,* now in its fourth revision; it provides for standardization of the classification of psychiatric diagnoses.[26] A second example, which was introduced in Chapter 5 and is one of the most widely used systems for the classification of diseases, is the *International Statistical Classification of Diseases and Related Health Problems,* now in its tenth revision (ICD-10).[27] The ICD is sponsored by the World Health Organization (Collaborative Centers for Classification of Diseases). It is designed for varied uses: for both clinical and general epidemiologic purposes and for the evaluation of health care. The ICD-10 spans three volumes; volume 1 provides classification of diseases into three- and four-character levels (an alphanumeric coding scheme replaces the previous numeric one).

Conclusion

This chapter discussed terminology related to the quality of measures employed in epidemiology. Measurement is a crucial issue because even the most carefully designed study may yield spurious results if premised upon faulty measures. Some of the topics covered in this chapter were reliability and validity, screening for disease, and methods for the classification of diseases. Formulas and examples for calculation of sensitivity, specificity, and predictive value were provided. The effect of prevalence of disease upon predictive value was discussed also.

Study Questions and Exercises

1. Are you able to define the following?
    a. reliability
    b. validity
    c. precision
    d. accuracy
    e. sensitivity
    f. specificity
    g. predictive value (+) and predictive value (−)
2. What factors should govern the selection and use of a screening instrument by a health clinic?
3. What is the relationship between reliability and validity? Is it possible for a measure to be reliable and invalid? Conversely, is it possible for a measure to be unreliable and valid?

4. Assume that the fasting blood level of a lipid is normally distributed in the population of people who do not have disease "X." There is a smaller distribution curve of the fasting blood levels of this lipid, which also is normal in shape, for the population of persons who have disease "X," and the curve overlaps the upper end (right side) of the curve for people without the disease. Draw distribution curves for the diseased and nondiseased populations and discuss the effects upon sensitivity and specificity of setting the cut point for disease and nondisease at various positions on the two overlapping curves.

5. How does the predictive value of a screening test vary according to the prevalence of disease?

6. A serologic test is being devised to detect a hypothetical chronic disease. Three hundred individuals were referred to a laboratory for testing. One hundred diagnosed cases were among the 300. A serologic test yielded 200 positives, of which one-fourth were true positives. Calculate the sensitivity, specificity, and predictive value of this test. (*Hint:* After setting up the appropriate 2 by 2 table, find missing data by subtraction. The numbers for the cells should then correspond to the numbers shown in Appendix 11.)

7. A new test was compared with a gold standard measurement with the following results:

	Gold Standard	
New Test	+	−
+	18	2
−	8	72

What are the sensitivity and specificity?

8. Using the data from question 6, what is the predictive value (+) and the predictive value (−)?

9. A test-retest reliability study of the new test was conducted with the following results:

	Test	
Retest	+	−
+	80	9
−	8	3

What is the percentage agreement (accuracy)?

10. The prevalence of undetected diabetes in a population to be screened is approximately 1.5%, and it is assumed that 10,000 persons will be screened. The screening test will measure blood serum glucose content. A value of 180 mg% or higher is considered positive. The sensitivity and specificity associated with this screening test are 22.9% and 99.8%, respectively.
    a. What is the predictive value of a positive test?
    b. What is the predictive value of a negative test?

References

1. Morrison AS. *Screening in Chronic Disease.* New York, NY: Oxford University Press; 1985.
2. Shapiro S, Venet W, Strax P, Venet L. *Periodic Screening for Breast Cancer: The Health Insurance Plan Project and Its Sequelae, 1963-1986.* Baltimore, MD: Johns Hopkins University Press; 1988.
3. Hurley SF, Kaldor JM. The benefits and risks of mammographic screening for breast cancer. *Epidemiol Rev.* 1992;14:101–129.
4. Fletcher SW, Black W, Harris R, Rimer BK, Shapiro S. Report of the International Workshop on Screening for Breast Cancer. *J Natl Cancer Inst.* 1993;85:1644–1656.
5. Haynes RB. How to read clinical journals, II: to learn about a diagnostic test. *Can Med Assoc J.* 1981;124:703–710.
6. Commission on Chronic Illness. *Chronic Illness in the United States: Prevention of Chronic Illness.* Cambridge, MA: Harvard University Press; 1957:1.
7. Last JM, ed. *A Dictionary of Epidemiology,* 3rd ed. New York, NY: Oxford University Press; 1995.
8. Wilson JMG, Jungner F. *Principles and Practice of Screening for Disease.* Public Health Paper 34. Geneva, Switzerland: World Health Organization; 1968.
9. Sackett DL, Holland WW. Controversy in the detection of disease. *Lancet.* 1975;2:357–359.
10. World Health Organization. *Mass Health Examinations.* Public Health Paper 45. Geneva, Switzerland: World Health Organization; 1971.
11. Halperin W, Baker EL Jr. *Public Health Surveillance.* New York, NY: Van Nostrand Reinhold; 1992.
12. Beaglehole R, Bonita R, Kjellström T. *Basic Epidemiology.* Geneva, Switzerland: World Health Organization; 1993.
13. Cochrane AL, Holland WW. Validation of screening procedures. *Br Med Bull.* 1971;27:3–8.
14. Thorndike RL, Hagen E. *Measurement and Evaluation in Psychology and Education,* 2nd ed. New York, NY: Wiley; 1961.
15. Abramson JH. *Survey Methods in Community Medicine,* 4th ed. New York, NY: Churchill Livingstone; 1990.
16. Weiss NS. *Clinical Epidemiology: The Study of the Outcome of Illness.* New York, NY: Oxford University Press; 1986.
17. Babbie E. *The Practice of Social Research,* 6th ed. Belmont, CA: Wadsworth; 1992.

18. McCunney RJ. Medical surveillance: principles of establishing an effective program. In: McCunney RJ, ed. *Handbook of Occupational Medicine.* Boston, MA: Little, Brown; 1988:297–309.

19. Myrowitz E. A public health perspective on vision screening. *Am J Optom Physiol Opt.* 1984;61:359–360.

20. MacMahon B, Pugh TF. *Epidemiology Principles and Methods.* Boston, MA: Little, Brown; 1970.

21. Catalona WJ, Smith DS, Ratliff TL, et al. Measurement of prostate-specific antigen in serum as a screening test for prostate cancer. *N Engl J Med.* 1991;324:1156–1161.

22. Oesterling JE, Jacobsen SJ, Chute CG, et al. Serum prostate-specific antigen in a community-based population of healthy men. *JAMA.* 1993;270:860–864.

23. Sheldon CA, Williams RD, Fraley EE. Incidental carcinoma of the prostate: review of the literature and critical reappraisal of classification. *J Urol.* 1980;124:626–631.

24. Oesterling JE, Jacobsen SJ, Cooner WH. The use of age-specific reference ranges for serum prostate specific antigen in men 60 years old or older. *J Urol.* 1995;153: 1160–1163.

25. Jacobsen SJ, Katusic SK, Bergstralh EJ, et al. Incidence of prostate cancer diagnosis in the eras before and after serum prostate-specific antigen testing. *JAMA.* 1995; 274:1445–1449.

26. American Psychiatric Association. *Diagnostic and Statistical Manual of Mental Disorders,* 4th ed. Washington, DC: American Psychiatric Association; 1994.

27. World Health Organization. *International Statistical Classification of Diseases and Related Health Problems,* 10th rev ed. Geneva, Switzerland: World Health Organization; 1992:1.

APPENDIX
11

Data for Problem 6

Given	Find by Subtraction			
Total = 300	Total − (TP + FN) = FP + TN	= 300 − 100 = 200
TP + FN = 100	FP = (TP + FP) − TP	= 200 − 50 = 150
TP + FP = 200	FN = (TP + FN) − TP	= 100 − 50 = 50
TP = 50	TN = (FP + TN) − FP	= 200 − 150 = 50

TP, true positive; FN, false negative; FP, false positive; TN, true negative.

CHAPTER 12

Epidemiology of Infectious Diseases

LEARNING OBJECTIVES

By the end of this chapter the reader will be able to:

- state modes of infectious disease transmission
- define categories of infectious disease agents
- identify the characteristics of agents, such as infectivity, pathogenicity, virulence, and incubation period
- define quantitative terms used in infectious disease outbreaks
- give examples of major infectious disease problems in the community

CHAPTER OUTLINE

Introduction

Controlling infectious diseases is one of the most familiar applications of epidemiology at work in the community. Although there have been many advances in the prevention and treatment of infectious diseases, they remain significant causes of morbidity and mortality for the world's population in developed as well as developing countries. For example, the human immunodeficiency virus (HIV) and pneumonia-influenza were the eighth and sixth leading U.S. causes of death in 1996. Outbreaks of infectious diseases may occur in institutional settings; estimates suggest that approximately 5 to 10 per 100 patients admitted to U.S. hospitals experience nosocomial, or hospital-acquired, infections, which range from wound infections to pneumonia to bloodstream infections.[1,2] Other institutions where infectious disease outbreaks occur are children's day care centers and residential settings for the developmentally disabled.

The epidemiologic triangle recognizes three major factors—agent, environment, and host—in the pathogenesis of disease. It is a venerable model that has been used for many decades, and epidemiologists still refer to it frequently.[3] The epidemiologic triangle (Fig. 12-1) provides one of the fundamental public health conceptions of disease causality.

This model is particularly well suited to an explanation of the etiology of infectious diseases, although the current view regarding etiology of infectious diseases involves more complex multivariate causality as well. This chapter will discuss how agent, host, and environment relate to the key topics in infectious disease epidemiology: methods for transmission of disease agents and specific outcomes, including food-borne illness and the major infectious diseases. Methods for investigation and control of epidemics also include examination of agent, host, and environment factors. Figure 12-2 presents one approach to categorizing the specific infectious diseases to be examined.

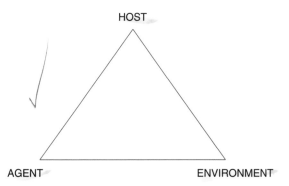

FIGURE 12-1 Epidemiologic triangle

Agents of Infectious Disease

The study of biologic agents is the province of microbiology and will not be reviewed in detail in this book. Rather, a brief overview of some of the major biologic agents and the diseases associated with them will be presented. The goal is to demonstrate how epidemiologists describe the frequency of diseases caused by infectious disease agents in populations and how they attempt to discover and control mechanisms of transmission. In relation to infectious diseases, an agent must be present for an infection to occur. Microbial agents include the following:

- *Bacteria:* In the United States and Europe, bacterial diseases were among the leading killers during the 19th century. Antibiotics and improvements in medical care have helped to control some of these killers. Nevertheless, bacteria remain significant causes of human illness. Examples of diseases caused by bacteria are tuberculosis, salmonellosis, and streptococcal infections (e.g., strep throat and necrotizing fasciitis). Of particular concern is the growing emergence of bacterial strains that are becoming resistant to antibiotics.
- *Viruses and rickettsia:* Examples of diseases caused by viruses include viral hepatitis A, herpes simplex, influenza, and viral meningitis (aseptic meningitis). Rickettsial agents produce Q fever, Rocky Mountain spotted fever, and rickettsialpox.
- *Mycoses (diseases caused by fungi):* Examples of fungal diseases are San Joaquin Valley fever (one of the endemic mycoses also called coccidioidomycosis), blastomycosis, ringworm (tinea capitis), and athlete's foot (tinea pedis). Opportunistic mycoses, which occur most commonly in immunocompromised patients, include candidiasis, cryptococcosis, and aspergillosis.[4]

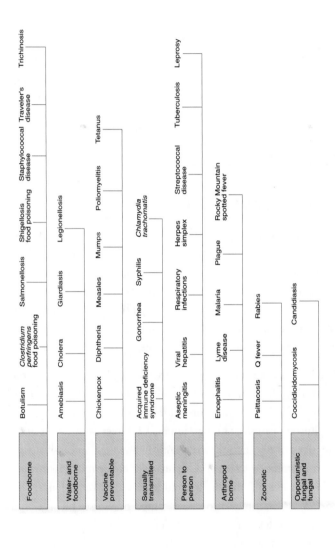

FIGURE 12-2 Epidemiologically significant infectious diseases (a partial list). The term *vaccine-preventable diseases* is used by the Centers for Disease Control and Prevention. Although some of the categories overlap, they are helpful for didactic purposes. *Source:* Data from JM Last and RB Wallace, eds, *Maxcy-Rosenau-Last: Public Health and Preventive Medicine,* 13th ed. pp xix–xxi, Appleton & Lange, 1992, and from Centers for Disease Control and Prevention, Reported vaccine-preventable diseases—United States, 1993, and the Childhood Immunization Initiative. *MMWR,* vol 43, p 57, February 4, 1994.

- *Protozoa:* These organisms are responsible for malaria, amebiasis, babesiosis, cryptosporidiosis, and giardiasis.
- *Helminths:* These organisms (found most frequently in moist, tropical areas) include intestinal parasites—roundworms (which produce ascariasis), pinworms, and tapeworms—as well as the organisms that cause trichinellosis (trichinosis; infectious agent *Trichinella spiralis*). Another well-known helminth, *Schistosoma mansoni* (and several other species), is responsible for schistosomiasis, sometimes known as snail fever, which occurs in Africa (e.g., along the Nile River) and in South America (Brazil, Surinam, and Venezuela), China, Japan, and many other areas. The infectious agents responsible for schistosomiasis are not indigenous to North America.[5]
- *Arthropods:* One of the largest classes of living things, arthropods act as insect vectors that carry a disease agent from its reservoir to humans. Mosquitos, ticks, flies, mites, and other insects of this type are examples of arthropod vectors that transmit a number of significant human diseases, such as malaria, encephalitis, Rocky Mountain spotted fever, trypanosomiasis, and leishmaniasis.

Characteristics of Infectious Disease Agents

- Infectivity
- Pathogenicity
- Virulence
- Toxigenicity
- Resistance
- Antigenicity

The following characteristics influence when an infectious disease agent will be transmitted to a host, whether it will produce disease, the severity of disease, and the outcome of infection.

- *Infectivity* refers to the capacity of the agent to enter and multiply in a susceptible host and thus produce infection or disease. Polio and measles are diseases of high infectivity. The secondary attack rate (discussed later in this chapter) is used to measure infectivity.
- *Pathogenicity* refers to the capacity of the agent to cause disease in the infected host. Measles is a disease of high pathogenicity (few subclinical

cases), whereas polio is a disease of low pathogenicity (most cases of polio are subclinical). A measure of pathogenicity is the proportion of infected individuals with clinically apparent disease.

- *Virulence* refers to the severity of the disease (i.e., whether severe clinical manifestations are produced). The rabies virus, which almost always produces fatal disease in humans, is an extremely virulent agent. A measure of virulence is the proportion of total cases that are severe. If the disease is fatal, virulence can be measured by the case fatality rate (CFR).
- *Toxigenicity* refers to the capacity of the agent to produce a toxin or poison. The pathologic effects of agents for diseases such as botulism and shellfish poisoning result from the toxin produced by the microorganism rather than from the microorganism itself.
- *Resistance* refers to the ability of the agent to survive adverse environmental conditions. Some agents are remarkably resistant, such as the agents responsible for coccidioidomycosis and hepatitis. Others are extremely fragile, such as the gonococcus and influenza viruses. Note: The term *resistance* also is applied to the host.
- *Antigenicity* refers to the ability of the agent to induce antibody production in the host. A related term is *immunogenicity,* which refers to an infection's ability to produce specific immunity.[3] Agents may or may not induce long-term immunity against infection. For example, repeated reinfection is common with gonococci, whereas reinfection with measles virus is thought to be rare.

Host

Although it was stated earlier that an agent must be present for an infectious disease to develop, it is not a sufficient cause. That is, the agent must be capable of infecting a host. The host, after exposure to an infectious agent, may progress through a chain of events leading from subclinical (inapparent) infection to an active case of the disease. The end result may be complete recovery, permanent disability, disfigurement, or death. For example, the common cold is usually self-limiting, and a complete recovery can be expected. Smallpox at one time was greatly feared because of its high morbidity and mortality. A small proportion of untreated cases of Group A streptococcal infection (β hemolytic) may produce the incapacitating sequelae of rheumatic fever and nephritis. Other examples of variation in the severity of illness are shown in Figure 12-3, which demonstrates that a high proportion of tuberculosis cases are inapparent and that a small proportion are fatal.

Measles virus produces a high proportion of cases with moderately severe illness. Some of the highly infectious virulent agents, such as the rabies virus, almost invariably cause death.

The ability to cause infection is determined by a number of factors; some are properties of the host. An important determinant of the degree of infection and the corresponding disease severity is the host's ability to fight off the infectious agent. This ability comprises two broad categories: nonspecific defense mechanisms and disease-specific defense mechanisms.

Nonspecific Defense Mechanisms

The human body is equipped with a number of means to reduce the likelihood that an agent will penetrate and cause disease. Most environmental agents are unable to enter the body because of the protection afforded by our skin. Similarly, the mucosal surfaces also afford protection against foreign invaders. Tears and saliva can be thought of as a means to wash away would-be infectious agents. The high pH of our gastric juices is lethal to many agents that manage to enter the body via ingestion. The immune system is also highly developed to ingest, via phagocytes and macrophages, infectious agents.

FIGURE 12-3 Variation in the severity of illness. Infectious diseases can result in a variety of effects ranging from no clinically detectable disease to fulminating symptoms and death. *Source:* Adapted from JS Mausner and S Kramer, *Epidemiology: An Introductory Text,* 2nd ed. p 265, with permission of WB Saunders, © 1985.

Although the foregoing examples of nonspecific mechanisms are important in determining host susceptibility, several other factors influence host responses to infectious agents. As we age, the ability of our nonspecific defense mechanisms to fend off agents may decrease (e.g., through reduced immune function). The nutritional status of the host also may be critical because, in comparison to those who have adequate nutrition, malnourished individuals may be less able to fight off infections. Genetic factors are involved also, as illustrated by the clear differences in individuals' reactions to a mosquito bite, for example. Some may demonstrate little or no reaction, whereas others may develop a large welt at the site.

Disease-Specific Defense Mechanisms

Disease-specific defenses include immunity against a particular agent. Immunity refers to the resistance of the host to a disease agent. Immunity to a disease may be either natural or artificial, active or passive:

- *Active:* All or part of a microorganism or a modified part of that microorganism is administered to invoke an immunologic response. The response mimics the natural infection but presents little or no risk to the recipient.[6]
- *Passive:* Preformed antibody is administered to a recipient; the immunity is usually of short duration (half-life, 3 to 4 weeks) for immune globulin (gamma globulin) derived from the pooled plasma of adults.[6]
- *Natural, active:* This type of immunity results from an infection by the agent. For example, a patient develops long-term immunity to measles because of a naturally acquired infection.
- *Artificial, active:* This type of immunity results from an injection with a vaccine that stimulates antibody production in the host.
- *Natural, passive:* Preformed antibodies during pregnancy are transferred across the placenta to the fetal bloodstream to produce short-term immunity in the newborn.
- *Artificial, passive:* Preformed antibodies against a specific disease are administered to an exposed individual to confer protection against a disease. An example is prophylaxis against hepatitis for individuals at risk.

The Environment

The environment refers to the domain in which the disease-causing agent may exist, survive, or originate. The external environment is the sum total of influences that are not part of the host and comprises physical, climatologic, biologic, social, and economic components. The physical environment includes weather, temperature, humidity, geologic formations, and similar physical dimensions. Contrasted with the physical environment is the social environment, which is the totality of the behavioral, personality, attitudinal, and cultural characteristics of a group of people. Both these facets of the external environment have an impact on agents of disease and potential hosts because the environment may either enhance or diminish the survival of disease agents and may serve to bring agent and host into contact.

The environment may act as a reservoir or niche that fosters the survival of infectious disease agents. The reservoir may be a part of the physical environment or may reside in animals or insects (vectors) or other human beings (human reservoir hosts). As an example of an environmental reservoir, contaminated water supplies or food may harbor infectious disease agents that cause typhoid, cholera, and many other illnesses. Fungal disease agents that may reside in the soil produce coccidioidomycosis (San Joaquin Valley fever). Infectious diseases that have vertebrate animal reservoirs and are potentially transmissible to humans under natural conditions are called the zoonoses.[7] Examples are rabies and plague. Some diseases have only humans as the reservoir; notable among these is smallpox, which has been successfully eradicated because the virus apparently does not survive outside the human reservoir. Other diseases, for example typhoid fever, may induce a chronic carrier state in some individuals who are not symptomatic for the disease but who have the capacity to transmit it to other susceptible individuals. A famous case was Typhoid Mary, a New York City area cook in the early 20th century who was a notorious and unwitting typhoid carrier.

Means of Transmission—Directly or Indirectly from Reservoir

Figure 12-4 illustrates the phases involved in the transmission of an infectious disease, which may be transmitted either directly or indirectly.

Direct Transmission

Direct transmission of diseases refers to spread of infection through person-to-person contact, as in the spread of sexually transmitted diseases, influenza, and acute respiratory infections. Portals of exit, defined as sites where infectious agents may leave the body, include the respiratory passages, the alimentary canal, the openings in the genitourinary system, and skin lesions (Table 12-1).

FIGURE 12-4 The chain of infection. *Source:* Centers for Disease Control and Prevention. *Principles of Epidemiology,* 2nd ed. Atlanta, GA: CDC; 1998, p 45.

Table 12-1 Correspondence Between Portal of Exit (Escape) Mode of Transmission and Portal of Entry

Portal of Exit	Mode of Transmission	Portal of Entry	Type of Disease
Respiratory secretions	Airborne droplets, fomites	Respiratory tract	Common cold, measles
Feces	Water, food, fomites, flies	Alimentary tract	Typhoid, poliomyelitis
Lesions, exudate	Direct contact, fomites, sexual intercourse	Skin, genital membranes	Carbuncles, syphillis, gonorrhea
Conjunctival exudate	Fomites, flies	Ocular mucous membrane	Trachoma
Blood	Bloodsucking arthropod vector	Skin (broken)	Malaria, yellow fever, epidemic typhus

Additional portals of exit may be made available through insect bites, the drawing of blood, surgical procedures, and accidents. For the chain of transmission to be continued, the portal of exit must be appropriate to the particular agent. To produce infection, the agent must exit the source in sufficient quantity to survive in the environment and to overcome the defenses surrounding the portals of entry in the new host. To be transmitted to a host, the agent requires a locus of access to the human body known as the portal of entry. The portals of entry consist of the respiratory system for such diseases as influenza and the common cold; the mouth and digestive system for diseases such as hepatitis A or staphylococcal food poisoning, and the mucous membranes or wounds in the skin for other types of disease.

Inapparent Infection

A subclinical or inapparent infection is one that has not yet penetrated the clinical horizon (i.e., does not have clinically obvious symptoms). Nevertheless, it is of epidemiologic significance because asymptomatic individuals could transmit the disease to other susceptible hosts. Isolation of infected individuals is more likely to occur when the infectious disease is clinically apparent (i.e., when the ratio of apparent to inapparent cases is high). To determine whether an infection has taken place in both symptomatic and asymptomatic individuals, one may search for serologic evidence of infection. An elevated blood antibody level suggests previous exposure and infection by the disease agent. For example, hepatitis A (infectious hepatitis) often is manifested as a subclinical infection in nursery school children, who may transmit the disease even though they do not have clinical symptoms. The infectious process may be tracked by monitoring blood antibody and enzyme responses to infection with hepatitis A virus. The epidemiologist and clinician may often conclude that infection has taken place by noting antibody and enzyme increases for hepatitis A after an appropriate incubation period.

Incubation Period

The incubation period is the time interval between exposure to an infectious agent and the appearance of the first signs or symptoms of disease. During this interval, the infectious organism replicates within the host. The incubation period is often a fixed period of hours, days, or weeks for each disease agent, and provides a clue to the time and circumstance of exposure to the agent. It is common practice for the epidemiologist to take into account the incubation period when attempting to fix the source of an infectious disease outbreak. For example, the incubation period for measles (rubeola) is most commonly 10 days, but it ranges from 7 to 18 days and requires about two weeks for a rash to appear. Another example is outbreaks of food-borne illness, in which the incubation period helps determine the etiologic agent.

Herd Immunity

The term *herd immunity* refers to the immunity of a population, group, or community against an infectious disease when a large proportion of individuals are immune (through either vaccinations or past infections). Herd immunity can occur when immune persons prevent the spread of a disease to unimmunized individuals; herd immunity confers protection to the population even though not every single individual has been immunized. For example, herd immunity against rubella may require that 85% to 90% of community residents are immune; for diphtheria it may be only 70%.

Generation Time

The term *generation time* relates to the time interval between lodgment of an infectious agent in a host and the maximal communicability of the host. The generation time for an infectious disease and the incubation time may or may not be equivalent. For some diseases, the period of maximum communicability precedes the development of active symptoms. An example of such a condition is mumps. The period of maximum comunicability precedes the swelling of salivary glands by about 48 hours.[3] There is another distinction between incubation period and generation time. The term *incubation period* applies only to clinically apparent cases of disease, whereas the term *generation time* applies to both inapparent and apparent cases of disease. Thus, *generation time* is utilized for describing the spread of infectious agents that have a large proportion of subclinical cases.

Colonization and Infestation

It is important to emphasize that not all exposures to agents lead to illness. Colonization refers to the situation where an infectious agent may multiply on the surface of the body without invoking tissue or immune response. Infestation describes the presence of a living infectious agent on the body's exterior surface, upon which a local reaction may be invoked. Thus, the full spectrum of disease in the community setting may involve much more than individuals presenting with clinical symptoms.

Iceberg Concept of Infection

The iceberg concept of infection posits that the tip of the iceberg, which corresponds to active clinical disease, accounts for a relatively small proportion of hosts' infections and exposures to disease agents. Figure 12-5 demonstrates that most infections are subclinical and that in a substantial number exposure to a disease agent may not produce any infection or cell entry.

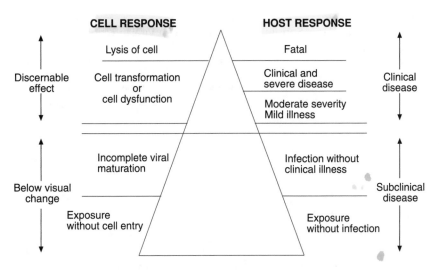

FIGURE 12-5 Iceberg concept of infection

Inapparent/Apparent Case Ratio

Table 12-2 illustrates the wide variation in clinical presentation of viral infections. Although the vast majority of polio infections do not produce severe disease, the opposite is true for rabies, where reportedly only one infected case (in the absence of timely administration of rabies prophylaxis) has survived. The percentage of apparent clinical cases for hepatitis A increases from childhood to adulthood. Epstein-Barr virus and influenza among young adults as well as childhood measles produce a high percentage of clinical cases.

Indirect Transmission

Indirect transmission involves the spread of infection through an intermediary source: vehicles, fomites, or vectors. Examples of vehicle transmission of disease are contaminated water, infected blood on used hypodermic needles, and food. A fomite is an inanimate object—such as a doorknob or clothing—that is laden with disease-causing agents. Contamination refers to the presence of a living infectious agent in or on an inanimate object. A vector is an animate, living insect or animal that is involved with transmission of the disease agent. Arthropod vectors, such as flies and mosquitos, may sometimes form a component of the life cycle of the disease agent. For example, the *Anopheles* mosquito is essential to the survival of infectious agents for malaria (e.g., *Plasmodium vivax*); if the former is eradicated, the frequency of malaria cases diminishes. Control of

Table 12-2 Examples of Subclinical/Clinical Ratio for Viral Infections (Inapparent/Apparent Ratio)

Virus	Clinical Feature	Age at Infection	Estimated Ratio	Clinical Cases
Polio	Paralysis	Child	± 1,000:1	0.1% to 1.0%
Epstein-Barr	Mononucleosis	1 to 5 years	>100:1	1%
		6 to15 years	10:1 to 100:1	1% to 10%
		16 to 25 years	2:1 to 3:1	50% to 75%
Hepatitis A	Icterus	<5 years	20:1	5%
		5 to 9 years	11:1	10%
		10 to 15 years	7:1	14%
		Adult	1.5:1	80% to 95%
Rubella	Rash	5 to 20 years	2:1	50%
Influenza	Fever, cough	Young adult	1.5:1	60%
Measles	Rash, fever	5 to 20 years	1:99	>99%
Rabies	Central nervous system symptoms	Any age	<1:10,000	>>>>99%

arthropod vectors may be an effective means of limiting outbreaks of vector-borne diseases, such as malaria.

Measures of Disease Outbreaks

Attack Rate

In Chapter 3, we defined an incidence rate as the number of new cases of disease per unit population per unit time. An attack rate is also an incidence rate. It is used when the occurrence of disease among a population at risk increases greatly over a short period of time, often related to a specific exposure. In addition, the disease rapidly follows the exposure during a fixed time period because of the nature of the disease process.[8] Thus, the term *attack rate* is frequently used to describe the occurrence of food-borne illness, infectious diseases, and other acute epidemics. The formula for attack rate is shown below. The numerator consists of people who are ill as a result of exposure to the suspected agent, and the denominator consists of all people, whether well or ill, who were exposed to the agent during a time period. A time interval during which exposure occurred is an important element of the definition. The attack rate is often expressed as a percentage.

$$\text{Attack rate} = \frac{\text{Ill}}{\text{Ill} + \text{Well}} \times 100 \text{ during a time period}$$

The example given in Table 12-3 provides for calculating attack rates for an outbreak of food-borne illness and for identifying food items that might have caused the outbreak. In a hypothetical outbreak of food-borne illness, several foods were implicated. Illustrated in Table 12-3 is the method to calculate the attack rate for a specific food item. Food X demonstrated 77% attack rates among those who ate and 64% attack rates among those who did not eat the food. In order to identify foods suspected of producing an outbreak, the following procedure is recommended.

First, a list of all foods consumed in the outbreak is compiled. Next, the persons involved in the outbreak are categorized in two columns: A (ate the food) and B (did not eat the food). One calculates the attack rate among those in categories A and B by dividing the number of ill persons by the total number of persons and multiplying the result by 100. For example, the attack rate in column A is $(10/13) \times 100 = 77\%$. After calculating the attack rate, one finds the difference

Table 12-3 Data to Illustrate Calculation of Attack Rates for Food X

A (ate the food)				B (did not eat the food)			
Ill	Not Ill	A Total	Attack Rate	Ill	Not Ill	B Total	Attack Rate
10	3	13	77%	7	4	11	64%

in attack rates (A − B) between those who ate and those who did not eat the food, in this case 13% (77% − 64%). One would repeat this process for each of the foods that were suspected in the outbreak of food-borne illness. The foods that have the greatest difference in attack rates may be the foods that were responsible for illness. To complete the investigation, additional studies, including cultures and laboratory tests, might be required. An example is given in the study questions and exercises at the end of the chapter.

Secondary Attack Rate

The secondary attack rate yields an index of the spread of a disease within a household or similar circumscribed unit (Exhibit 12-1). The secondary attack

EXHIBIT 12-1

Secondary Attack Rate

The secondary attack rate refers to the spread of disease in a family, household, dwelling unit, dormitory, or similar circumscribed group.

$$\text{Secondary attack rate (\%)} = \frac{\text{Number of new cases in group} - \text{initial case(s)}}{\text{Number of susceptible persons in the group} - \text{initial case(s)}} \times 100$$

Initial case(s) = Index case(s) + coprimaries

Index case(s) = Case that first comes to the attention of public health authorities

Coprimaries = Cases related to index case so closely in time that they are considered to belong to the same generation of cases

Source: Adapted from JS Mausner and S Kramer. *Epidemiology: An Introductory Text,* 2nd ed. WB Saunders, © 1985, with permission from Elsevier.

rate is defined as "the number of cases of an infection that occur among contacts within the incubation period following exposure to a primary case in relation to the total number of exposed contacts; the denominator is restricted to susceptible contacts when these can be determined. The secondary attack rate is a measure of contagiousness and is useful in evaluating control measures."[7(p165)] For example, a case of measles brought into a family may spread from the initial case to other members. Table 12-4 provides data for calculation of a secondary attack rate for the hypothetical spread of measles (rubeola) in a military barracks housing ROTC summer cadets. The two initial cases occurred at the beginning of the military summer program and were presumed to have resulted from exposure outside the military base. Of the two initial cases, the case that came to the attention of public health authorities is called the index case.[3] The other case could be considered a coprimary case. This term refers to a case that is related to the index case so closely in time that it is thought to belong to the same generation of cases as the index case. The eight secondary cases occurred approximately 10 to 12 days after measles symptoms were observed in the index cases. The total number of new cases in the group was 10 (initial cases plus secondary cases). The secondary attack rate was $[(10 - 2)/(14 - 2)] \times 100 = 66.7\%$.

Here is a second example of how to calculate a secondary attack rate:

"Seven cases of hepatitis A occurred among 70 children attending a child care center. Each infected child came from a different family. The total number of persons in the 7 affected families was 32. One incubation period later, 5 family members of the 7 infected children also developed hepatitis A."[9(p89)] By applying the formula shown in Exhibit 12-1 to these data, we obtain the following information:

Numerator = 5 (number of cases of hepatitis A among family contacts with hepatitis)

Denominator = 25 = 32 − 7 (total number of family members − children already infected)

Note: In this example, no subtraction is necessary in calculating the numerator because the initial cases have already been removed from the number of new cases in the group; the problem specified that five family members developed hepatitis one incubation period later.

Table 12-4 Hypothetical Secondary Attack Rate Data for Military Cadets

Number of Cadets In Barracks		Number of Initial Cases		Number of Secondary Cases	
Unimmunized	Immunized	Unimmunized	Immunized	Unimmunized	Immunized
14	6	2	0	8	0

For diseases such as measles, which confer prolonged immunity, the index cases (and coprimaries) are excluded from the denominator.[10] If means are available to determine immune status, any other immune persons also would be excluded from the denominator (as implied by the definition).[11] In addition to assessing the infectivity of an infectious disease agent, the secondary attack rate may be used to evaluate the efficacy of a prophylactic agent (e.g., a vaccine or gamma globulin). It also may be used to trace the secondary spread of a disease of unknown etiology to determine whether there is a transmissible agent.[11]

Case Fatality Rate

The CFR is different from the mortality rate, or death rate, for a disease. We have already discussed the crude death rate (refer to Chapt. 3), which is defined as the number of deaths that occur in a population of interest during a time period. The CFR refers to a proportion formed by the number of deaths caused by a disease among those who have the disease during a time interval (Exhibit 12-2). It provides an index of the deadliness of a particular disease within a specific population.

Let us compare the kinds of information yielded by the death rate and the CFR. Recent epidemiologic surveillance demonstrates that mortality from human rabies is very uncommon in the United States. The fact that rabies is uncommon in humans may be attributed to its confinement to wildlife (epizootic rabies) and to postexposure prophylaxis (passive immunization and vaccines) among those who have been potentially exposed to rabies. Therefore, the cause-specific death rate for any given recent year due to rabies, which has a small numerator and the total population as a denominator, would be low. The cause-specific mortality rate due to rabies therefore would be a small number. In contrast, the CFR for rabies would be high. The CFR reflects the fatal outcome of disease, which is affected by efficacy of treatment. Among the cases of human rabies that may occur as a result of failure to receive postexposure prophylaxis, mortality remains almost invariably certain, as has been historically true.

Case Fatality Rate (CFR)

$$CFR\,(\%) = \frac{\text{Number of deaths due to disease "X"}}{\text{Number of cases of disease "X"}} \times \begin{array}{l}\text{100 during a}\\\text{time period}\end{array}$$

Note that the numerator and denominator refer to the same time period.

Sample calculation: Assume that an outbreak of plague occurs in an Asian country during the month of January. Health authorities record 98 cases of the disease, all of whom are untreated. Among these, 60 deaths are reported.

$$CFR = (60/98) \times 100 = 61.2\%$$

Examples of diseases with a high CFR are rabies, untreated bubonic plague, and acquired immune deficiency syndrome.

Procedures Used in the Investigation of Infectious Disease Outbreaks

These include many of the techniques developed by John Snow[12]: mapping and tabulation of cases, identification of agents, and clinical observation. The investigation of an outbreak can be logically divided into five basic steps:

1. *Define the problem.* It is important to determine from the outset whether the epidemic is real.
2. *Appraise existing data.* This step includes evaluation of known distributions of cases with respect to person, place, and time. Examples of activities performed at this stage include case identification, making clinical observations, and generation of tables and spot maps.

   - *Case identification.* This step includes all cases of disease potentially involved in the outbreak, for instance, in a mass occurrence of food-borne illness. Examples of food-borne illnesses include staphylococcal food poisoning and trichinosis. For communicable diseases, such as tuberculosis, contacts of cases need to be identified.

- *Clinical observations.* The epidemiologist records the number, types, and patterns of symptoms associated with the disease (e.g., whether the symptoms are primarily gastrointestinal, respiratory, or febrile). Additional clinical information may come from stool samples, cultures, or antibody assays.
- *Tabulation and spot maps.* Cases of disease may be plotted on a map to show geographic clustering (as in an outbreak of tuberculosis in a high school). Cases may be tabulated by date or time of onset of symptoms, by demographic characteristics (i.e., age, sex, and race), or by risk categories (e.g., intravenous drug use or occupational exposure). This method is similar to Snow's mapping of cholera cases in the Broad Street district of London in the mid-1800s.[12] It remains an important epidemiologic technique. Graphing cases according to time of onset helps determine the modal incubation period or other aspects of the outbreak.
- *Identification of responsible agent.* The epidemiologist may be able to determine the agent or other factors responsible for the disease outbreak by estimating the incubation period, by reviewing the specific symptoms, and by noting evidence from cultures and other laboratory tests. In some outbreaks of food-borne illness, it may be possible to link an etiologic agent to cultures of food specimens and stool samples.

3. *Formulate a hypothesis.* What are the possible sources of infection? What is the likely agent? What is the most likely method of spread? What would be the best approach for control of the outbreak?

4. *Test the hypothesis.* Collect the data that are needed to confirm or refute your initial suspicions. At this stage it is important to continue to search for additional cases, evaluate alternative sources of data, and begin laboratory investigations to identify the causative agent.

5. *Draw conclusions and formulate practical applications.* Based on the results of your investigation, it is likely that programs, policies, or procedures will need to be implemented to facilitate long-term surveillance and ultimate prevention of the recurrence of similar outbreaks.

Epidemiologically Significant Infectious Diseases in the Community

The following discussion illustrates major outbreaks of infectious diseases and demonstrates how the foregoing methods are utilized. A partial list of epidemiologically significant infectious diseases is shown in Figure 12-2. These include the broad categories of food-borne, water-borne, vaccine preventable, sexually transmitted, person to person, arthropod-borne, zoonotic, and fungal diseases.

Food-borne Illness in the Community

Table 12-5 provides examples of agents and diseases that are associated with food contamination, which is one of the most common infectious disease problems in the community. Among the agents of food-borne illness noted in Table 12-5 is *Staphylococcus aureus*. Figure 12-6 illustrates a mass episode of food-borne illness that was transmitted from *Staphylococcus*-infected lesions to passengers on an international flight. There were 144 cases of illness among 343 passengers. Storage of the food at improper temperatures contributed to development of the *Staphylococcus* toxin. Another food-borne illness is trichinosis (Exhibit 12-3). Trichinosis is most commonly associated with consumption of pork products that have not been adequately cooked.

Table 12-5 Partial List of Infectious Agents That Cause Food-borne Illness

Disease/Agent	Incubation Period and Syndrome	Mode of Transmission
Classic botulism/ *Clostridium botulinum*	12–36 hours, classic syndrome compatible with botulism	Contaminated food containing toxins (e.g., home-canned foods)
Salmonellosis/various species of *Salmonella* (e.g., *S. typhimurium* and *S. enteritidis*)	12–36 hours, gastro-intestinal syndrome	Contaminated food that contains *Salmonella* organisms (e.g., undercooked chicken, eggs, meat; raw milk)
Staphylococcal food poisoning/*Staphylococcus aureus* (see Fig. 12-6)	1–7 hours, gastrointestinal syndrome; majority of cases with vomiting	Contaminated food that contains staphylococcal enterotoxin
Cholera/*Vibrio cholerae*	2–3 days, profuse watery diarrhea (painless)	Contaminated water that contains infected feces or vomitus; also contaminated food
Clostridium perfringens food poisoning	6–24 hours, diarrhea	Heavily contaminated food (e.g., meats and gravies inadequately heated or stored at temperatures that permit multiplication of bacteria)
Campylobacter enteritis/ *Campylobacter jejuni*	2–5 days, diarrhea, abdominal pain, malaise, fever	Undercooked chicken or pork, contaminated food and water, raw milk

Source: Data from AS Benenson. *Control of Communicable Diseases in Man.* American Public Health Association, 1990.

The classic pattern of cause and effect in an outbreak of mass illness is often postulated but not proven. Recently, the actual sequence involved in food poisoning on an international jet flight was traced by epidemiologists, and their findings fit the textbook pattern. Here is what took place:

1. On the weekend of Feb. 1, a cook in Alaska preparing ham and omelet breakfasts for International Inflight Catering has blisters on two fingers. The blisters are infected with staphylococcus, a common contagious bacteria. The cook handles at least 205 portions of ham, which are kept at room temperature for 6 hours during preparation of the food trays.

2. The 543 passengers board a Japan Air Lines jumbo jet in Tokyo. While the plane flies to its scheduled refueling stop in Anchorage, the contaminated food trays are stored overnight at 50 degrees. Staph multiply at temperatures over 40; as they multiply, they produce a toxin which is a common cause of food poisoning.

3. Food trays are loaded on the 747 at Anchorage. The trays have been labeled for distribution on the plane: The contaminated trays go to Galley 1, which serves 40 first class seats, and Galley 2, which serves 93 seats in the forward portion of the coach cabin; 72 of them go to Galleys 3 and 4 to the rear. A fresh crew boards, and the plane takes off for Copenhagen, the next refueling stop on its polar route to Paris.

4. Six to seven hours later, the passenger breakfasts are heated in 300-degree ovens for 15 minutes, treatment which cannot inactivate the toxin. The passengers are served. For the crew it is dinner time and only one stewardess takes a ham and omelet tray. As the plane approaches Copenhagen, those who ate contaminated food begin to experience staph food-poisoning symptoms: nausea, vomiting, cramps, and diarrhea.

5. The sick; 144 of them disembark at Copenhagen the morning of February 3. The rest, 51 of whom later become ill, go on to Paris.

The pattern of contagion was reconstructed through laboratory analysis that matched bacterial samples from the cook's blisters, uneaten tainted food, and the victims' vomit and stool. Dr. Mickey S. Eisenberg, the U.S. Public Health Service officer in Anchorage who had pinpointed the probable source of infection, completed the picture by comparing passenger interviews with the galley plan.

FIGURE 12-6 Textbook case of food-borne illness. *Source: The New York Times.* February 16, 1975, p7. Drawings by Oliver Williams. Copyright © 1975 by The New York Times Company. Reprinted by permission.

EXHIBIT 12-3

Trichinosis Associated with Meat from a Grizzly Bear—Alaska

Eight cases of trichinosis reported recently from Barrow, Alaska, were associated with a dinner on December 20, 1980. The 12 persons who attended were served a meal that included *maktak* (whale blubber), *ugruk* (bearded-seal meat, dried and stored in seal oil) fresh raw whitefish and grayling and *quaq* (raw frozen meat), thought by the participants to be caribou but later discovered to have been grizzly bear.

Five men and three women, ranging in age from 32 to 76 years, became ill 2 to 16 days after the meal (mean, 8.6 days). All eight reported eating *quaq;* the four who denied doing so remained well, a statistically significant difference. *Quaq* was the only meat eaten by all the persons who became ill. Thirty other family members who were not present at the dinner also remained well, again a statistically significant difference. Signs and symptoms of illness included edema (100%), fatigue (100%), myalgia (87.5%), rash (87.5%), fever (87.5%), chills (75%), periorbital edema (62.5%), headache (50%), visual disturbance (37.5%), diarrhea (37.5%), abdominal cramps (25%), nausea (25%) and vomiting (25%). None of the ill persons had notable pulmonary, neurologic, or cardiac complications. Five were hospitalized. Five received steroids, and two received anthelmintic therapy.

The grizzly bear from which the meat came had been shot the previous autumn at the family's summer camp, 140 miles inland from Barrow. At that time, parts had been cooked thoroughly and consumed without adverse effects. The hindquarters were included in a large cache of moose and caribou meat that was returned to Barrow and stored frozen in the family's cold cellar. None of the bear meat had been eaten in Barrow before the dinner on December 20, and none had been given away. The remains of the hindquarter eaten at the dinner were fed to dogs; the other hindquarter remained in cold storage. A sample taken from the digestive tract of one of the patients contained 70 *Trichinella* larvae per gram of meat.

Source: Adapted from Centers for Disease Control and Prevention. Trichinosis associated with meat from a grizzly bear—Alaska. *MMWR*, vol 30, pp 115–116, March 20, 1981.

Water- and Food-borne Diseases

Diseases associated with food or water include amebiasis, cholera, giardiasis, legionellosis, and schistosomiasis. The following example describes the transmission of schistosomiasis in Africa along the Nile River. Transmission of schistosomiasis requires *Biomphalaria glabrata*, the intermediate snail host for *Schistosoma mansoni*, the species that is the major cause of schistosomiasis in Africa. The life cycle of schistosomes entails a complex cycle involving alternate human and snail hosts. According to the U.S. Department of Health and Human Services:

> Upon reaching fresh water, parasite eggs, voided in the urine and feces, hatch immediately into larvae called miracidia, which swim about until they find a suitable snail host. After penetrating the snail, miracidia develop into another larval form called cercariae. The cercariae are the forms capable of infecting [humans]. They do this after emerging from the snail host, burrowing through the skin of persons exposed to the contaminated water. Once inside the body, the cercariae develop into adult worms.[13(p13)]

The Nile River is used for a wide variety of common activities, including sewage disposal, personal hygiene, and recreation. Deposition of human wastes into the river water causes contamination by the agent. Those who come into contact with the water are at increased risk of exposure to the cercariae. After the building of the Aswan Dam, there was an increase in rates of schistosomiasis, attributable to human intervention in the life cycle of the schistosome. Figure 12-7 illustrates the life cycle of *Schistosoma mansoni*.

Cholera is another example of a water- or food-borne disease. It is characterized as an acute enteric disease with sudden onset, occasional vomiting, rapid dehydration, acidosis, and circulatory collapse.[5] Caused by the bacterial agent *Vibrio cholerae*, it still occurs in many parts of the developing world. In the early 1990s, epidemic cholera continued to spread throughout Central and South America. The Centers for Disease Control and Prevention tallied more than 300,000 cholera cases and more than 200 deaths from cholera-related causes in 1992. In that same year, 102 cholera cases were reported in the United States.[14] Figure 12-8 illustrates the spread of cholera from South America to Central America and Mexico during the epidemics of 1991 and 1992.

A third example of a water- or food-borne disease agent is *Entamoeba histolytica*, a fairly common parasitic organism associated with amebiasis, which in many cases manifests as intestinal disease. The following excerpt from a report by the Centers for Disease Control and Prevention demonstrates the transmission of *E. histolytica* through colonic irrigation:

The Colorado State Department of Health has reported an outbreak of amebiasis that occurred in the period December 1977–November 1980 and was associated with a chiropractic clinic. All of the cases had received colonic irrigation—a series of enemas performed by machine to "wash out" the colon—a practice that has been gaining popularity recently among some chiropractors, naturopaths, and nutritional counselors. Thirteen cases were confirmed by biopsy review or serologic tests. Seven cases were fatal.[15(p101)]

Stool cultures, blood tests, and biopsy studies strongly suggested amebas as the etiologic agent. Specimens from the colonic irrigation machine were heavily contaminated with fecal bacteria.

Sexually Transmitted Diseases

A major public health problem from this category is the acquired immunodeficiency syndrome (AIDS) epidemic, which has had major consequences for the economic activities and health resources of many nations. According to the Centers for Disease Control and Prevention (CDC), "The greatest impact of the epidemic is among men who have sex with men (MSM) and among racial/ethnic minorities, with increases in the number of cases among women and of cases attributed to

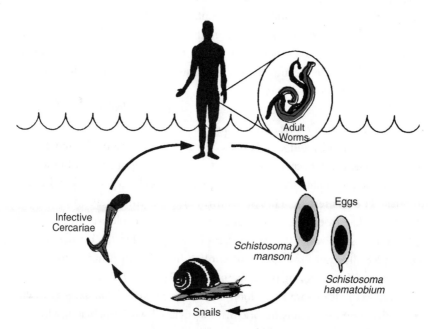

FIGURE 12-7 Life cycle of *Schistosoma mansoni*. *Source:* Reprinted from Centers for Disease Control and Prevention. Schistosomiasis in US Peace Corps Volunteers—Malawi, 1992. *MMWR*, vol 42, p 568, July 30, 1993.

FIGURE 12-8 Spread of epidemic cholera—Latin America, 1991–1992. *Source:* Reprinted from Centers for Disease Control and Prevention, Update: Cholera—Western Hemisphere, 1992. *MMWR,* vol 42, p 89, February 12, 1993.

heterosexual transmission. The number of persons living with AIDS has increased as deaths have declined."[16(p430)] In addition, the CDC notes that "As of December 31, 2000, 774,467 persons had been reported with AIDS in the United States; 448,060 of these had died; 3,542 persons had unknown vital status. The number of persons living with AIDS (322,865) is the highest ever reported. Of these, 79% were men, 61% were black or Hispanic, and 41% were infected through male-to-male sex."[16(p430)] Table 12-6 lists information regarding the characteristics of AIDS cases in the United States over four periods of observation.

Table 12-7 reports the estimated number of persons living with AIDS by age group, sex, exposure category, and year from 1993 through 2001 in the United

Table 12-6 Number and percentage of persons with AIDS, by selected characteristics and period of report—United States, 1981–2000

Characteristic	1981–1987 No.	(%)	1988–1992 No.	(%)	1993–1995 No.	(%)	1996–2000 No.	(%)
Sex								
Male	46,251	(92.0)	177,132	(87.5)	211,909	(82.4)	204,730	(77.4)
Female	4,029	(8.0)	25,387	(12.5)	45,353	(17.6)	59,672	(22.6)
Age Group (yrs.)								
0–4	649	(1.3)	2,763	(1.4)	2,105	(0.8)	1,355	(0.5)
5–12	101	(0.2)	667	(0.3)	650	(0.3)	618	(0.2)
13–19	199	(0.4)	759	(0.4)	1,381	(0.5)	1,722	(0.7)
20–29	10,523	(20.9)	38,507	(19.0)	43,445	(16.9)	36,252	(13.7)
30–39	23,239	(46.2)	92,178	(45.5)	116,335	(45.2)	114,072	(43.1)
40–49	10,472	(20.8)	46,922	(23.2)	67,475	(26.2)	78,032	(29.5)
50–59	3,684	(7.3)	14,494	(7.2)	19,153	(7.4)	23,980	(9.1)
≥60	1,413	(2.8)	6,230	(3.1)	6,718	(2.6)	8,373	(3.2)
								(34.0)
Race/Ethnicity								
White, Non-Hispanic	30,033	(59.7)	102,130	(50.4)	109,101	(42.4)	88,896	(44.9)
Black, Non-Hispanic	12,796	(25.5)	63,319	(31.2)	97,742	(38.0)	118,665	(44.9)
Hispanic*	7,044	(14.0)	35,116	(17.3)	47,442	(18.4)	52,092	(19.7)
Asian/Pacific Islander	312	(0.6)	1,342	(0.7)	1,927	(0.8)	2,147	(0.8)
American Indian/ Alaska Native	68	(0.1)	437	(0.2)	870	(0.3)	962	(0.4)
Region†								
Northeast	19,541	(38.9)	62,102	(30.7)	78,000	(30.3)	81,466	(30.8)
North Central	3,772	(7.5)	20,416	(10.1)	25,778	(10.0)	25,532	(9.7)
South	12,933	(25.7)	65,754	(32.5)	89,559	(34.8)	102,576	(38.8)
West	13,502	(26.9)	46,303	(22.9)	55,586	(21.6)	45,574	(17.2)
U.S. territories	524	(1.0)	7,883	(3.9)	8,812	(3.2)	8,829	(3.3)

continued

Table 12-6 *continued*

Characteristic	1981–1987		1988–1992		1993–1995		1996–2000	
	No.	(%)	No.	(%)	No.	(%)	No.	(%)
Vital Status								
Living	2,103	(4.2)	20,572	(10.2)	96,998	(37.7)	203,192	(76.9)
Deceased	47,993	(95.5)	181,212	(89.5)	159,048	(61.8)	59,807	(22.6)
Total§	50,280	(6.5)	202,520	(26.2)	257,262	(33.2)	264,405	(34.1)

* Persons of Hispanic origin may be of any race.

† *Northeast* = Connecticut, Maine, Massachusetts, New Hampshire, New Jersey, New York, Pennsylvania, Rhode Island, and Vermont; *North Central* = Illinois, Indiana, Iowa, Kansas, Michigan, Minnesota, Missouri, Nebraska, North Dakota, Ohio, South Dakota, and Wisconsin; *South* = Alabama, Arkansas, Delaware, District of Columbia, Florida, Georgia, Kentucky, Louisiana, Maryland, Mississippi, North Carolina, Oklahoma, South Carolina, Tennessee, Texas, Virginia, and West Virginia; *West* = Alaska, Arizona, California, Colorado, Hawaii, Idaho, Montana, Nevada, New Mexico, Oregon, Utah, Washington, and Wyoming.

§ Includes persons for whom sex, age, race/ethnicity, region, or vital status are missing.

Source: Reprinted from HIV/AIDS--United States 1981–2000, *MMWR*, vol 50, No. 21, p 431, 2001, Centers for Disease Control and Prevention.

Table 12-7 Estimated number of persons living with AIDS by age group, sex, exposure category, and year, 1993 through 2001, United States[1]

	Year								
	1993	1994	1995	1996	1997	1998	1999	2000	2001
Male adult/adolescent exposure category									
Men who have sex with men	86,074	94,249	100,131	109,335	120,951	131,184	141,080	151,212	162,151
Injecting drug use	34,157	39,646	43,635	47,754	52,599	56,450	60,075	63,756	67,366
Men who have sex with men and inject drugs	14,038	15,128	16,007	16,885	18,227	19,265	20,107	20,756	21,520
Hemophilia/coagulation disorder[2]	1,607	1,687	1,710	1,718	1,771	1,803	1,830	*	*
Heterosexual contact	6,141	7,952	9,812	12,247	15,021	17,725	20,500	23,412	26,660
Receipt of blood transfusion, blood components, or tissue[2]	865	883	922	987	1,070	1,176	1,281	*	*
Other/risk not reported or identified[3]	964	912	900	928	968	1,015	1,061	4,348	4,553
Male subtotal	143,846	160,457	173,117	189,854	210,607	228,618	245,934	263,484	282,250
Female adult/adolescent exposure category									
Injecting drug use	13,843	16,244	18,311	20,279	22,557	24,307	25,737	27,395	29,145
Hemophilia/coagulation disorder[2]	91	109	133	160	196	224	243	*	*
Heterosexual contact	11,837	15,172	18,498	22,596	27,016	31,225	35,366	40,111	45,128
Receipt of blood transfusion, blood components, or tissue[2]	732	812	843	923	1,010	1,107	1,206	*	*
Other/risk not reported or identified[3]	365	366	367	400	445	483	520	2,183	2,423
Female subtotal	26,868	32,703	38,152	44,358	51,224	57,346	63,072	69,689	76,696
Pediatric (<13 years old) exposure category	3,057	3,292	3,440	3,522	3,632	3,745	3,798	3,845	3,881
Total[4]	173,772	196,452	214,711	237,735	265,464	289,709	312,804	337,017	362,827

continues

Table 12-7 *continued*

[1] These numbers do not represent the actual number of persons living with AIDS. Rather, these numbers are point estimates of the number of persons living with AIDS derived by subtracting the estimated cumulative number of deaths in persons with AIDS from the estimated cumulative number of persons diagnosed with AIDS. Estimated AIDS incidence and estimated deaths are adjusted for reporting delays and for redistribution of cases initially reported with no identified risk, but not for incomplete reporting. The year 2000 is the most recent year for which reliable estimates are available. Refer to Technical Notes in original source.

[2] Statistical estimates for AIDS prevalence in 2000 and 2001 among persons exposed to HIV through hemophilia/coagulation disorder or receipt of blood transfusion, blood components, or tissue are not presented, but are included in the exposure category "other." The relatively small number of AIDS cases in these categories in recent years does not provide information that results in reliable annual estimates of prevalence (* = data not available); only cumulative estimates are presented. CDC is evaluating and revising the algorithm for estimating AIDS prevalence among persons infected in the early 1980s through these exposure categories.

[3] For 2000 and 2001, estimates of "other" include cases exposed through hemophilia/coagulation disorder and receipt of blood transfusion, blood components, or tissue.

[4] Because column totals were calculated independently of the values for the subpopulations, the values in each column may not sum to the column total.

Source: Adapted from Centers for Disease Control and Prevention. *HIV/AIDS Surveillance Report.* 13(2). Available at: http://www.cdc.gov/hiv/stats/hiv/hasr1302/table30.htm. Accessed June 16, 2003.

States. The CDC indicated that "Male-to-male sex has been the most common mode of exposure among persons reported with AIDS (46%), followed by injection drug use (25%) and heterosexual contact (11%). The incidence of AIDS increased rapidly in all three of these risk categories through the mid-1990s; however, since 1996, declines in new AIDS cases have been higher among MSM and injection drug users than among persons exposed through heterosexual contact. . . ."16(p430)

Vaccine-Preventable Diseases

In the United States, health care providers administer routine vaccinations to children for the prevention of nine diseases: diphtheria, *Haemophilus influenzae* type b infections, hepatitis B, measles, mumps, pertussis, paralytic poliomyelitis, rubella, and tetanus. According to provisional data reported by the Centers for Disease Control and Prevention, for 1993,[17] the following numbers of cases for several conditions reached low frequency:

- congenital rubella syndrome, 7 reported cases
- rubella, 195 reported cases
- diphtheria, 0 reported cases
- poliomyelitis, 4 cases suspected

In 1997, there were 138 measles cases. This figure represented a dramatic drop after a major resurgence of measles occurred during the period 1989 to 1990. Subsequently, the reported numbers of cases declined. The respective numbers were 27,786 (1990); 9,643 (1991); and 2,231 (1992).[18] The measles rate continued to decline thereafter. Figure 12-9 illustrates the reported cases of measles from 1950 to 1997. Measles outbreaks may occur in institutional settings, such as universities or colleges, if there is a significant proportion of unimmunized individuals. Measles outbreaks are also a potential health problem on military bases. Exhibit 12-4, which typifies measles outbreaks that can occur in contemporary times, describes a measles outbreak at an international gymnastics competition in 1991.

Diseases Spread by Person-to-Person Contact

Tuberculosis, a significant cause of morbidity and mortality throughout the world, was uncommon in many developed countries, including the United States, until the late 1980s, when it began to increase in frequency. Reasons for the resurgence of tuberculosis include the increasing prevalence of human immunodeficiency

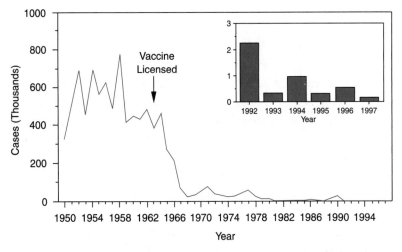

FIGURE 12-9 Reported measles cases, by year—United States, 1950–1997. *Source:* Reprinted from Measles—United States; 1997. *MMWR,* vol 47, No 14, p 273, 1998. Centers for Disease Control and Prevention.

EXHIBIT 12-4

Measles at an International Gymnastics Competition—Indiana, 1991

On September 7, 1991, the Indiana State Department of Health (ISDH) was notified of three suspected measles cases among athletes from New Zealand (NZ) participating in an international gymnastics competition September 6–15 in Indianapolis (Marion County). Among those potentially at risk for measles were approximately 700 athletes and 1200 coaches, trainers, and managers from 51 countries; an estimated 2500 volunteers and staff; international media, families, and employees; and approximately 60,000 spectators attending the competition. This report summarizes the epidemiologic investigation of these cases.

Sixteen NZ delegation members arrived August 29 and stayed on one floor of a hotel. Throughout the following week, they practiced in a curtain-divided area shared with three other teams and visited nearby shopping and eating establishments. On August 30, two 15-year-old female ath-

continues

EXHIBIT 12-4 *continued*

letes (patients 1 and 2) developed cough, coryza, and conjunctivitis, followed by onset of rash on September 4. Patient 2's symptoms were mild and improved within 24 hours of onset of rash. A third athlete (patient 3), a 16-year-old female, developed symptoms on September 5 and rash on September 7. All three patients had measles IgM antibody in their acute serum specimens (greater than or equal to 1:40 by indirect fluorescent antibody [IFA] test). Complement-fixation testing of both the acute and convalescent specimens collected 7 weeks later demonstrated fourfold or greater rise in IgG measles antibody for patients 1 and 3 and a fourfold decline in measles IgG antibody for patient 2. The three patients had documented histories of live-virus measles vaccination in NZ at 11, 13, and 14 months of age and reported exposure to a person with physician-diagnosed measles at their NZ practice gymnasium approximately 2 weeks before onset of rash.

Following onset of rash, patients 1 and 3 were isolated in their hotel rooms for at least 4 days. Remaining NZ delegation members born after 1956 were isolated until serologic evidence of measles immunity could be determined; within 12 hours, all were demonstrated to be seropositive (measles IgG greater than or equal to 1:40 by IFA).

An investigation by the ISDH identified numerous groups with probable measles exposure. Because of the large-scale exposure, the seriousness of measles illness . . ., the extreme infectiousness of the measles virus . . ., and the difficulty in obtaining timely evidence of measles immunity from throughout the world, the ISDH recommended that all participants, volunteers, staff, and hotel employees born after 1956 receive live-virus measles vaccine. . . .

During September 8–12, six vaccination clinics were held. The vaccine was administered using an automatic hypodermic injection apparatus. Among the 1300 persons vaccinated were 608 international delegates, 264 Indianapolis and 139 other Indiana residents, 152 out-of-state volunteers, and 137 hotel employees. More than 1100 (85%) persons were vaccinated within 72 hours after the opening ceremonies on September 6 when most widespread exposure occurred.

Three persons experienced adverse events following vaccination; all were local reactions at the injection site and resolved without serious con-

continues

EXHIBIT 12-4 *continued*

sequences. Two of these three patients were treated with antibiotics and improved promptly; the third was thought to have had an allergic reaction and was treated with corticosteroids.

Surveillance for secondary cases included (1) twice-daily reports from delegations on whether any member had prodromal measles symptoms; (2) daily review of visits to the competition's medical station and observation of the venue for persons with measles symptoms; (3) letters to participants, volunteers, and staff advising them of the outbreak and control measures, signs and symptoms of measles, the need to seek health care, and the importance of notifying local public health officials if symptoms occurred; (4) daily telephone calls to all emergency rooms and urgent-care centers in Marion County during September 16–23; and (5) notification of states whose residents attended the competition. No additional cases associated with the outbreak have been reported.

Source: Reprinted from Measles at an International Gymnastics Competition—Indiana, 1991, *MMWR*, vol 41, No 7, pp 109–111, 1992, Centers for Disease Control and Prevention.

virus infection, the increase in the homeless population, and the importation of cases from endemic areas. As an illustration of current trends in the occurrence of tuberculosis, Exhibit 12-5 shows data from migrant farm workers and the homeless population, two high-risk groups. From 1984 to 1992, there was an upward trend in the number of reported tuberculosis cases from 22,201 to 26,673. For this time period, 51,700 excess cases were reported, according to statistical models of expected cases in comparison to observed cases (Fig. 12-10). The number of cases increased in all racial/ethnic groups except non-Hispanic whites and Native Americans. All age groups except for the over-65 age group showed increases, with the largest increase occurring among the 25- to 44-year age group.[19]

Zoonotic Diseases

Q fever, the agent for which is *Coxiella burnetii*, is an example of a zoonosis, a disease that, under natural conditions, can be spread from vertebrate animals to humans. Zoonotic diseases may be either enzootic (similar to endemic in human diseases) or epizootic (similar to epidemic in human diseases).[5] The reservoir for the agent in Q fever is infected livestock (cattle, sheep, and goats). The spectrum of infection in humans ranges from mild to severe, debilitating illness with

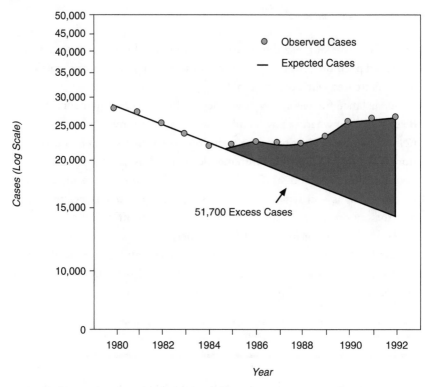

FIGURE 12-10 Expected and observed number of tuberculosis cases—United States, 1980–1992. *Source:* Reprinted from Centers for Disease Control and Prevention. Tuberculosis morbidity—United States, 1992. *MMWR,* vol 42, p 696, September 17, 1993.

EXHIBIT 12-5

Tuberculosis Among Migrant Farm Workers and the Homeless Population

Farm workers are approximately six times more likely to develop tuberculosis (TB) than the general population of employed adults. ... The following services, listed by priority, that should be available for migrant and seasonal farm workers and their family members are: a) detection and diagnosis of those with current symptoms of active TB; b) appropriate treatment and monitoring for those who have current disease; c) contact investigation and appropriate preventive therapy for those exposed to infectious persons; d) screening and appropriate

continues

EXHIBIT 12-5 *continued*

preventive therapy for asymptomatically infected workers who may be immunosuppressed, such as those with human immunodeficiency virus (HIV) infection; e) screening and appropriate preventive therapy for children of migrant and seasonal farm workers; and f) wide- spread tuberculin test screening for workers and families with preventive therapy prescribed, as appropriate. Health-care providers should immediately perform appropriate diagnostic studies for persons with a productive, prolonged cough, or other symptoms suggestive of tuberculosis. Health departments should be immediately notified when TB is suspected or diagnosed to enable examination of contacts and initiation of other health department diagnostic, preventive, or patient management services.

Homeless persons suffer disproportionately from a variety of health problems, including tuberculosis. Although there is no generally agreed upon definition of homelessness, the homeless can be defined, on a general level, as those who do not have customary and regular access to a conventional dwelling or residence. . . . Since 1984, three outbreaks of tuberculosis in shelters for the homeless have been reported to CDC . . . , and recent investigations have shown a prevalence of 1.6%–6.8% for clinically active tuberculosis among selected homeless populations. . . . These prevalence rates are 150 to 300 times higher than the nationwide prevalence rate. The prevalence of asymptomatic tuberculosis infection among the homeless has been reported to be as high as 22%–50% (3–5), thus indicating that a large reservoir of infection may exist from which future cases will emerge unless large-scale preventive measures are undertaken.

Source: Data from Prevention and control of tuberculosis in migrant farm workers recommendations of the Advisory Council for the Elimination of Tuberculosis. *MMWR,* vol 41 (RR10), 1992, Centers for Disease Control and Prevention; and Perspectives in disease prevention and health promotion tuberculosis control among homeless populations. *MMWR,* vol 36, No 17, pp 257–260, 1987, Centers for Disease Control and Prevention.

symptoms similar to those of influenza or pneumonia. Those at high risk for infection include workers and others who come into contact with infected livestock: veterinarians, farmers, agricultural employees, and laboratory personnel. For example, Q fever occurred among laboratory personnel who used sheep in their research at a medical center in San Francisco, California. A more ordinary source of transmission is infected raw milk.

Mycoses

Coccidioidomycosis (San Joaquin Valley fever) often manifests as a lung disease and is caused by a fungus, *Coccidioides immitis*. The agent is endemic to the San Joaquin Valley in California and to the lower Sonoran life zone, which covers parts of California, Arizona, Texas, and Mexico. Cases of infection have been associated with those occupations or activities that bring susceptible persons in contact with contaminated soil (e.g., construction, archeology, and dirt bike riding). Merely driving through an endemic area may result in infection. The following excerpt describes an epidemic that occurred after exposure to a severe dust storm at a naval air station in Lemoore, California:

> Eighteen new cases of symptomatic valley fever were diagnosed at the Naval Hospital, Lemoore . . . following a severe natural dust storm that occurred from December 20 to 22, 1977. This storm arose from the southeast near Bakersfield, California, an area of high endemicity. The storm lasted approximately 48 hours. Visibility during the storm decreased to approximately 0.25 mile. The wind velocity rose to 34 mph. The dust was ubiquitous. It seeped through windows, depositing a layer of soot on car seats and household furniture, making it virtually impossible to avoid exposure to the dust.[20(p566)]

The authors of the report concluded that a temporal relationship existed between the dust storm and the marked increase in the incidence of symptomatic San Joaquin Valley fever.

In 1991, an outbreak of coccidioidomycosis (1,208 cases) was reported in California. The majority of cases (80%) occurred in Kern County, where coccidioidomycosis is endemic.[21] The numbers of reported cases of coccidioidomycosis by year are shown in Figure 12-11.

Arthropod-Borne Diseases

Arthropod-borne diseases include arboviral diseases. These are a diverse group of diseases that involve transmission of arboviruses between vertebrate hosts (for example, from animal to animal or from animal to human) by blood-feeding arthropod vectors.[7] Examples of these vectors are sand flies, ticks, and mosquitos, the last of which are responsible for transmission of the encephalitis virus. During 1992, the following types and numbers of cases of encephalitis were reported: St Louis encephalitis, 26 reported cases; La Crosse encephalitis, 29 reported cases; Eastern equine encephalitis and Western equine encephalitis, 0 reported cases. Enzootic (referring to diseases that afflict animals in a particular locality) viral activity was reported in 1992; viral isolates or antigens of arboviruses were found in wild birds, sentinel birds, and captured mosquitos; epizootic cases were documented in horses.[22]

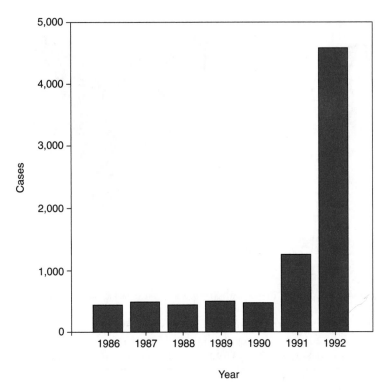

FIGURE 12-11 Reported cases of coccidioidomycosis, by year—California, 1986–1992. *Source:* Reprinted from Centers for Disease Control and Prevention, Coccidioidomycosis—United States, 1991–1992. *MMWR,* vol 42, p 22, January 22, 1993.

Lyme disease, a second example of a vector-borne illness, is transmitted by ticks. Cases, which are distributed across the United States, showed a steady increase from 1982 to 1991, during which time period 40,195 cases were reported. In 1992, a total of 9,677 cases were reported, representing an incidence rate of 3.9 per 100,000 population. The highest incidence occurred in Nantucket County, Massachusetts, where the incidence rate was 449.1 cases per 100,000 population.[23] Figure 12-12 shows a map of the distribution of cases during 1992.

Emerging Infections

The emergence of seemingly new infections presents a challenge to epidemiologists worldwide. When a young man and his fiancée appeared in an emergency room in New Mexico with fever and acute respiratory distress, a whole chain of events

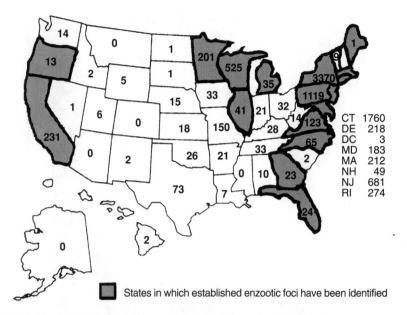

FIGURE 12-12 Reported cases of Lyme disease—United States, 1992. *Source:* Reprinted from Centers for Disease Control and Prevention. Lyme disease—United States, 1991–1992. *MMWR,* vol 42, p 346, May 14, 1993.

began, which eventually led to the definition of U.S. hantaviral syndrome.[24] This syndrome, identified initially in the Four Corners region of the United States, claimed 20 lives out of 36 patients—a greater than 50% case fatality rate. Subsequently it has been identified in California and other states. Hantavirus infection had been previously described in other parts of the world, but appeared suddenly in a slightly altered form in several locations in the United States.

"Emerging infections are those that erupt suddenly, like the U.S. hantaviral pulmonary syndrome, or that suddenly increase in incidence or geographic scope. Recent examples range from Lyme Disease to AIDS."[24(p85)] Also included in this category is food-borne illness caused by *E. coli.* Many emerging infections are not caused by sudden mutations in a pathogen; instead they appear when an existing pathogen gains access to new host populations. Changes in climate, human activities such as farming or reforestation, technologic changes such as air travel and organ transplantation, and demographic changes such as migration to cities may all contribute to the emergence of seemingly new and deadly infections. Table 12-8 shows a summary of recent examples of emerging infections.

Escherichia coli: An Emerging Food-borne Pathogen

E. coli food-borne illness outbreaks have received dramatic and continuing attention in the media. Two outbreaks were associated with the same fast food restaurant chain in 1982. A multistate outbreak in the western United States produced 700 cases of illness and four deaths in 1993.[25] The pathogen responsible for the vast majority of cases of illness that present as severe bloody diarrhea (hemolytic uremic syndrome) is called *E. coli* O157:H7. This organism is regarded as an emerging pathogen because of the occurrence of major food-borne illness outbreaks that have been distributed over a wide geographic area. Such large-scale outbreaks were not generally recognized before the early 1980s. The most frequent vehicle implicated in *E. coli* O157:H7 food-borne illness outbreaks is ground beef. When hamburgers made with contaminated ground beef are eaten rare or are inadequately cooked, infections may occur.

One of these infections is caused by hepatitis C virus (Exhibit 12-6), for which a routine vaccination is not presently available. Another example is West Nile virus infection (refer to case study shown in box).

Conclusion

Infectious disease epidemiology has developed a body of methods for investigating and controlling infectious diseases in the community. The reservoir for infectious diseases may consist of humans, animals, arthropods, or the physical environment. Transmission of disease may be direct (person to person) or indirect. Noteworthy terms used to describe infectious disease outbreaks include *attack rate, secondary attack rate,* and *CFR.* Agents for infectious disease encompass a broad range of microbial agents, from bacteria to viruses to protozoa. Infectious diseases remain major causes of morbidity and mortality. Examples of significant problems include food-borne illness, vaccine-preventable diseases such as measles, diseases spread from person to person such as tuberculosis, and sexually transmitted diseases, notably AIDS.

Table 12-8 Recent Examples of Emerging Infections

Pathogen	Disease	Distribution	Natural Host	Transmission	Notable Factors in Emergence
Bunyaviridae/ (Hantaviruses)	Hemorrhagic fever	Asia	Rodents	Inhalation of infected excreta	Contact with rodent host during rice harvest, dissemination by ship-borne infected rats
	Respiratory distress syndrome	U.S., probably Europe and South America	Rodents	Inhalation of infected excreta	Ecologic changes causing increased contact with rodents
Cryptosporidium	Cryptosporidiosis	Probably worldwide	?Ungulates*	Ingestion of contaminated water	Faulty water purification
Filoviridae (Ebola, Marburg)	Hemorrhagic fever	Africa	Unknown	Contact with unknown host, nosocomial (infected needles)	Unknown (in Europe and U.S., importation of monkeys)
Group A strepococci	Necrotizing fasciitis; other invasive infections	Probably worldwide	?Humans	Inhalation (classic strep), wound infection; skin contamination	Unknown, possibly new strain or strain not recently prevalent
Hepatitis C virus	Hepatitis	Worldwide	?Humans	Contaminated IV needles, transfusions, organ transplantation, probably sexual	Transfusions
Lassa virus	Lassa fever	West Africa	Rodents	Contact with infected secretions (of natural host or infected persons)	Urbanization
Vibrio cholerae	Cholera	Asia; recently reintroduced to South America, Africa	?Zooplankton	Ingestion of infected human excreta in food or water	Transoceanic shipping, lapsed public health measures, travel

*Hoofed mammals such as sheep, goats, and reindeer.

Source: Reproduced with permission, SS Morse. Patterns and predictability in emerging infections. *Hospital Practice*, 1996, 31(4), p 85. © 1996 The McGraw-Hill Companies, Inc.

EXHIBIT 12-6

Hepatitis C Fact Sheet

Clinical features

- 80% of infections asymptomatic
- Jaundice
- Fatigue
- Abdominal pain
- Loss of appetite
- Intermittent nausea
- Dark urine

Etiologic agent

- Hepatitis C virus (HCV)

Incidence in the United States

- From 240,000 in the 1980s to about 25,000 in 2001

Sequelae

- Chronic infection 75-85% of infected persons
- Chronic liver disease: 70% of infected persons
- Deaths from chronic liver disease <3%
- Leading indication for liver transplantation

Prevalence

- Estimated 3.9 million (1.8%) Americans have been infected with HCV, of whom 2.7 million are chronically infected.

Transmission

- Primarily blood-borne; also sexual and perinatal

Recommendations for testing based on risk for HCV infection

Persons	Risk of Infection	Testing Recommended?
Injecting drug users	High	Yes
Recipients of clotting factors made before 1987	High	Yes
Hemodialysis patients	Intermediate	Yes
Recipients of blood and/or solid organs before 1992	Intermediate	Yes
People with undiagnosed liver problems	Intermediate	Yes
Infants born to infected mothers	Intermediate	After 12–18 months old
Healthcare/public safety workers	Low	Only after known exposure
People having sex with multiple partners	Low	No
People having sex with an infected steady partner	Low	No

continues

EXHIBIT 12-6 *continued*

> **Trends**
> - Transfusion-associated cases occurred prior to donor screening, now very rare
> - Most infections due to illegal injection drug use
>
> **Prevention**
> - Screening of blood/organ/tissue donors
> - Counseling to reduce/modify high-risk practices
>
> *Source:* Adapted from Centers for Disease Control and Prevention, *Hepatitis C Fact Sheet.* Available at: http://www.cdc.gov/ncidod/diseases/hepatitis/c/fact.htm. Accessed June 15, 2003.

Case Study—West Nile Virus

West Nile (WN) virus infection is a mosquito-borne illness that in most cases does not produce symptoms. The incubation period is approximately 3 to 15 days after the bite of an infected mosquito. Evidence suggests that a minority of infected persons will develop a mild illness with fever, headache, body aches, and sometimes skin rash and swollen glands. Infection infrequently results in severe illness, known as WN encephalitis. A small number of cases have been fatal. The principal transmission cycle of WN virus involves several species of mosquitos and various species of birds.

WN virus first was recognized in 1999 as the cause of severe and fatal human illness in metropolitan New York City. WN virus is commonly found in Africa, West and Central Asia, and the Middle East. It is not known how the virus first was introduced into the United States, but since the initial appearance it has spread rapidly, and by 2001 was found throughout the eastern half of the country. ■

Source: Adapted from Centers for Disease Control and Prevention. *West Nile Virus.* Available at: http://www.cdc.gov/ncidod/dvbid/westnile. Accessed June 16, 2003.

Study Questions and Exercises

1. Define and give the formulas for attack rates, secondary attack rates, and case fatality rates.

2. A flu outbreak occurred in a military barracks that housed 20 soldiers. Case A began on October 1, and case B was diagnosed on October 2. After approximately 10 days, 12 additional cases occurred during approximately a one-week time span. Military epidemiologists believed that this second group of cases represented the same generation of cases, and was in the second incubation period after the occurrence of cases A and B; none of the 20 soldiers was known to be immune. Calculate the secondary attack rate using the foregoing data.

3. Explain the etiology of tuberculosis, measles, and rabies by applying the epidemiologic triangle (Fig. 12-1).

4. Give one example of each type of prevention—primary, secondary, and tertiary—for food-borne salmonellosis, malaria, and AIDS. To answer this question, you will need to review the chapters where the three types of prevention are discussed and apply the methods to a new situation.

5. What is the epidemiologic importance of an inapparent infection?

6. Name two examples of a disease spread from person to person, and suggest methods for the control of such a disease in the community.

7. When is isolation for an infectious disease not likely to be an effective means of control of the disease in the community?

8. Discuss host responses to infectious disease agents. Be sure to include herd immunity as a community health concept.

9. Discuss the following statement: High cooking temperature will sanitize food even after it has been stored improperly (e.g., at room temperature for 6 hours); one can be certain that there will be no remaining hazard to human health and that all the pathogenic material has been destroyed. (Refer to Fig. 12-6, the illness outbreak on a 747 jetliner.)

10. A local health department epidemiologist investigated an outbreak of gastrointestinal illness thought to be associated with a college cafeteria. There were many complaints about the quality of the cafeteria's offerings, and it appeared that the students' worst expectations were confirmed when several students visited the college's infirmary during the middle of the night and the following day complaining of nausea, diarrhea, fever, vomiting, and cramps. The health department's investigation revealed that 24 students had eaten in the cafeteria immediately before the out-

break. The times between eating in the cafeteria and the development of active symptoms ranged from 20 to 36 hours. A list of foods eaten, the number of persons eating the foods, and tabulations of illness are presented in Appendix 12. Fill in the attack rates where indicated. On the basis of your calculations, answer the following questions:

a. What food or foods would you suspect caused the problem?

b. Based on the description of the clinical symptoms and the list of infectious disease agents presented in Table 12-5, which agent(s) do you think was (were) responsible?

References

1. Doebbeling BN. Nosocomial infections. In: Last JM, Wallace RB, eds. *Maxcy-Rosenau-Last: Public Health and Preventive Medicine,* 13th ed. Norwalk, CT: Appleton & Lange; 1992:203–207.

2. Osterholm MT. Infectious diseases and child day care. In: Last JM, Wallace RB, eds. *Maxcy-Rosenau-Last: Public Health and Preventive Medicine,* 13th ed. Norwalk, CT: Appleton & Lange; 1992:207–212.

3. Mausner JS, Kramer S. *Epidemiology: an Introductory Text,* 2nd ed. Philadelphia, PA: Saunders; 1985.

4. Pfaller MA. Opportunistic fungal infections. In: Last JM, Wallace RB, eds. *Maxcy-Rosenau-Last: Public Health and Preventive Medicine,* 13th ed. Norwalk, CT: Appleton & Lange; 1992:287–293.

5. Benenson AS. *Control of Communicable Diseases in Man.* Washington, DC: American Public Health Association; 1990.

6. American Academy of Pediatrics, Committee on Infectious Diseases. *Report of the Committee on Infectious Diseases,* 22nd ed. Elk Grove Village, IL: American Academy of Pediatrics; 1991.

7. Last JM, ed. *A Dictionary of Epidemiology,* 4th ed. New York, NY: Oxford University Press; 2001.

8. Hennekens CH, Buring JE. *Epidemiology in Medicine.* Boston, MA: Little, Brown; 1987.

9. Centers for Disease Control and Prevention. *Principles of Epidemiology,* 2nd ed. Atlanta, GA: CDC; 1992.

10. MacMahon B, Pugh TF. *Epidemiology Principles and Methods.* Boston, MA: Little, Brown; 1970.

11. Lilienfeld AM, Lilienfeld DE. *Foundations of Epidemiology,* 2nd ed. New York, NY: Oxford University Press; 1980.

12. Snow J. *Snow on Cholera.* Cambridge, MA: Harvard University Press; 1965.

13. U.S. Department of Health and Human Services. Center supplies etiological agents of schistosomiasis. *Res Resour Rep.* 1981;5:12–13.

14. Centers for Disease Control and Prevention. Update: cholera—Western Hemisphere, 1992. *MMWR.* 1993;42:89–91.

15. Centers for Disease Control and Prevention. Amebiasis associated with colonic irrigation—Colorado. *MMWR.* 1981;30:101–102.

16. Centers for Disease Control and Prevention. HIV and AIDS—United States, 1981–2000. *MMWR.* 2001;50:429–455.

17. Centers for Disease Control and Prevention. Reported vaccine-preventable diseases—United States, 1993, and the Childhood Immunization Initiative. *MMWR.* 1994;43:57–60.

18. Centers for Disease Control and Prevention. Measles surveillance—United States, 1991. *MMWR.* 1992;41:1–11.

19. Centers for Disease Control and Prevention. Tuberculosis morbidity—United States, 1992. *MMWR.* 1993;42(36):696–697, 703–704.

20. Williams PL, Mendez P, Smyth LT. Symptomatic coccidioidomycosis following a severe natural dust storm. *Chest.* 1979;76:566–569.

21. Centers for Disease Control and Prevention. Coccidioidomycosis—United States, 1991–1992. *MMWR.* 1993;42(02):21–24.

22. Centers for Disease Control and Prevention. Arboviral diseases—United States, 1992. *MMWR.* 1993;42(24):467–468.

23. Centers for Disease Control and Prevention. Lyme disease—United States, 1991–1992. *MMWR.* 1993;42(18):345–348.

24. Morse SS. Patterns and predictability in emerging infections. *Hosp Pract.* 1996;31:85–91, 96–101, 104.

25. Armstrong GL, Hollingsworth J, Morris JG. Emerging foodborne pathogens: *escherichia coli* O157:H7 as a model of entry of a new pathogen into the food supply of the developed world. *Epidemiol Rev.* 1996;18:29–51.

APPENDIX
12

Data from a Food-borne Illness Outbreak in a College Cafeteria

Food Items Served	Number of Persons Who Ate				Number Who Did Not Eat			
	Ill	Not Ill	Total	Percent Ill	Ill	Not Ill	Total	Percent Ill
Three-bean salad	10	3	13		7	4	11	
Beef, rare	17	6	23		0	1	1	
Beef, specified well cooked	3	6	9		5	10	15	
Potato salad	12	6	18		4	2	6	
Macaroni salad	11	5	16		5	3	8	
Tuna salad*	13	1	14		3	7	10	
Cold cuts and cheese plate	10	6	16		5	3	8	
Rolls and butter	13	4	17		4	3	7	

*The tuna salad was prepared from fresh ingredients approximately 1 hour before consumption and stored under refrigeration.

CHAPTER 13

Epidemiologic Aspects of Work and the Environment

LEARNING OBJECTIVES

By the end of this chapter the reader will be able to:

- define the term *environmental epidemiology*
- give examples of environmental agents that are associated with human health effects
- provide examples of study designs used in environmental epidemiology
- state methodologic difficulties with research on environmental health effects
- list some of the terms used to characterize environmental exposure and human responses to exposure
- cite health outcomes studied in relation to environmental agents

CHAPTER OUTLINE

I. Introduction
II. Health Effects Associated with Environmental Hazards
III. Study Designs Used in Environmental Epidemiology
IV. Toxicologic Concepts Related to Environmental Epidemiology

Introduction

This chapter will focus on epidemiologic studies of health outcomes linked to the environment and the work setting. During the past few decades, environmental health hazards have become a concern not only for epidemiologists, but for society at large because of their enormous social, health, and economic ramifications. The adverse impacts of toxic chemicals found in the environment, although a major source of morbidity and mortality, are potentially preventable.[1] Through epidemiologic research, it may be possible to control or prevent diseases by identifying exposures to the relevant environmental hazards. Among the more notable of human exposures to environmental hazards are the following:

- chemical agents (from chemical spills, pesticides, and hazardous wastes)
- electromagnetic radiation from high-tension wires
- ionizing radiation from natural and synthetic sources
- heavy metals
- air pollution

The health effects associated with these hazards are the domain of environmental epidemiology, which is defined by the Committee on Environmental Epidemiology of the U.S. National Research Council as "the study of the effect on human health of physical, biologic, and chemical factors in the external environment, broadly conceived. By examining specific populations or communities exposed to different ambient environments, it seeks to clarify the relationship between physical, biologic, or chemical factors and human health."[2(p28)]

Health Effects Associated with Environmental Hazards

Health effects (both morbidity and mortality) attributed to environmental exposures encompass a wide range of conditions, including cancer and reproductive impacts, such as congenital malformations and low birth weight. In the work environment, ionizing radiation, infectious agents, toxic substances, and drugs may pose unique health risks for pregnant workers and the unborn fetus.[3] Other adverse health outcomes are linked potentially to the occupational environment. They include lung diseases (byssinosis, coal workers' pneumoconiosis, and asbestosis), dermatologic problems, neurotoxicity, coronary heart disease, injuries and trauma, and various psychologic conditions (e.g., work absenteeism and stress at work). Researchers have been concerned about the possible link between environmental exposure to carcinogenic agents and cancer. Occupational exposure to toxic substances is known to be responsible for certain forms of cancer (e.g., bladder cancer in dye workers and leukemia among workers exposed to benzene). Between 1950 and 1988 (among U.S. whites), the age-adjusted incidence for all forms of cancer rose by 43.5%, and the age-adjusted cancer mortality increased by 2.9%, a trend that needs to be evaluated systematically in the context of increasing worldwide use of chemicals.[1]

Study Designs Used in Environmental Epidemiology

Environmental epidemiology employs a wide range of study designs, including both descriptive and analytic approaches. Wegman offered definitions of descriptive and etiologic studies applied to the epidemiology of occupational diseases that apply equally well to the broader category of environmental epidemiology. "*Descriptive studies* provide information for setting priorities, identifying hazards, and formulating hypotheses for new occupational risk."[4(p944)] A historical example is William Farr's work showing that Cornwall metal miners had higher mortality from all causes than the general population.[4] "Etiologic studies are planned examinations of causality and the natural history of disease. These studies have required increasingly sophisticated analytic methods as the importance of low-level exposures is explored and greater refinement in exposure-effect relationships is sought."[4(p945)] Examples of different study designs that may be employed in environmental epidemiology are introduced below in an effort to present a broad overview of the field.

Retrospective Cohort Studies

In evaluating the health effects of occupational exposures to toxic agents, researchers may study various end points. For example, in some studies self-reported symptom rates are used as a measure of the effects of low-level chemical exposure. Occupational health investigators can design and administer self-report questionnaires inexpensively. Self-reports to questionnaires, however, may not always be reliable, and although they often correlate with clinical diagnoses they also may differ markedly.[5] Physiologic or clinical examinations are other means to evaluate adverse health effects. For example, in a study of respiratory diseases, pulmonary function tests, such as forced expiratory volume, may be an appropriate indicator. While clinical examinations may provide "harder" evidence of health effects than self-reports, they may be expensive or impractical to collect in the case of workers who have left employment. In other studies, mortality is the outcome of interest; research on mortality frequently uses a retrospective cohort study design.[6] Mortality experience in an employment cohort can be compared with the expected mortality in the general population (national, regional, state, or county) by using the standardized mortality ratio (see Chapt. 3). One also can contrast the mortality experience of exposed workers with the mortality rate of nonexposed workers in the same industry. For example, production workers might be compared with drivers or office workers. Another option is to identify a second industry or occupation that is comparable in terms of skill level, educational requirements, or geographic location, but in which the exposure of interest is not present.

The use of mortality as a study end point has several advantages, including the fact that it may be relevant to agents that have a subtle effect over a long time period. Although any fatal chronic disease may be investigated, mortality from cancer is often studied as an outcome variable in occupational exposures. According to Monson, "cancer specifically tends to be a fatal illness; its presence is usually indicated on the death certificate. Also, cancer is a fairly specific disease and is less subject to random misclassification than, say, one of the cardiovascular diseases."[6(p106)]

Methods for Selection of a Research Population and Collection of Exposure Data

The investigator may select a study population from personnel records maintained by a company. If the records of former and retired workers are retained by the company, a complete data set spanning long time periods may be available.

Ideally, every previous and current worker exposed to the factor should be included. Selection bias may occur if some workers are excluded because their records have been purged from the company's database.[6] Data collected from employment records may include:

- personal identifiers to permit record linkage to Social Security Administration files and retrieval of death certificates
- demographic characteristics, length of employment, and work history with the company
- information about potential confounding variables, such as the employee's medical history, smoking habits, lifestyle, and family history of disease

The Healthy Worker Effect

One of the factors that may reduce the validity of exposure data (introduced in Chapt. 10) is the healthy worker effect. Monson states that the healthy worker effect refers to the "observation that employed populations tend to have a lower mortality experience than the general population."[6(p114)] The healthy worker effect may have an impact on occupational mortality studies in several ways. People whose life expectancy is shortened by disease are less likely to be employed than healthy persons. One consequence of this phenomenon would be a reduced (or attenuated) measure of effect for an exposure that increases morbidity or mortality. That is, because the general population includes both employed and unemployed individuals, the mortality rate of that population may be somewhat elevated compared with a population in which everyone is healthy enough to work. As a result, any excess mortality associated with a given occupational exposure is more difficult to detect when the healthy worker effect is operative. The healthy worker effect is likely to be stronger for nonmalignant causes of mortality, which usually produce worker attrition during an earlier career phase, than for malignant causes of mortality, which typically have longer latency periods and occur later in life. In addition, healthier workers may have greater total exposure to occupational hazards than those who leave the work force at an earlier age because of illness.

Ecologic Study Designs

Studies of the health effects of air pollution have used ecologic analyses to correlate air pollution with health effects. Instead of correlating individual exposure to air pollution with mortality, the researcher measures the association between average exposure to air pollution within a census tract and the average mortality in that census tract. Other types of geographic subdivisions besides census tracts may be used as well. This type of study attempts to demonstrate that mortality is higher in more polluted census tracts than in less polluted census tracts. A major problem of the ecologic technique for the study of air pollution, however, stems from uncontrolled factors. Examples include individual levels of smoking and smoking habits, occupational exposure to respiratory hazards and air pollution, differences in social class and other demographic factors, genetic background, and length of residence in the area.[7] Nonetheless, ecologic studies may open the next generation of investigations. Future studies will probably attempt to measure the relevant potential confounders in more rigorous analytic study designs.

Case-Control Studies

In comparison with cross-sectional study designs, case-control studies may provide more complete exposure data, especially when the exposure information is collected from the friends and relatives of cases who died of a particular cause. Nevertheless, some unmeasured exposure variables as well as confounding variables may remain in case-control studies. For example, in studies of health and air pollution, precise quantitation of air pollution exposure and unobserved confounding factors, including smoking habits and occupational exposure to air pollution, may be difficult to achieve.[7]

Toxicologic Concepts Related to Environmental Epidemiology

The terms *dose response, threshold, latency,* and *synergism,* which are from toxicology, characterize exposure to hazardous agents. The following definitions are from Gochfeld.[8]

Dose-Response Curve

The dose-response curve is used to assess the effect of exposure to a chemical or toxic substance upon an organism (e.g., an experimental animal). A typical dose-response curve is shown in Figure 13-1. The dose is indicated along the x-axis, and the response is shown along the y-axis. The response could be measured as the percentage of exposed animals showing a particular effect, or it could reflect the effect in an individual subject. The dose-response curve, which has a sigmoid shape, is also a cumulative percentage response curve. At the beginning of the curve, there is a flat portion suggesting that at low levels an increase in dosage produces no effect.

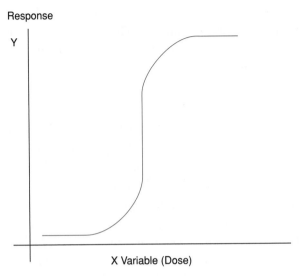

Response

Y

X Variable (Dose)

Figure 13-1 Illustration of the dose-response curve

This is also known as the subthreshold phase. After the threshold is reached, the curve rises steeply and then progresses to a linear phase, where an increase in response is proportional to the increase in dose. When the maximal response is reached, the curve flattens out. A dose-response relationship is one of the indicators used to assess a causal effect of a suspected exposure upon a health outcome.

Threshold

The threshold refers to the lowest dose at which a particular response may occur. It is unclear whether exposure to toxic chemicals at low (subthreshold) levels may produce any health response. Although society's concern about the health effects of exposure to environmental pollutants has increased, it still remains unclear whether chronic exposures to toxic chemical agents in the environment occur at a high enough dose to affect human health.[9] There also have been increasing concerns over the long-term effects of low-level exposures to toxic substances in the workplace.[6]

Latency

Latency refers to the time period between initial exposure and a measurable response. The latency period can range from a few seconds (in the case of acutely toxic agents) to several decades. For example, mesothelioma (a rare form of cancer) has a latency period as long as 40 years between first exposure to asbestos and subsequent development of the condition. The long latency for many of the health events studied in environmental research makes detection of hazards a methodologically difficult problem.

Synergism

Synergism refers to a situation in which the combined effect of several exposures is greater than the sum of the individual effects. The synergistic relationship between asbestos and smoking in causing lung cancer is an example. A classic study of lung cancer risk among asbestos insulation workers was reported by Selikoff and colleagues.[10] A total of 370 workers were studied between 1963 and 1967. The occurrence of lung cancer in this occupational group was seven to eight times greater than that expected for the general white population of the United States. It was apparent that exposure to asbestos was not the entire explanation, however. No lung cancer deaths were observed among the 87 workers who did not smoke, but 24 of 283 workers who smoked died of lung cancer, a 92-fold greater risk than that for workers who did not smoke and were not exposed to asbestos as part of their occupation.

Types of Agents

A partial list of potential disease agents found in the environment (work, home, and external) is shown in Table 13-1. The nature and significance of these agents are discussed below. Although there are thousands of possible agents of environmental disease, the broad categories include toxic chemicals, metals (especially heavy metals, such as lead), electric and magnetic radiation, ionizing radiation, dusts (such as silica and coal dust), asbestos, and mechanical and physical energy.

Chemical Agents

Chemical substances have potential effects on human health through acute toxicity, direct skin irritation, contact dermatitis, or long-term effects, such as cancer. Chemical agents are found in the home, in foodstuffs that contain chemical additives, and in the external environment. Vastly higher concentrations of chemical exposure may occur among workers than among the general population. Exposure to chemicals in the occupational setting averages 1 to 100 times higher than in the ambient environment.[1] Each year, an estimated 50,000 to 70,000 U.S. workers develop chronic occupational disease produced by exposure to toxic chemicals in the workplace.[1]

Table 13-1 Selected List of Environmental Disease Agents

Type of Agent	Examples	Health Effects Studied
Chemical	Pesticides, organochlorides	Cancers
	Vinyl chloride	Angiosarcoma
	Benzene	Leukemia
Heavy metals and metallic compounds	Mercury	Minamata disease
	Lead	Neurologic Impairment
	Cadmium, manganese	Cancers
	Arsenic	Cancers
Electric and magnetic radiation	Radiation from high-tension power lines	Leukemia
Ionizing radiation	γ-rays	Cancers
	X-rays	Cancers
	Radon	Lung cancer
Allergens and molds	Animal fur, pollen	Allergic responses
Asbestos	Brake linings, construction materials	Lung cancer, mesothelioma
Dusts	Coal dust	Pneumoconiosis
	Silica	Silicosis
Physical/mechanical energy	Industrial machinery, high ambient temperature	Noise-induced hearing loss, mortality

Pesticides

Examples are the organochloride family, which includes dichlorodiphenyltri-cloroethane (DDT), polychlorobiphenyls, and atrazine. Direct exposure may follow mishandling, improper disposal, accidents, or spills; indirect pesticide exposure may result from ground water contamination through agricultural use of pesticides. Benarde wrote, "many believe that the accumulation of pesticides in the environment causes actual and potential harm in the form of residues ingested in food and water or inhaled with each breath; others maintain that the effects of long-term low-level exposure are unknown."[11(p97)] Data from one small study suggest, however, that women with breast cancer have higher serum concentrations of DDT residues than women who are free from cancer.[12]

Occupational exposure to pesticides, such as organophosphates, is a problem of great potential concern for up to five million farm workers in the United States. The long-term effects of pesticide exposure include several types of cancer, teratogenic effects, sterility, spontaneous abortions, and cognitive deficits. Blood cholinesterase depression occurs among farm workers actually and possibly exposed to pesticides over a long time period, although the pathophysiologic significance of such depression is unclear.[13]

Vinyl Chloride

Vinyl chloride, used in the plastics industry, has been associated with angiosarcoma of the liver and is described also as a carcinogenic substance related to lung and central nervous system tumors.[14] Workers in employment settings who are occupationally exposed to vinyl chloride have experienced the specific hazard of hepatic angiosarcoma. However, research evidence has not supported vinyl chloride as responsible for other cancers or nonmalignant disease.[15]

Asbestos

Asbestos was once widely used in shipbuilding, construction, insulation, and automobiles. As a result, numerous schools, homes, and public buildings are contaminated. Before the 1980s, billions of tons of asbestos were used in the United States.[1] Asbestos exposure is associated with asbestosis, malignant mesothelioma, and lung cancer. Selikoff et al.[16] reported unexpectedly high death rates due to cancer of the lung or pleura, mesothelioma, and cancer of the stomach, colon, or rectum among building trade insulation workers who had relatively light exposure to asbestos.

Metallic Compounds

Metallic compounds that pose an environmental hazard include aluminum, arsenic, antimony, beryllium, cadmium, chromium, lead, mercury, nickel, and tin. Three of these, arsenic, mercury, and lead, merit elaboration.

Arsenic

Arsenic in its pure form is a crystalline metalloid, an element with properties that are intermediate between those of a metal and a nonmetal. It is able to combine with other substances, metallic and nonmetallic, and also to form stable organic compounds.[17] A poisonous material that is ubiquitous in nature—in soils and water—arsenic varies in toxicity depending upon its chemical form; it is also the byproduct of refining gold and other metals. In olden days, arsenic was used as an acute poison and also for medicinal purposes; at present it is no longer widely used as a medicine, but has commercial applications as a pesticide and wood preservative, and in manufacturing processes.[18]

Several massive arsenic poisoning incidents, due to the contamination of foodstuffs with arsenic, have been documented.[17] Arsenic-contaminated beer killed 6,000 people in England in 1900; several thousand people were poisoned in Japan in the mid-twentieth century due to arsenic contaminated dry milk and soy sauce. Particularly at risk of arsenic exposure are some groups of mining and smelter workers as well as agricultural workers who come into contact with pesticides.

Accumulated evidence suggests that arsenic is a carcinogen. It is a cause of skin and lung cancer, when ingested or inhaled, and has been linked to internal cancers, such as bladder, kidney, and liver cancers.[19] Geographic regions that have high levels of naturally occurring arsenic in the drinking water (e.g., Taiwan and Argentina) also have elevated levels of bladder cancer mortality.[20] There may be a dose-response relationship between exposure to inorganic arsenic in drinking water and bladder cancer. Because many of the findings of an association between arsenic in drinking water and bladder cancer have used ecologic study designs, there is a need for additional analytical research on this topic.

Mercury

A naturally occurring chemical that is highly toxic, mercury has been used medically to treat syphilis, as an agricultural fungicide, and in dental amalgams. Canned tuna fish at one point was suspected of containing unhealthful levels of mercury. In 1956, an environmental catastrophe occurred in Minamata Bay, Japan, where approximately 3,000 cases of neurologic disease resulted among people who ate fish contaminated with methyl mercury.[21] The neurologic condition, which became known as Minamata disease, was characterized by numbness of the extremities, deafness, poor vision, and drowsiness; the condition was unresponsive to medical intervention and frequently culminated in death. The cause was attributed to discharges of mercury compounds into the bay by a plastics factory.

Lead

Exposure to lead, which was once widely used in paint and gasoline, is associated with serious central nervous system effects, even at low levels. Lead poisoning is one of the most common environmental pediatric health problems of the United States. In 1984, approximately 3 to 4 million American preschool children had blood lead levels sufficiently high to have an adverse effect on intelligence, behavior, and development.[22] One study found that among children who had blood lead levels above 15 µg/dL, lead toxicity was associated with maladaptive behavior.[23] A second study of inner-city pregnant women, nonpregnant women of childbearing age, and their children found a high prevalence of elevated blood lead levels compared with the general U.S. population of whites and African Americans.[24]

Electric and Magnetic Fields

Some sources of electric and magnetic fields are high-voltage electric lines, microwave ovens, stoves, clocks, electric blankets, toasters, and cellular telephones. Epidemiologic research has found an association between residential proximity to high-tension wires and childhood cancers.[25-27] London et al.[28] conducted a case-control study of leukemia risk among children in Los Angeles as a function of measured magnetic or electric fields and wiring configuration (e.g., overhead electric transmission and distribution facilities). They reported an association for wiring configuration and childhood leukemia risk but not for measured magnetic and electric fields. A second case-control study investigated everyone in Sweden under age 16 years who had lived on property within 300 m of high-tension power lines during a 25-year period.[29] A total of 142 cancer cases were identified (including 39 leukemia cases and 33 central nervous system tumors) from the Swedish Cancer Registry. Models of historical exposure to magnetic fields were used. The estimated relative risk for childhood leukemia increased at higher magnetic field exposure levels. Other research found no significant association between childhood leukemia and power lines.[30] Regarding other carcinogenic effects of exposure to electromagnetic radiation, research conducted in the United States and Norway reported an increased risk of male breast cancer (which is rare) among male electrical workers potentially exposed to electromagnetic fields.[31]

This field of epidemiologic inquiry, which has numerous methodologic challenges, provides a rich opportunity to address an important public policy issue. Among the methodologic issues is the precise measurement of residential exposure to electromagnetic radiation.[32]

Ionizing Radiation

Ionizing radiation consists of either particle energy (e.g., highly energetic protons, neutrons, α and β particles, etc.) or light energy in the form of photons (e.g., γ-rays and X-rays). U.S. radiation sources comprise two main categories: natural radiation, which is responsible for the majority of the annual radiation exposure of the human population, and synthetic radiation, which is responsible for a minority of the total annual exposure. Natural radiation consists of radon, cosmic rays from outer space, and radiation from geologic sources. Synthetic sources are medical X-rays and agents used in nuclear medicine, consumer products, nuclear generators, and nuclear weapons explosions. Health effects associated with ionizing radiation from nuclear facilities are discussed later in this chapter. Studies of the long-term consequences of exposure to radiation from the atomic bombs dropped in Japan confirmed increases in the risk of breast cancer, especially if exposure occurred between the ages of 10 and 19 years.[33]

Radon is an inert gas produced by the decay of radium and uranium, which are found universally in the earth's crust in varying amounts. Environmental radon produces one of the largest sources of human exposure to ionizing radiation. Up to 20% of U.S. lung cancers may be caused by radon despite evidence that cigarette smoking, asbestos exposure, and urban air pollution are the leading causes of lung cancer. Radon exposure found in residential areas may be linked to cancer. Both lifetime risk of lung cancer and years of life lost show a dose-response increase with increasing radon exposure.[34]

Allergens and Molds

Allergens, which are found in the environment (e.g., the ambient air), are substances that provoke an allergic reaction in susceptible individuals, who may demonstrate a great deal of variation in responsiveness. The allergenic stimulus may consist of fur, pollen, or any of numerous other substances in the environment. Allergic reactions range from dermatitis, asthma, itchy eyes, and other uncomfortable sensations to anaphylactic shock.

While employed by a local health department, Robert Friis once investigated a community outbreak of respiratory disease symptoms alleged to be an allergy associated with molds that were growing in a certain housing tract. A visit to the area disclosed a large number of expensive homes that had been constructed with elegant sunken living rooms. After intense rainfall, the sunken areas flooded and remained permanently saturated with water. Molds of four different colors flourished on the nearby walls and carpets and resisted all attempts at elimination. Some of the residents began to complain of increased numbers of colds, respiratory illnesses, and allergic symptoms. The health department's serologic tests and questionnaire studies, however, did not reveal any increase in illness or symptoms above what might be usually expected. Investigators concluded that, in this instance, there was no statistically significant relationship between exposure to molds and lung diseases or other health conditions examined.

Physical and Mechanical Energy

These agents are associated with accidental injury, as in automobile accidents or accidents in the home and workplace. In addition to traumatic forces, other examples include noise, vibration, and extremes of temperature. Morbidity and mortality from the effects of physical and mechanical energy (e.g., extremely high temperatures) may be studied epidemiologically, as Exhibit 13-1 demonstrates. Another example is from the July 1995 heat wave in Chicago. An excess of at least 700 deaths occurred at the same time as a record-breaking heat wave; most of this excess mortality was classified as heat-related. Semenza et al. conducted a case-control study of risk factors associated with heat-related and cardiovascular mortality.[35] They reported that those at greatest risk of dying from heat-related causes did not have access to air conditioning or were socially isolated.

Environmental Hazards Found in the Work Setting

Monitoring and Surveillance of Exposure to Occupational Hazards

Surveillance programs aid in the prevention of occupational illness. They can be used to identify occurrence of illness or injury in the workplace and to monitor trends in illnesses or injuries. The trends may vary by industry, geographic area, and over time, and may suggest specific industries to be targeted for further investigation or intervention. Hazard surveillance refers to the characterization of known chemical, physical, and biologic agents in the workplace. If measurements demonstrate that the hazards are present in sufficient quantity to affect health, strategies can be used to reduce exposure of workers to them.[36] Related to hazard surveillance is the concept of the sentinel health event, popularized by Rutstein and colleagues.[37] This concept facilitates the recognition of unhealthful workplaces. Seligman and Frazier stated, "A sentinel health event is a case of unnecessary disease, unnecessary disability, or untimely death whose occurrence is a warning signal that the quality of preventive or medical care may need to be improved."[38(p16)]

Biologic Hazards

Hospital employees, sewage workers, and agricultural workers are examples of persons who are potentially exposed to hazards from biologic agents of disease. Physicians and nurses come into direct contact with patients who may be affected by a communicable disease, sewage workers may be exposed to the hazards of disease carried in raw sewage, and agricultural workers are at increased risk of exposure to zoonotic diseases and disease agents contained in the soil.

EXHIBIT 13-1

High Temperature and Mortality in the United States

Hot weather is a significant cause of morbidity and mortality in the United States. On the average, high ambient temperature is associated with the deaths of more than 200 Americans annually. However, summers with sustained periods of very hot weather (heat waves) are associated with even more widespread health effects. Advanced age is a characteristic strongly associated with risk of heat-related illness. High-risk groups include infants under one year of age and certain groups of young adults (e.g., military recruits and those occupationally exposed to high temperatures). Low socioeconomic status has also been associated with high risk of heatstroke, probably functioning not as a cause but as a correlate of a cause or group of causes of heatstroke. Studies of race and sex as predisposing factors for heat-related illness have yielded inconsistent results. Other high-risk groups include the chronically ill or bedfast, the mentally ill, those taking antipsychotic or anticholinergic drugs, and alcoholics. ■

Source: Adapted from Centers for Disease Control and Prevention. Heatstroke—United States, 1980. *MMWR,* vol 30, pp 277–278, June 19, 1981.

One study showed increased risk of hepatitis B among employees at a major urban hospital center.[39] Sources of infection included possible accidental needle punctures and errors in routine laboratory procedures. The hospital also had a large dialysis center that brought employees into direct contact with blood and blood products. Of great concern is the possible transmission of the human immunodeficiency virus (HIV) through accidental needle sticks.

Mineral and Organic Dusts

Prolonged, and even short-term, exposure to dusts in the work environment may pose a major health hazard to workers. Among the notorious examples of occupational diseases resulting from exposure to dusts are black lung disease, also known as coal miners' pneumoconiosis, and silicosis, which occurs among sandblasters and others exposed to silica dust. Another example is the association between exposure to rubber dust and chronic obstructive pulmonary disease.[40] Rochette[41] found that the standardized mortality ratio for overall mortality was higher among coal miners than among the total U.S. male population. Mortality from nonmalignant respiratory disease, accidents, and stomach cancer also was higher than expected. Milham[42] reported an association between lung cancer and pulmonary emphysema among aluminum workers.

Vapors

Vapors and fumes represent a significant occupational hazard in many types of work. Given the yearly increase in the numbers of chemical substances and solvents that are utilized in the work environment, fumes and vapors are likely to become an increasing hazard to the health of workers. Various organic solvents, such as benzene, may act as carcinogenic agents. Buffler et al.[14] discussed the relationship between exposure to vinyl chloride and angiosarcoma. In addition to being potential carcinogenic agents, organic solvents may damage internal organs of the body, the liver being especially vulnerable.

Psychosocial Aspects of Employment and Health

Stresses and other psychosocial aspects of the work environment represent an important area of investigation for occupational health epidemiologists. Some of the findings related to this field of inquiry are reported in Chapter 15. Researchers have probed the psychosocial aspects of the job environment in great depth. Examples of research topics include work overload and coronary heart disease, job stresses and absenteeism due to infectious and chronic diseases, shift work and physical and mental health, health effects of physical activity at work, and variations in chronic disease mortality according to occupational status. A representative study reported that stress-related characteristics of work (e.g., level of mental demand) were associated with periodontal health status.[43] Work stress included high mental demands and excessive work and time pressure.

Noteworthy Community Environmental Health Hazards

Environmental hazards are not restricted to the workplace. Examples of such potential hazards in the community include chemicals from industrial sources and toxic waste dumps, air pollution, emissions of ionizing radiation from nuclear power facilities, and degradation of water quality. Two specific environmental health incidents are the sick building syndrome and Gulf War syndrome (see Exhibits 13-2 and 13-3, respectively).

EXHIBIT 13-2

The Sick Building Syndrome (SBS)

SBS has enormous potential for great economic impact from lost workdays, litigation, and workers' compensation claims. It is a condition that has several hypothesized etiologies, one being poor indoor air quality, which may affect health adversely. Indoor air quality became an issue during the 1970s when, in response to an energy crisis, buildings were made more airtight and ventilation rates were reduced.[44] Cases of SBS frequently occur in heavily populated, carpeted, and poorly cleaned buildings.

The term *sick building syndrome* was coined in 1983 at a World Health Organization meeting in Geneva to describe illnesses of office employees that included "dryness of the skin and mucous membranes, mental fatigue, headaches, general pruritis, and airway infections."[45] The prevalence of SBS has not been determined accurately because of the lack of a precise case definition and the absence of specific biologic markers.

Not only is the precise definition of SBS unclear, it also bears some similarity to three other controversial disorders: multiple chemical sensitivity, chronic fatigue syndrome, and fibrositis. For example, all have fatigue as a component as well as sharing a nonspecific quality. One of the noteworthy features of SBS, in contrast to these other disorders, is temporality of symptoms; they begin when the affected person enters the building and diminish when the person leaves. One study showed that the prevalence of SBS symptoms decreased greatly when employees were exposed to an improved ventilation system.[46]

In addition to poor indoor air quality and inadequate ventilation, other proposed causes of SBS include exposure to volatile organic compounds (e.g., solvents), low humidity, airborne microbial agents—bacterial endotoxins, molds, dust mites—and tobacco smoke and odors.[44] Several psychosocial factors for SBS have been linked to the nature of some work environments: monotonous, authoritarian, and overly demanding.[44] Organizational stress—poor worker cooperation and physical and mental stress—may be an important component of the SBS.[47] ■

EXHIBIT 13-3

The Gulf War Syndrome (GWS)

Following the conclusion of the 1991 war in the Persian Gulf, veterans began to report symptoms of GWS.[48] As of the late 1990s, nearly 15% of the almost 700,000 U.S. veterans who served in this conflict complained of health conditions that they believed were the result of the war. Some of the veterans' health problems could be accounted for by standard medical or psychiatric diagnoses that were not connected with the war. Nevertheless, for many of the remaining ill veterans, GWS emerged as a common pattern or array of nonspecific, vague symptoms with uncertain etiology.[49]

An influential Presidential Advisory Committee of Gulf War Veterans' Illnesses suggested that GWS might be explained by wartime stress. GWS appeared to bear similarities to the posttraumatic stress disorder that was said to follow other wars. However, some reports have been critical of this explanation.[49]

Among other causes suggested for GWS were the chronic fatigue syndrome, fibromyalgia, or exposure to nerve gas, which is known to be a cholinesterase inhibitor.[48] Possible contact with nerve gas might have occurred when U.S. troops destroyed an ammunition dump that was later found to contain traces of mustard gas and the potent nerve agent, sarin.[50] A large number of troops were downwind from the dump. Many of the symptoms of GWS would be consistent with neurotoxicity from low-grade nerve gas poisoning, pesticides, or other cholinesterase inhibitors. Exposure to these agents might account for the muscle weakness, sweating, wheezing, and other symptoms that the affected Gulf War veterans reported. ■

Hazardous Waste Sites

Hazardous waste sites represent a potential source of human exposure to toxic chemicals. It has been estimated that more than 750 million tons of toxic chemical substances have been discarded into as many as 50,000 hazardous waste sites.[51] Notorious toxic waste sites in the United States include Love Canal, New York; the Valley of the Drums in Kentucky; Times Beach, Missouri; and the Stringfellow acid pits in California. A major public health concern is the potential impact upon human health of waste leachates emitted by disposal sites into community water supplies. Most communities in the United States receive water supplies from underground aquifers and surface water, which are at potential risk of contamination by toxic wastes. One study reported a statistically significant excess of some forms of cancer mortality among residents of counties that contain hazardous waste sites.[51]

Epidemiologic research into the health effects associated with hazardous waste sites confronts several methodologic difficulties. Because hazardous wastes involve a complex mixture of substances, it is difficult not only to sort out which chemicals affect human health, but also to determine how best to measure specific exposures in a valid and reliable manner. Some studies may not control adequately for potentially confounding factors and thus need to be interpreted with caution.[52] Measurement of the long-term effects of continuous exposure is difficult. Some of the research in this field is based upon small study samples, relatively few health events, statistically nonsignificant findings, and inadequate assessment of exposures. A technique for reducing the danger of misinterpretation inherent in a single study is the use of meta-analysis, which allows for the pooling of the results of all available research.[2]

Possible adverse effects of hazardous waste exposure include birth outcomes (low birth weight and occurrence of congenital malformations or other birth defects), neurologic disease, cancer, synergistic effects, illness symptoms, and other adverse health conditions.[2] A study of residents of Love Canal (which is located in upstate New York near Niagara Falls) showed an excess of low birth weights as well as growth retardation for those exposed compared with the general population and an excess of birth defects in residents closest to the site. The rate of respiratory cancer was similar to that for the Niagara Falls area, however.[52] An extensive case-control study of over 9,000 newborns with congenital malformations living in proximity to hazardous waste sites in New York state found a small but statistically significant risk for birth defects.[9]

Air Pollution

Air pollution lowers quality of life by obscuring the natural environment and by being malodorous. Among the constituents of air pollution (although these vary from one location to another depending upon the types of fuels in use) are sulfur oxides, particulates, oxidants (including ozone, carbon monoxide, hydrocarbons, and nitrogen oxides), lead, and some other heavy metals.[53] Indoor air pollution from cigarette smoke, gas stoves, and formaldehyde may pose risk for respiratory illness.[54] Another example is the sick building syndrome,[55,56] which was noted earlier in this chapter.

Major lethal air pollution episodes include those in Donora, Pennsylvania (1948); London, England (1952); and Meuse Valley in Western Europe (1930).[2] Air pollution levels, which in many urban areas (e.g., Mexico City) are alarmingly high, are related to human mortality. Individuals who have preexisting heart and lung disease may be at particular risk for the fatal or aggravating effects of air pollution. Cigarette smoking and air pollution may act synergistically in aggravation of lung diseases, such as emphysema.[53]

An example of research on air pollution's health effects is that conducted by Henderson et al.[57] Census tracts in Los Angeles were aggregated into 14 study areas that represented homogeneous air pollution profiles. The study reported a correlation between the geographic distribution of lung cancer cases and the general location of emission sources for hydrocarbons.

Other epidemiologic analyses have shown a correlation between increases in total daily mortality and increased air pollution in New York City.[58] Daily mortality also was related to gaseous and particulate air pollution in St. Louis, Missouri, and the counties in eastern Tennessee.[59] Researchers estimated the daily mortality rate associated with inhalable particles, fine particles, and aerosol acidity. The total mortality rate was found to have increased by 16% in St. Louis, Missouri, and by 17% in the eastern Tennessee counties. The data further suggested that the mass concentrations of particles have an association with daily mortality.

Carbon monoxide arises from cigarette smoking, automobile exhaust, and certain types of occupational exposures. An investigation into the possible association between angina pectoris and heavy freeway traffic found no direct association between myocardial infarction and ambient carbon monoxide. It was hypothesized that there was an indirect association between exposure to carbon monoxide in the ambient air and acute myocardial infarction through smoking, which is associated with elevated blood carbon monoxide levels.[60]

The air of one large metropolitan city exposed pedestrians and outside workers to carbon monoxide levels that ranged from 10 to 50 ppm; there were even higher levels in poorly ventilated areas of the city.[61] The recommended standard for carbon monoxide in occupational settings is a maximum of 50 ppm. Pedestrians and workers who have heart problems may be at increased risk of aggravation of their condition when exposed to high levels of ambient carbon monoxide in the urban environment.

A major investigation, the Tucson Epidemiological Study of Airways Obstructive Diseases, has tracked the etiology and natural history of obstructive lung disease.[62] Based on a multistage stratified cluster sample of white households in the Tucson, Arizona, area, it has generated many important findings, including the effects of passive smoking in children.[63]

The term *passive smoking,* also known as sidestream exposure to cigarette smoke, refers to the involuntary breathing of cigarette smoke by nonsmokers in an environment where there are cigarette smokers present. In restaurants, waiting rooms, international airliners, and other enclosed areas where there are cigarette smokers, nonsmokers may be unwillingly (and, perhaps, unwittingly) exposed to a potential health hazard. The effects of chronic exposure to cigarette smoke in the work environment were examined in a cross-sectional study of 5,210 cigarette smokers and nonsmokers. Nonsmokers who did not work in a smoking environment were compared with nonsmokers who worked in a smoking environment as well as with smokers. Exposure to smoke in the work environment among the nonsmokers was associated with a statistically significant reduction in pulmonary function test measurements in comparison with the nonsmokers in the smoke-free environment.[64] A 1992 report from the U.S. Environmental Protection Agency concluded that environmental tobacco smoke is a human lung carcinogen responsible for approximately 3,000 lung cancer deaths annually among U.S. nonsmokers.[65] Among children, passive smoking is associated with bronchitis, pneumonia, fluid in the middle ear, asthma incidence, and aggravation of existing asthma.

Research on passive smoking presents several methodologic difficulties. Eleven studies conducted in the United States have shown an average relative risk of death of 1.19 among nonsmoking spouses of smokers.[66] Relatively small increases in risk of death from passive smoking are difficult to demonstrate, given the use of questionnaires to quantify smoking by spouses, the long- and short-term variability in exposures to cigarette smoke from sources other than the spouse (e.g., those at work, restaurants, and entertainment venues), and the long latency period between exposure to cigarette smoke and onset of disease. Additional research will require improved methods for assessing exposure to cigarette smoke, such as the use of biologic markers (e.g., cotinine).

Nuclear Facilities

Nuclear facilities include weapons production plants, test sites, and nuclear power plants. In the United States, nuclear weapons have been produced at Oak Ridge, Tennessee; Hanford, Washington; and Rocky Flats in Denver, Colorado. Epidemiologists have studied the health effects of a nuclear accident at Three Mile Island, Pennsylvania, that occurred on March 26, 1979. One study reported that there was a modest association between postaccident cancer rates and proximity to the power plant. There was a postaccident increase in cancer rates during 1982 and 1983, which subsequently declined. Radiation emissions from the plant did not appear to account for the observed increase in cancer rates, however.[67]

The nuclear power plant accident at Chernobyl, Ukraine, in April 1986 was a major public health disaster that produced massive exposure of European populations to ionizing radiation. Radioactive materials, primarily iodine and cesium, were dispersed over the eastern part of the former Soviet Union, Sweden, Austria, Switzerland, and parts of Germany and northern Italy.[68] A considerable time interval will need to pass before it is possible to observe the carcinogenic effects of the accident in geographic areas that are at a distance from the Chernobyl power plant. Preliminary epidemiologic research has investigated the association between cases of childhood cancers (leukemia and lymphoma) and the accident. Although one study found a statistically significant increase in childhood cancers after the mishap, it is unclear whether these are linked to radiation from Chernobyl.[68] Furthermore, it may never be possible to determine whether there was any increase in cancer incidence due to radiation exposure from this untoward event. There is no method to distinguish between leukemia resulting from the Chernobyl disaster and leukemias of other origins. Natural background radiation and medical radiation may exceed the radiation levels from the Chernobyl release.

Closer to the Chernobyl nuclear facility, however, there have been marked increases in thyroid cancer as soon as four to five years after the accident. The Gomel region of Belarus in the former Soviet Union lies immediately to the north of Chernobyl. There was a sharp increase in thyroid cancer cases among children in Gomel from 1 to 2 per year during 1986–1989 to 38 in 1991.[69] These increases in the number of thyroid cancer cases suggest that the carcinogenic effect of radioactive fallout is much greater than previously believed.[70]

Another health effect of the Chernobyl accident could be the production of birth defects, such as congenital anomalies. Data from the EUROCAT epidemiologic surveillance of congenital anomalies have not suggested an increase in central nervous system anomalies or Down's syndrome in Western Europe.[71]

In terms of cancer rates and proximity to other nuclear installations, studies with conflicting results have emerged. One study reported an excess of leukemia in a five-town area in Massachusetts in which one of the towns was the site of a commercial nuclear power plant. The excess cases were found mostly in adults and the elderly, but the authors believed that the results from this descriptive study were suggestive and warranted additional, more intensive follow-up investigations.[72] In contrast, no excess of cancer deaths was found among populations near the Rocky Flats nuclear weapons plant in Colorado[73] or the San Onofre nuclear power plant in California.[74] A systematic literature review concluded that, although many studies of the health effects of community exposure to radiation were statistically sound, they did not provide adequate quantitative estimates of radiation dose that could be used to assess dose-response relationships.[75]

There have been many studies of the health effects of above-ground atmospheric testing of nuclear weapons at the Nevada test site in the United States during the period from 1951 to 1958. Among the components of fallout from weapons testing is radioactive iodine, which may become concentrated in the thyroid gland, producing thyroid cancer. An ongoing epidemiologic project is a cohort study of young people who lived in proximity to the test site during infancy and childhood.[76] Three cohorts, similar in demographic and lifestyle characteristics, were selected. Two cohorts were from Washington County, Utah, and Lincoln County, Nevada, both on the west side of the test site, close to the site, and in the pathway of the heaviest fallout. A third unexposed cohort was selected from Graham County, far to the south of the test site. At 12 to 15 years and 30 years after the heaviest fallout, there was a slight but nonsignificant increase in rates of thyroid cancer among the two exposure cohorts in comparison with the control cohort. Thus, it was concluded that living near the Nevada test site did not produce a statistically significant increase in thyroid neoplasms.

Drinking Water

Recently, public health experts have been concerned about possible degradation of the quality of water supplies in the United States due to increasing industrialization, urbanization, and population growth. Sources of contamination of ground water include chemical plants and nuclear facilities, which may threaten permanent contamination of ground water with pesticides, carcinogens, and radioactivity.

A summary report assessed the quality of drinking water in the United States.[77] Five classes of contaminants were examined in the report: microorganisms, particulate matter, inorganic solutes, organic solutes, and radionuclides. Although the use of chlorination and standard drinking water treatments adopted early in the 20th century have led to a decline in the incidence of gastroenteric diseases, the report noted that more than 10,000 cases of water-borne enteric disease were reported in one year in the mid-1970s. This finding questions the effectiveness of methods of water disinfection currently in use. The report stated that finely divided solid particles are commonly found in drinking water supplies, especially those not treated by filtration. Although most of these particulate contaminants are not believed to pose a hazard to health, asbestos fibers constitute a clear exception. The evidence regarding the toxicity of asbestos particles is not conclusive, however. The report concluded that the inorganic contaminant with the greatest potential for toxicity is lead in water supplies. Much is unknown about the effects of organic compounds, such as pesticides, in the water. Radiation found in water supplies was small in proportion to the normal background level of radiation to which all human beings are exposed. It would appear that the problem of health hazards associated with low water quality is one that requires much additional epidemiologic study.

Conclusion

Environmental epidemiology is the study of the impact of the environment on human health in populations. Epidemiologic methods can be used to investigate a wide variety of conditions that are thought to be associated with the physical environment and the work environment. Suspected health outcomes include morbidity and mortality from cancer, lung disease, birth defects, injuries and trauma, neurologic disease, and dermatologic problems. Many of the traditional study designs are used to conduct epidemiologic research into environmentally associated health problems. Toxicologic concepts also play a central role in this field of research. Suspected agents of environmentally associated disease include toxic chemicals, dusts, metals, and magnetic and ionizing radiation. Workers in many occupational settings are at risk of exposure to a wide variety of hazardous agents. Environmental health hazards that may affect the community include toxic waste dumps, air pollution, ionizing radiation from power plants and weapons testing, and polluted drinking water. Increases in the human population and urbanization are certain to maintain society's concern about health hazards potentially associated with the environment.

Study Questions and Exercises

1. Define the following terms:
   a. environmental epidemiology
   b. retrospective cohort study

    c. ecologic analysis

    d. ecologic fallacy

    e. dose-response curve

    f. synergism

    g. threshold

2. A hypothetical community located near a large military base is suspected of having a toxic chemical present in the ground water. Propose a study design from each of the categories—cross-sectional, case-control, and cohort—to study the impacts on humans of exposures to the toxic chemicals.

3. An ecologic study reports an increase in mortality in census tracts that have high levels of air pollution in comparison with less polluted census tracts. What are some possible alternative explanations for the findings of the study?

4. What is meant by end points in occupational health studies? Discuss the advantages and disadvantages of using each of the following end points: self-reported symptoms, results of clinical examinations, and mortality.

5. How does the "healthy worker effect" influence the interpretation of findings from occupational health research? An epidemiologic researcher finds that mortality for assembly line workers in an automobile factory is slightly higher than the mortality of the general population. Assume that the healthy worker effect is operative. Would it tend to decrease or increase mortality differences between the workers and the general population?

6. Which pesticides are included in the organophosphate family? What hazards do they present to agricultural workers and to the general population?

7. List examples of metallic compounds that pose environmental hazards. What are some examples of health effects thought to be associated with arsenic, mercury, and lead?

8. Discuss the possible health effects that have been associated with exposure to electric and magnetic fields and ionizing radiation.

9. Examples of environmental hazards found in the work setting include biologic agents, mineral and organic dusts, vapors, and occupational stress. What are possible roles for epidemiologists in designing research studies to investigate and control exposures to these hazards?

10. Identify challenges and opportunities for epidemiology from the following environmental health problems: hazardous waste sites, air pollution, and nuclear electricity generating plants.

References

1. Landrigan PJ. Commentary: environmental disease—a preventable epidemic. *Am J Public Health.* 1992;82:941–943.
2. National Research Council, Committee on Environmental Epidemiology. *Environmental Epidemiology, Volume 1: Public Health and Hazardous Wastes.* Washington, DC: National Academy Press; 1991.
3. Lehmann P. *Women Workers and Job Health Hazards.* Washington, DC: US Department of Labor, Occupational Safety and Health Administration; 1993.
4. Wegman DH. The potential impact of epidemiology on the prevention of occupational disease. *Am J Public Health.* 1992;82:944–954.
5. Lebowitz MD, Burrows B, Traver GA, et al. Methodological considerations of epidemiological diagnoses in respiratory diseases. *Eur J Epidemiol.* 1985;1:188–192.
6. Monson RR. *Occupational Epidemiology.* Boca Raton, FL: CRC Press; 1990.
7. Lave LB, Seskin EP. Air pollution and human health. *Science.* 1970;169:723–733.
8. Gochfeld M. Principles of toxicology. In: Last JM, Wallace RB, eds. *Maxcy-Rosenau-Last Public Health and Preventive Medicine,* 13th ed. Norwalk, CT: Appleton & Lange; 1992:315–341.
9. Geschwind SA, Stolwijk JAJ, Bracken M, et al. Risk of congenital malformations associated with proximity to hazardous waste sites. *Am J Epidemiol.* 1992;135:1197–1207.
10. Selikoff IJ, Cuyler HE, Chung J. Asbestos exposure, smoking, and neoplasia. *JAMA.* 1968;204:106–112.
11. Benarde MA. *Our Precarious Habitat,* rev ed. New York, NY: W.W. Norton & Company; 1973.
12. Wolff MS, Tonido PG, Lee EW, Rivera M, Dubin N. Blood levels of organochlorine residues and risk of breast cancer. *J Natl Cancer Inst.* 1993;85:648–652.
13. Ciesielski S, Loomis DP, Mims SR, Auer A. Pesticide exposures, cholinesterase depression, and symptoms among North Carolina migrant farmworkers. *Am J Public Health.* 1994;84:446–451.
14. Buffler PA, Wood S, Eifler C, et al. Mortality experience of workers in a vinyl chloride monomer production plant. *J Occup Med.* 1979;21:195–203.
15. Doll R. Effects of exposure to vinyl chloride: an assessment of the evidence. *Scand J Work Environ Health.* 1988;14:61–78.
16. Selikoff IJ, Chung J, Hammond EC. Asbestosis exposure and neoplasia. *JAMA.* 1964;188:142–146.
17. Peters GR, McCurdy RF, Hindmarsh JT. Environmental aspects of arsenic toxicity. *Crit Rev Clin Lab Sci.* 1996;33:457–493.
18. Jager JW, Ostrosky-Wegman P. Arsenic: a paradoxical human carcinogen. *Mutat Res.* 1997;386:181–184.
19. Cantor KP. Arsenic in drinking water: how much is too much? *Epidemiology.* 1996;7:113–115.
20. Hopenhayn-Rich C, Biggs ML, Fuchs A, Bergoglio R, Tello EE, Nicolli-Smith AH. Bladder cancer mortality associated with arsenic in drinking water in Argentina. *Epidemiology.* 1996;7:117–124.
21. Powell PP. Minamata disease: a story of mercury's malevolence. *South Med J.* 1991;84:1352–1358.
22. Centers for Disease Control and Prevention. Surveillance of children's blood lead levels—United States, 1991. *MMWR.* 1992;41(34):620–622.

23. Sciarillo WG, Alexander G, Farrell KP. Lead exposure and child behavior. *Am J Public Health.* 1992;82:1356–1360.

24. Flanigan GD, Mayfield R, Blumenthal HT. Studies on lead exposure in patients of a neighborhood health center, part II: a comparison of women of child bearing age and children. *J Natl Med Assoc.* 1992;84:23–27.

25. Wertheimer N, Leeper E. Electrical wiring configurations and childhood cancer. *Am J Epidemiol.* 1979;109:273–284.

26. Tomenius L. 50-Hz electromagnetic environment and the incidence of childhood tumors in Stockholm County. *Bioelectromagnetics.* 1986;7:191–207.

27. Savitz DA, Wachtel H, Barnes FA, et al. Case-control study of childhood cancer and exposure to 60-Hz magnetic fields. *Am J Epidemiol.* 1988;128:21–38.

28. London SJ, Thomas DC, Bowman JD, et al. Exposure to residential electrical and magnetic fields and risk of childhood leukemia. *Am J Epidemiol.* 1991;134:923–937.

29. Feychting M, Ahlbom A. Magnetic fields and cancer in children residing near Swedish high-voltage power lines. *Am J Epidemiol.* 1993;138:467–481.

30. Fulton JP, Cobb S, Preble L, et al. Electrical wiring configurations and childhood leukemia in Rhode Island. *Am J Epidemiol.* 1980;111:292–296.

31. Thomas DB. Breast cancer in men. *Epidemiol Rev.* 1993;15:220–231.

32. Savitz DA, Pearce N, Poole C. Update on methodological issues in the epidemiology of electromagnetic fields and cancer. *Epidemiol Rev.* 1993;15:558–566.

33. Tokunaga M, Norman JE, Asano M, et al. Malignant breast tumors among atomic bomb survivors, Hiroshima and Nagasaki, 1950–1974. *J Natl Cancer Inst.* 1979;62:1347–1359.

34. Vonstille WT. Radon and cancer. *J Environ Health.* 1990;53:25–27.

35. Semenza JC, Rubin CH, Falter KH, et al. Heat-related death during the July 1995 heat wave in Chicago. *N Engl J Med.* 1996;335:84–90.

36. Baker EL, Matte TP. Surveillance of occupational illness and injury. In: Halperin W, Baker EL Jr, Monson RR, eds. *Public Health Surveillance.* New York, NY: Van Nostrand Reinhold; 1992.

37. Rutstein DD, Mullan RJ, Frazier TM, et al. Sentinel health events (occupational): a basis for physician recognition and public health surveillance. *Am J Public Health.* 1983;73:1054–1062.

38. Seligman PJ, Frazier TM. Surveillance: the sentinel health event approach. In: Halperin W, Baker EL Jr, Monson RR, eds. *Public Health Surveillance.* New York, NY: Van Nostrand Reinhold; 1992:16–25.

39. Schneider WJ. Hepatitis B: an occupational hazard of health care facilities. *J Occup Med.* 1979;21:807–810.

40. Lednar WM, Tyroler HA, McMichael AJ, Shy CM. The occupational determinants of chronic disabling pulmonary disease in rubber workers. *J Occup Med.* 1977;19: 263–268.

41. Rochette HE. Cause specific mortality of coal miners. *J Occup Med.* 1977;19: 795–801.

42. Milham S. Mortality in aluminum reduction plant workers. *J Occup Med.* 1979;21: 475–480.

43. Marcenes WS, Sheiham A. The relationship between work stress and oral health status. *Soc Sci Med.* 1992;35:1511–1520.

44. Horvath EP. Building-related illness and sick building syndrome: from the specific to the vague. *Cleve Clin J Med.* 1997;64:303–309.

45. Bardana EJ. Sick building syndrome—a wolf in sheep's clothing. *Ann Allergy Asthma Immunol.* 1997;79:283–293.

46. Bourbeau J, Brisson C, Allaire S. Prevalence of the sick building syndrome symptoms in office workers before and six months and three years after being exposed to a building with an improved ventilation system. *Occup Environ Med.* 1997;54:49–53.

47. Ooi P, Goh K. Sick building syndrome: an emerging stress-related disorder. *Int J Epidemiol.* 1997;26:1243–1249.

48. Roberts J. New U.S. theory on Gulf War syndrome. *BMJ.* 1996;312:1058.

49. Haley RW. Is Gulf War syndrome due to stress?: the evidence reexamined. *Am J Epidemiol.* 1997;146:695–703.

50. Roberts J. US responds to new suggestion of Gulf War syndrome. (News) *BMJ.* 1996;312:1629.

51. Griffith J, Riggan WB. Cancer mortality in U.S. counties with hazardous waste sites and ground water pollution. *Arch Environ Health.* 1989;44:69–74.

52. Najem GR, Cappadona JL. Health effects of hazardous chemical waste disposal sites in New Jersey and in the United States: a review. *Am J Prev Med.* 1991;7:352–362.

53. Mitchell RS, Judson FN, Moulding TS, et al. Health effects of urban air pollution. *JAMA.* 1979;242:1163–1168.

54. Lebowitz MD, Holberg CJ, Boyer B, Hayes C. Respiratory symptoms and peak flow associated with indoor and outdoor air pollutants in the southwest. *J Air Pollut Control Assoc.* 1985;35:1154–1158.

55. Jaakkola JJK, Tuomaala P, Seppänen O. Air recirculation and sick building syndrome: a blinded crossover trial. *Am J Public Health.* 1994;84:422–428.

56. Mendell MJ, Fine L. Building ventilation and symptoms—where do we go from here? *Am J Public Health.* 1994;84:346–348.

57. Henderson BE, Gordon RJ, Menck H, et al. Lung cancer and air pollution in south-central Los Angeles County. *Am J Epidemiol.* 1975;101:477–488.

58. Schimmel H, Greenberg L. A study of the relation of pollution to mortality: New York City, 1963–1968. *J Air Pollut Control Assoc.* 1972;22:607–616.

59. Dockery DW, Schwartz J, Spengler JD. Air pollution and daily mortality: associations with particulates and acid aerosols. *Environ Res.* 1992;59:362–373.

60. Kuller LH, Radford EP, Swift DP, et al. Carbon monoxide and heart attacks. *Arch Environ Health.* 1975;30:477–482.

61. Wright GR, Jewizyk S, Onrot J, et al. Carbon monoxide in the urban atmosphere. *Arch Environ Health.* 1975;30:123–129.

62. Lebowitz MD, Holberg CJ, Knudson RJ, Burrows B. Longitudinal study of pulmonary function development in childhood, adolescence, and early adulthood. *Am Rev Respir Dis.* 1987;136:69–75.

63. Lebowitz MD. The relationship of socio-economic factors to the prevalence of obstructive lung diseases and other chronic conditions. *J Chronic Dis.* 1977;30:599–611.

64. White JR, Froeb HF. Small-airways dysfunction in nonsmokers chronically exposed to tobacco smoke. *N Engl J Med.* 1980;302:720–723.

65. US Environmental Protection Agency (EPA). *Respiratory Health Effects of Passive Smoking: Lung Cancer and Other Disorders.* EPA publication 600/6-90/006F. Washington, DC: EPA; 1992.

66. Boyle P. The hazards of passive—and active—smoking. *N Engl J Med.* 1993;328:1708–1709.

67. Hatch M, Wallenstein S, Beyea J, et al. Cancer rates after the Three Mile Island nuclear accident and proximity of residence to the plant. *Am J Public Health.* 1991;81:719–724.

68. Vanchieri C. Chernobyl has no early effect on childhood leukemia. (News) *J Natl Cancer Inst.* 1992;84:1616.

69. Kazakov VS, Demidchik EP, Astakhova LN. Thyroid cancer after Chernobyl. (Letter) *Nature.* 1992;359:21.

70. Beaverstock K, Egloff B, Pinchera A, Ruchti C, Williams D. Thyroid cancer after Chernobyl. (Letter) *Nature.* 1992;359:21–22.

71. Dolk H, Lechat MF. Health surveillance in Europe: lessons from EUROCAT and Chernobyl. *Int J Epidemiol.* 1993;22:363–368.

72. Clapp R, Cobb S, Chan C, Walker B. Leukemia near Massachusetts nuclear power plant. (Letter) *Lancet.* 1987;2:1324–1325.

73. Johnson CJ. Cancer incidence in an area contaminated with radionuclides near a nuclear installation. *Ambio.* 1981;10:176–182.

74. Enstrom JE. Cancer mortality patterns around the San Onofre nuclear power plant, 1960–1978. *Am J Public Health.* 1983;73:83–91.

75. Shleien B, Ruttenber AJ, Sage M. Epidemiologic studies of cancer in populations near nuclear facilities. *Health Phys.* 1991;61:699–713.

76. Rallison ML, Lotz TM, Bishop M, et al. Cohort study of thyroid disease near the Nevada test site: a preliminary report. *Health Phys.* 1990;59:739–746.

77. Safe Drinking Water Committee. *Drinking Water and Health.* Washington, DC: National Academy of Sciences; 1977.

Molecular and Genetic Epidemiology

LEARNING OBJECTIVES

By the end of this chapter the reader will be able to:

- state the fundamental differences between molecular and genetic epidemiology
- describe the basic principles of inheritance and sources of genetic variation
- identify at least three reasons for the familial aggregation of a given disease
- define epidemiologic approaches for the identification of genetic components to disease
- explain the basic principles of segregation and linkage analysis
- state research applications of molecular and/or genetic epidemiology in infectious diseases, cancer, and other chronic diseases

CHAPTER OUTLINE

Introduction

The mapping of the human genome and the tremendous advances in molecular biology will forever change epidemiologic research on disease etiology. (Refer to Fig. 14-1 for a picture of the deoxyribonucleic acid [DNA] helix.) Gone are the days when measurement of exposure is limited to simple interview

FIGURE 14-1 Helix model. *Source:* Photodisc.

data, mailed questionnaires, inspection of secondary data, and surrogate measures of the primary exposure of interest. The value of descriptive epidemiology and disease monitoring and surveillance remain important applications of epidemiology. However, modern epidemiologists find themselves armed with several new strategies to assess precursors of disease, identify biologic markers of exposure, and search for the biologic bases for responses. The wide differential in human responses to the same environmental exposure is an intriguing issue for epidemiology that may be explored by using these advanced techniques.

The traditional epidemiologic approach—characterized by examination of the distribution of health conditions in populations and discerning risk factors for them—has proved useful for generating hypotheses and unraveling disease etiologies. However, suppose that it were possible to go beyond these methods and look inside the "black box" of disease processes. If this black box were to become transparent, epidemiologists would be able to change the definition of risk factors or clarify their location in a causal model.[1]

This chapter presents an overview of this rapidly growing area of epidemiology. For readers without a strong background in biology, we begin with a review of basic principles of human genetics (Exhibit 14-1). This review will be followed by definitions of the terms *genetic epidemiology* and *molecular epidemiology* and an attempt to distinguish one from the other. We then present several epidemiologic approaches to identify genetic components of disease, as well as an overview of the strategies that geneticists use to identify genes in studies of families. The chapter will provide examples of this exciting new frontier, and conclude with an overview of how the field of genetics has and will continue to influence the practice of public health.

Definitions and Distinctions: Molecular Versus Genetic Epidemiology

It is becoming increasingly fashionable to be a hyphen-epidemiologist. That is, rarely is it sufficient to describe oneself as a "simple country epidemiologist" anymore. Many folks in the field add some sort of modifier to their title, for example, pharmaco-epidemiologist, behavioral-epidemiologist, or neuro-epidemiologist. To this partial list we must add molecular-epidemiologist and genetic-epidemiologist, terms that many people use interchangeably. The authors will describe in which respects these two fields overlap, and how they differ.

EXHIBIT 14-1

Basic Principles of Human Genetics

Readers with a prior background in molecular biology and genetics (MBG) may wish to skip this section. It is a refresher for readers who have some familiarity with MBG or who have been away from the topic. For readers with limited grounding in MBG, this brief review may be insufficient. You are encouraged to pursue additional details in one of several fine textbooks on human genetics. In order of simplest to most complex, we recommend the following texts:

Mange EJ, Mange AP. *Basic Human Genetics.* Sunderland, MA: Sinauer Associates, Inc; 1994.

Vogel F, Motulsky AG. *Human Genetics: Problems and Approaches,* 3rd ed. Heidelberg, Germany: Springer; 1997.

Singer M, Berg P. *Genes & Genomes: A Changing Perspective.* Mill Valley, CA: University Science Books; 1991.

The Genetic Code

The genetic code is the blueprint of instructions to make our body. These instructions, coded in the form of DNA (deoxyribonucleic acid), are passed on from parents to their children at the time of conception, and are recorded using a very simple "alphabet" of only four "letters." The letters are A, C, G, and T, which represent the symbols for four different nucleic acids: adenine, cytosine, guanine, and thymine. These "letters" are used to spell "words," called *codons.* Each "word" contains only three "letters." The "words" or codons represent the codes to construct amino acids.

Although the genetic alphabet contains only four letters (deoxyribonucleic acids), they can be combined to code for 64 different words (amino acids). However, the human body is composed of only 20 amino acids, some of which can be encoded in more than one way. This possibility means that our genetic code is *degenerate* and that most amino acids can be specified in several ways. The only exceptions are methionine (TAC) and the least frequent amino acid, tryptophan (ACC). In fact, nine amino acids can be coded in two different ways, one can be coded three different ways, five can be coded four different ways, and three can be coded with six different

continues

EXHIBIT 14-1 *continued*

codons. Three codons do not code for an amino acid, but rather signal the end of the gene (ACT, ATT, ATC).

The "words" (amino acids) are strung together in long sequences to form "sentences." These sentences are the complete instructions to make a specific protein in a part of our body—such as skin, hair, red blood cells, bone, nerve spindles—or the enzymes, hormones, and growth factors that regulate our body and make us what we are. A *gene* is the genetic code corresponding to one "sentence."

Physical Arrangement of DNA

Although the coded instructions for making our body are contained in linear sequences of DNA (representing roughly 3 billion bases), it is not one long garbled string of genes. Rather, the units of DNA themselves are organized onto chromosomes. Each human should have 23 pairs of chromosomes—one pair to determine sex and 22 pairs of *autosomes*. Each chromosome differs in size and is numbered from 1 to 22. Women have two X chromosomes (one from the mother and one from the father) and men have one X from their mother and a Y chromosome from their father. Transmission of chromosomes from parents to offspring occurs through the formation of gametes during a process called *meiosis*. For men, meiosis is the production of sperm, and occurs throughout life. For women, meiosis leads to the production of oocytes, or eggs. As opposed to men, women are born with their full complement of oocytes, but only one or two are allowed to mature each month during their years of reproductive potential. Normal sperm and oocytes contain only one copy of each chromosome, so at the time of conception a full complement of 23 pairs of chromosomes is formed.

From DNA to Protein

There are several important things to know about the human genome. Not all DNA contained in our cells is transcribed into protein. Also, within a region of DNA on a particular chromosome that codes for a gene, only certain segments are *transcribed*—the process by which DNA is copied into RNA (ribonucleic acid)—and *translated*—the process by which RNA is read and proteins are

continues

EXHIBIT 14-1 *continued*

assembled. That is, the sequence of nucleic acids that determine the order and length of amino acids needed to build a certain protein is not necessarily a straight run. Certain stretches of DNA will be copied (called *exons* or *expressed sequences*) and other stretches of DNA will be essentially ignored (called *introns* or *intervening sequences*). As an extreme example, the gene that codes for clotting factor VIII (and is mutated in persons with hemophilia) has 26 exons that code for about 2,000 amino acids. However, these codes represent only about 4% of the total length of the gene! The final, and most important, point is that individuals differ from one another in terms of their DNA. Although all humans can be thought of as having essentially the same number of genes, they clearly do not have identical sequences of DNA.

Genetic Variation

How is DNA different from one person to the next? Although the complete story is beyond the scope of this chapter, suffice it to say that changes can occur in a wide variety of ways. A *mutation* is defined as a change in DNA that may adversely affect the host. One category of mutations, known as *frameshift mutations,* is the result of deletions or insertions of one or more DNA bases. These mutations not only alter the codon in which they occur, but also may shift the *reading frame* of all successive three-letter words.

Another type of mutation is one that changes the chemical structure of one nucleic acid to that of another. Because most amino acids can be formed from more than one combination of nucleic acids, sometimes mutations can be "silent" and not result in a change in amino acid. For example, a mutation from AAA to AAG would still lead to the incorporation of phenylalanine. Thus, although the sequence of DNA has changed, the amino acid sequence of the transcribed protein has not. Alternatively, the alteration of a single codon can have a profound effect. For example, a mutation of T to A in the middle base of the sixth codon for the β chain of hemoglobin changes the amino acid from glutamine to valine. The result is a change in the shape of hemoglobin from smooth and rounded to distorted, and ultimately a disease known as sickle-cell anemia.

Mutations also can occur within introns, the noncoding regions of DNA, which would be expected to have little effect on the protein product

continues

EXHIBIT 14-1 *continued*

of that gene. Recent evidence suggests that even mutations in introns can sometimes have a profound effect on the protein product of a gene. The most serious, and easiest to recognize, mutations are ones in which a mutation in a nucleic acid produces an inadvertent "stop" codon that signals the end of transcription before the full-length gene product can be transcribed. The result is a protein that is shorter than normal, or truncated, with a corresponding effect on its function or integrity.

Review of Genetic Terminology

Having finished this brief review of DNA and genetic variation, a few more discrete definitions are in order. The basic unit of heredity is a *gene,* the particular segment of a DNA molecule on a chromosome that determines the nature of an inherited trait. An *allele* is one of two or more alternate forms of a gene that occurs at the same locus. Of course, we have not yet defined a *locus,* either. It is the site or location on a chromosome occupied by a gene (i.e., a particular set of alleles). The *genotype* of an individual refers to his or her genetic constitution, often stated in reference to a specific trait or at a particular locus. The *phenotype* is the realized expression of the genotype, or the observable physical appearance or functional expression of a gene. A critical domain where genetics intersects with epidemiology is when genotype is modified (or interacts with environment) to affect phenotype (disease). Another important term is *mendelian inheritance* (named for 19th century Austrian monk Gregor Mendel), which denotes the transmission of a disease or trait from parents to offspring according to simple laws of inheritance. ■

Genetic Epidemiology

The field of genetic epidemiology is devoted to the identification of inherited factors that influence disease, and how variation in the genetic material interacts with environmental factors to increase (or decrease) risk of disease. A popular textbook on the subject defines it as a "discipline that seeks to unravel the role of genetic factors and their interactions with environmental factors in the etiology of diseases, using family and population study approaches."[2] An important premise of the field is that a better understanding of the genetic etiology of disease can facilitate early detection in high-risk subjects and the design of more effective intervention strategies.[3] The unifying theme of genetic epidemiology is the focus on genes and evidence for genetic influences.

Genetic epidemiology can be thought of as a collection of methodologies designed to answer four questions:

1. Does the disease of interest cluster in families?
2. Is the clustering a reflection of shared lifestyle, common environment, or similar risk factor profiles?
3. Is the pattern of disease (or risk factor for a disease) within families consistent with the expectations under mendelian transmission of a major gene?
4. Where is the chromosomal location of the putative gene?

Note that to answer questions two through four, families (or at least pairs of relatives) are required. This approach is quite different from traditional epidemiology, which assumes that the subjects under study are independent. When study subjects share genetic factors, by definition they are no longer independent. Lack of independence necessitates special rules in selection of subjects and analytic approaches that are not only appropriate for this situation, but in fact capitalize on it to improve our understanding of disease etiology.

The epidemiologic approach to identify genetic factors that influence disease does not require prior knowledge about the pathophysiologic process that underlies the inherited susceptibility. Rather, given that a disease clusters in families, is not due to shared environment, and is consistent with mendelian transmission of a major gene, the goal is to identify regions of DNA that cosegregate (are inherited in the same pattern) with the disease of interest. Once the chromosomal region is narrowly defined, the torch is passed to molecular geneticists to identify the appropriate gene using highly specialized techniques. This approach, called *positional cloning* or *physical mapping*, is in contrast to a more traditional laboratory approach called *functional cloning* or *functional mapping*. The latter does not require epidemiology or families, and is based instead on identification of proteins that are involved in a disease process. Once a protein has been identified, scientists can determine its amino acid sequence. Working backward, the researcher is able to decipher the DNA code for the sequence of amino acids. Finally, the investigator finds where this DNA sequence occurs in the human genome. Note that physical mapping works well only when the genetic influence on disease is great enough that there will be a mendelian pattern of disease in the family. These contrasts in approaches are depicted in Figure 14-2, adapted from a review on the subject by Dr. Francis Collins.[4]

Molecular Epidemiology

The basic premise of molecular epidemiology is that greater precision in estimation of exposure-disease associations can be made by using molecular biology to improve the measurement of exposures and disease. The term *molecular epidemiology* has been attributed to researchers Perera and Weinstein. Molecular epidemiology has the possibility of providing early warnings for disease by flagging preclinical effects of exposure.[5] The field is much broader than genetic epidemiology and includes a wide variety of biological measures of exposure and disease. As it relates to her research on the causes of cancer, Perera noted that molecular epidemiology combines "advances in the molecular biology and molecular genetics of cancer with epidemiology to understand the molecular dose of specific agents, their preclinical effects, and the biologic factors that modulate susceptibility to their exposure."[6(p233)] Many definitions of molecular epidemiology include the concept of biomarkers.[7] Consider the following examples:

- Rather than rely on individual recall of usual diet to classify individuals according to intake of fruits and vegetables, assess serum levels of micronutrients to obtain more precise measurements.

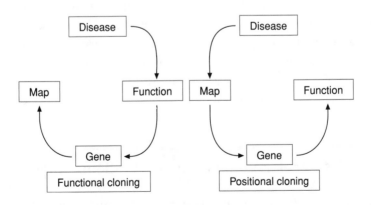

FIGURE 14-2 Strategies to identify human genes. *Source:* Adapted from FS Collins, Positional Cloning Moves from Perditional to Traditional, as published in *Nature Genetics,* vol 9, pp 347–350, 1995.

- Rather than conduct a clinical trial with colon cancer as the end point, use an intermediate marker (an accepted precursor lesion: the adenomatous polyp).
- Rather than treat all cases of breast cancer as the same disease, use tumor markers to identify potentially more heterogeneous subsets.
- In trying to identify whether clusters of cases of infectious disease are from a common source, characterize the agents according to their DNA fingerprint.

From these examples, the reader should notice that the markers (exposures) are based on biological specimens (e.g., blood, tissue, urine, and sputum) rather than questionnaire or medical records data. As stated earlier, the terms *molecular epidemiology* and *genetic epidemiology* are sometimes used interchangeably. One reason for this confusion is that another common application of molecular epidemiology is the use of inherited variation in DNA (as opposed to acquired variation—mutations—in our DNA) to classify subjects. Thus, when genes are involved, there is an overlap between molecular and genetic epidemiology. One distinction between the two is that molecular epidemiology does not involve studies of biologically related individuals. Another distinction is that most molecular epidemiologic studies are conducted to evaluate the significance of variation in genes that would not necessarily manifest as mendelian patterns of disease in a family. As molecular biologists and molecular geneticists work to unravel disease processes, they discover various proteins that are involved. Genes determine these proteins; if individuals differ from one another in the genetic sequence of a protein that is functionally involved in the disease process, then evaluation of this genetic variation in epidemiologic studies could yield important insights into disease etiology. Molecular epidemiology evaluates the association of variation in *known* genes with risk of disease, whereas genetic epidemiology includes the identification of *unknown* genes that influence risk of disease.

Molecular Versus Genetic Epidemiology

Genetic epidemiology: concerned with inherited factors that influence risk of disease

Molecular epidemiology: uses molecular markers to establish exposure-disease associations

Epidemiologic Evidence for Genetic Factors

If a disease has a genetic component, at the very least one might expect to observe the occurrence of the same disease among close family members, the rationale being that, because close relatives of a case have a certain probability of sharing the same gene that influences risk of disease, there should be an excess occurrence of disease in that family. From an etiologic perspective, measurement and evaluation of family history as a risk factor may shed light on the contribution of "familial" factors on the pathogenesis of the outcome of interest. A simple definition of a positive family history is the occurrence of the same disease or trait within a family.

Several epidemiologic designs might be employed to evaluate the association of family history with disease. A cross-sectional survey of a representative sample of the population could assess the frequency of respondents with a positive history. However, if the frequency of the disease of interest was rare, this method would not provide a good basis for assessing the association of family history with disease. A more common strategy is to conduct a case-control study and compare the frequency of family history in both groups. If there was a genetic component to the disease, one would expect the odds of a positive family history of the disease to be greater among the cases than among the controls.

As with any case-control study, recall bias is always a potential problem with family studies. *Family recall bias* is the special situation where cases are more likely to be informed about their family history than are controls.[8] It is not difficult to imagine that, as a consequence of having the disease, one learns much greater detail about affected family members than had been known prior to disease onset. An approach to overcome this bias is to perform a cohort study in which assessment of family history occurs at baseline, prior to the onset of disease. The cohort is then followed prospectively for the development of the outcome under investigation. A disadvantage, of course, is that the length of the follow-up period could be extensive before sufficient cases accrue for meaningful analysis. In addition, family history is not a static characteristic, but a dynamic risk factor that can change with time as unaffected relatives develop the outcome under investigation. Assessment of family history at a single point in time cannot capture such changes.

Causes of Familial Aggregation

Although demonstration that a disease or trait clusters in families is certainly acceptable evidence that genetics may be important, several alternative explanations must be considered. The explanations include the operation of chance and the influence of environmental factors. Zhao and colleagues have presented the case that the series of inquiries that characterize genetic epidemiology can be considered as part of a sequence of studies, built upon a common epidemiologic framework.[9]

Bad Luck

The first of the explanations for the familial aggregation of disease is simply chance. Given that there is a finite probability for the development of a particular disease or adverse health phenomenon, even in the absence of any genetic contribution at all, the disease may afflict several members of the same family. This occurrence is especially prevalent for the common diseases of major public health importance, such as obesity, mental illness, heart disease, and cancer. For example, an early study of the aggregation of cancer used cancer mortality rates for the adult British population to show that half of all families with more than five adults would have at least one case of cancer by chance alone.[10]

Two other factors—not necessarily a simple reflection of "bad luck"—would affect the likelihood that someone reports a positive family history: age and family size. Although every person has at least two first-degree biologic relatives (our parents), the person's numbers of siblings, aunts, uncles, cousins, and children are clearly random variables. For example, someone who has 15 close relatives at risk for a common chronic disease is almost certainly more likely to have a relative with the disease than a person with only two relatives at risk. Similarly, because age is the single most important risk factor for many diseases of public health importance, an older person (with older relatives) is more likely than a younger person (with corresponding younger relatives) to have a family history for nongenetic reasons. Consequently, adjustment for age and family size in the analysis may be important when one is trying to assess the association of family history with risk of a particular disease.

Bad Environment

Epidemiologists have historically devoted their energies and attention to the identification of nongenetic risk factors for disease. As illustrated throughout the earlier chapters of this book, history is replete with many success stories. This information on exposure-disease relationships must be considered as explanations for any observed clustering of disease in families. For example, although roughly 95% of all lung cancer cases are smokers, fewer than 20% of heavy smokers ever develop the disease.[11] This observation has caused some to hypothesize that host factors might influence response to environmental agents (tobacco). A complicating factor in the study of a disease with such a strong environmental risk factor is the extent to which family members also smoke cigarettes. Twin studies conducted in the 1930s provided strong evidence that smoking habits clustered in families.[12] Therefore, if family members of cases were more likely to smoke than family members of controls, a greater proportion of cases would be expected to report a positive family history of lung cancer. In this situation, however, clustering of cases in families could be due to shared lifestyle, rather than shared genes.

We know that diet relates to disease risk in a variety of ways: high-fat diets, particularly saturated fat, are associated with coronary heart disease and cancer. Diets low in complex carbohydrates and fruits and vegetables are associated with diabetes and cancer. Several studies suggest the familial nature of dietary intake patterns.[13,14] To the extent that family members share dietary habits that increase risk for a given disease, familial clustering of disease may occur. Similarly, behaviors and personality traits, such as exercise habits, alcohol intake, and use of sunscreen, may be learned within a family and indirectly relate to clustering of disease. Some of these behavioral factors in disease are discussed in Chapter 15.

Many risk factors shared by family members are a reflection of shared environment, such as water supply, radon from the soil, air quality, pesticides, lead paints, and even occupation. A case report of a family with four members with mesothelioma, a rare cancer of the lining of the peritoneal cavity, was traced back to a common occupational exposure to asbestos.[15] Infectious diseases also may be included in this category, and there are a number of published examples in which familial clustering of hepatitis or tuberculosis occurs from common exposures.

Shared Family Environment and Familial Aggregation

A difficulty in interpretation of "family history" data is the inability to determine the influence of nongenetic risk factors on any observed familial clustering. From an etiologic perspective, measurement and evaluation of risk factors are necessary in order to answer the question, "Is the observed clustering due to (shared) environmental factors?" A family study can be defined as one in which data on phenotype and risk factors are measured on individual family members.

Design of Case-Control Family Studies

As with all epidemiologic studies, there are several issues that must be considered regarding selection of case and control families. In genetic jargon, a *proband* is the individual in a family that brings a disease of interest to the attention of the investigator. In a case family, the proband is likely to be a person affected with the disease (although one can select families on the basis of an unusual family history among healthy study participants). The proband in a control family is the subject matched to the case. The definition of family also must be clearly stated: three-generation families (or more) are most valuable for elucidation of genetic mechanisms, but this comes at the expense of less complete data and greater difficulty validating medical histories. For diseases with late ages at onset, parents might be deceased and offspring will not be informative, owing to their youth. Therefore, some study designs include only siblings of probands as families.

> As opposed to most types of epdiemiologic study designs, two steps (rather than only one) are required to establish the sampling frame for a case-control family study:
> - Step 1: Ascertainment of cases (probands) and controls
> - Step 2: Enumeration of the relatives of the probands and controls

The *ascertainment* considerations might include:

1. Where will probands be drawn from? A random sample of the population might be considered for a common condition (high prevalence), but is inefficient for rare diseases. If the researcher is fortunate, there might be a disease registry that contains all incident cases in a defined geographic region. In many situations one is restricted to ascertainment of probands from hospitals and clinics, which raises questions about the representativeness of the probands if only specialized facilities are canvassed. Probands may be identified also through death certificates,16 although this selection method would prohibit the collection of biologic samples from the index case.

2. Does the disease or trait require medical attention? It is not difficult to envision a number of important public health problems that may have a significant genetic component (e.g., alcohol or drug abuse) but the condition either does not require medical attention or required medical care is not sought. In those situations, it is virtually impossible to determine whether all eligible probands have been identified.

3. Is the prevalence of the disease known? When the incidence or prevalence of the condition under study is known, one has a much greater likelihood of evaluating whether or not the sampling frame of probands includes all eligible cases with the disease.

The purpose of control families derives from the need to be able to evaluate whether familial clustering among cases is greater than can be expected. This consideration is especially important when there are no population-based rates to calculate the expected number of disease events in case families. Control families also are needed to be able to rule out common familial (measured) exposure as an explanation for any observed familial aggregation. Control families must be as similar as possible to the case families for all other (unmeasured) environmental exposures in order to determine properly whether or not a disease or trait truly has a genetic component (Exhibit 14-2).

EXHIBIT 14-2

Family Study of Lung Cancer Risk in Southern Louisiana

Carcinoma of the lung has been traditionally cited as an example of a malignancy solely determined by the environment.[17] Indeed, the risks associated with cigarette smoking are well documented. Numerous studies also have found that lung cancer cases are significantly more likely than controls to report a positive family history of the disease.[13] Before concluding that lung cancer clusters in families as a result of a genetic predisposition, it is important to control for the fact that smoking itself "runs in families."[18] Southern Louisiana has some of the highest lung cancer mortality rates in the country.[19] Epidemiologic studies designed to identify the basis for these high rates were unable to attribute the excess rates to high prevalence of tobacco exposure or industrial exposures, such as shipbuilding,[20] oil refining,[21] and sugarcane farming.[22]

To investigate the hypothesis that a genetic predisposition was operative, Ooi and colleagues conducted a case-control family study.[16] Probands were deceased lung cancer patients identified from a listing of all deaths attributed to lung cancer in a 10-parish (county) area over a four-year period (1976–1979). A total of 440 case probands were identified. Control probands were identified as the spouse of the case if he or she had ever been married. Telephone interviews were conducted to construct pedigrees of parents, siblings, offspring, and half-siblings of the cases and

continues

EXHIBIT 14-2 *continued*

controls. Interviews also collected data on cancer history, current age (or age at death), age at onset for affected persons, smoking histories, and occupational exposures. Participation rates were equivalent for case and control families (76%). The study reported that cases were 2.4 times more likely than controls to have a first-degree relative with lung cancer. After excluding the probands and spouses, statistical models were fitted to predict the risk of lung cancer in relatives. The models adjusted for age, sex, pack-years of cigarette smoking, occupational/industrial exposures, and a variable to reflect whether or not a study participant shared genes with the lung cancer proband (i.e., was a case relative or a control relative). After adjusting for the established risk factors for lung cancer, relationship to a lung cancer proband remained a significant predictor of risk (odds ratio [OR] = 2.4). Risk was especially elevated for parents (OR = 4.4) and non-smoking sisters of the probands (OR = 4.6). Further analysis of the data suggested that susceptibility to cancer included sites besides the lung, notably other smoking-associated cancers.[23] ∎

Control families can be identified from several possible sources. One would be the same disease registry, clinic, or hospital from which the probands were drawn, but with sampling based on a different disease. Another choice is random selection from the general population (e.g., neighborhood controls). Relatives of the proband's spouse have been used as controls since the turn of the twentieth century. This clever approach "matches" families on unmeasured lifestyle, economic status, education, and even religious influences, because likes tend to marry likes.[24]

Although the primary focus of this section has been on the selection of families through a proband with a disease of interest, other strategies may be considered. For example, a random sample of families from a cross-sectional study might be considered if one is interested in the genetic epidemiology of a common biologic trait or process, such as steroid hormone levels or eating behaviors.

Gene Mapping: Segregation and Linkage Analysis

If a disease or trait is demonstrated to cluster in families and shown to persist even after controlling for shared nongenetic risk factors, then sufficient evidence has accumulated to begin to explore the hypothesis that the familial aggregation may be the reflection of an underlying genetic influence. For studies of this type, families or pairs of related individuals are required. Ideally, one would want a population-based sample of families ascertained through probands diagnosed in a defined geographic area over a specific time period. If one had conducted a case-control family study to rule out shared environment as the cause of familial aggregation, then the case families from that investigation could be subjected to further analysis. *Segregation analysis* is an approach to determine, from a sample of families, whether a particular disease or trait is inherited in mendelian fashion. By mendelian, we mean the situation in which the mode of transmission of a disease or trait from parents to offspring is consistent with simple laws of inheritance, as first discovered by the Austrian monk, Gregor Mendel.

Modes of Inheritance

The mode of inheritance refers to the association between the number of mutated alleles at a locus and a given phenotype (disease or trait) and whether or not the locus is situated on one of the 22 autosomes or on a sex chromosome. Consider the simple situation in which there are only two possible alleles at a locus, B and b. Furthermore, suppose that allele B is associated with disease. Because humans have two alleles at a locus, the three possible genotypes are therefore BB, Bb, or bb. An individual's genotype is determined by the genotypes of his or her parents and the particular two alleles that were passed on at meiosis. According to the principles of mendelian inheritance, the alleles transmitted from parents to offspring are randomly determined. Consequently, a parent whose genotype is Bb will transmit, on average, the B allele 50% of the time and the b allele the other 50%. Parents who are either BB or bb are capable of transmitting only the B and b alleles, respectively. Another way of stating mendelian transmission is in terms of the probability that the deleterious gene is passed from a parent to child. The expectations that BB, Bb, and bb parents transmit a B allele are 1.0, 0.5, and 0.0, respectively.

Some diseases are referred to as autosomal dominant or recessive. The term *autosomal dominant* refers to the situation in which only a single copy of an altered gene located on a non-sex chromosome is sufficient to cause an increased risk of disease. In these situations, one typically expects to see an affected parent and, on average, half of his or her offspring affected with the same disease or condition. *Autosomal recessive* diseases denote those for which two copies of an altered gene are required to increase risk of disease. Carriers, individuals who have only one copy of the altered gene (heterozygotes) are typically not thought to be at increased risk of the disease. Matings of two carriers will produce, on average, affected children one-fourth of the time.

Traits are said to be genetically additive or codominant when heterozygotes have a phenotype that is distinguishable from the two homozygous states. Codominance may occur for both quantitative and qualitative traits. Codominance is easy to imagine for a quantitative trait—such as blood pressure or enzyme activity—that facilitates categorizing individuals into one of three levels (say high, medium, or low enzyme activity). For a qualitative trait (e.g., presence or absence of a type of cancer), the effect may be on the age at onset of disease. Homozygous carriers would have an earlier mean age at onset than heterozygotes, who in turn have an earlier mean age at onset than noncarriers of an altered allele. Although disease-predisposing genes may be carried on the X or the Y chromosome, there are very few known examples of the latter. X-linked traits are passed from women to sons or daughters, but from men only to daughters (because fathers pass their Y chromosome to sons). X-linked recessive traits affect men much more frequently than women, because men need only have the gene on their one X chromosome mutated to be in the recessive state at that locus.

Determining the Mode of Inheritance

Elucidation of the potential mode of inheritance of susceptibility to a complex disease is determined by comparing how well different hypotheses (genetic and nongenetic) fit the observed pattern of disease in a collection of families.[25] A variety of computer software programs are available to perform this analysis (e.g., some acronyms are SAGE, PAP, and POINTER). Coverage of these various options is beyond the scope of this chapter, as is the mathematical underpinnings showing how the various hypotheses are constructed. The concept, however, is basically as follows. In the traditional realm of science, hypotheses are generated and data are collected and analyzed to accept or refute the hypothesis. With segregation analysis, the outcome of the experiment (random mating and assortment of genes from parents to offspring) has already occurred (individuals who inherit the deleterious gene have an increased risk for disease). Thus, one is essentially asking the question, "Given the pattern of disease in these families, what is the likelihood that the underlying cause was transmission of an altered allele in a mendelian fashion?" Models representing possible modes of transmission (genetic and nongenetic) are fit to the data. The goodness-of-fit is compared for the various models to determine which is the most likely explanation for the observed pattern of disease. Exhibit 14-3 describes the findings of a segregation analysis of breast cancer.

EXHIBIT 14-3

Genetic Epidemiology of Early-Onset Breast Cancer in the CASH Study

The Cancer and Steroid Hormone (CASH) study is a multicenter, population-based case-control study conducted by the Centers for Disease Control and Prevention. Researchers studied a total of 4,730 histologically confirmed cases of breast cancer among patients (aged 20 to 54 years) and 4,688 controls. Initial analyses confirmed that cases were significantly more likely than controls to have a family history of the disease, especially the earlier the age at onset.[26] Segregation analysis of the case families provided evidence that the pattern of breast cancer was consistent with mendelian dominant transmission of a rare allele (carrier frequency of 3 women per 1,000) associated with increased breast cancer risk.[27] The proportion of cases predicted to carry the allele was highest (36%) among women aged 20 to 29 years, but decreased to only 1% of cases aged 80 or older. The cumulative lifetime risk among carriers was predicted by the model parameters to be high: approximately 92%. For noncarriers the predicted lifetime risk was roughly 10%, essentially the same as the lifetime risk for the general population. ∎

LOD Score Linkage Analysis

The results of the Claus et al[27] analysis (Exhibit 14-3) provided strong evidence, but not definitive proof, for the existence of a gene that influenced risk of breast cancer. Linkage analysis is an attempt to identify a DNA marker that cosegregates with the disease of interest, and is considered strong evidence for the existence of a gene.[25] The basis for linkage analysis is the simple concept that there are exceptions to Mendel's law of independent assortment of traits. Specifically, genes that are in close physical proximity to each other on the same chromosome tend to be *linked* (i.e., inherited together). Two genes on different chromosomes are unlinked, and will be inherited together roughly 50% of the time. It is important to emphasize that two genes on the same chromosome will be linked only if they are close together on the chromosome. That is because during meiosis (the formation of gametes), homologous pairs of chromosomes can undergo *recombination* through "crossing over" of the DNA strands. Although earlier in the chapter we said that parents assort half of their chromosomes to their offspring, the shifting of genetic material across homologous chromosomes often modifies the chromosomes. If genes are far apart on the same chromosome, there is a high probability that a crossover event will occur, and the genes will end up on different chromosomes. Genes that are close together on the same chromosome have a much lower probability of being separated during meiosis by a recombination (crossover) event. Therefore, the probability of a recombination event is a function of the distance between two loci. In a given number of meioses, the proportion that yields a recombinant chromosome is defined as the *recombination fraction* (θ). If the number of recombinants between two loci is estimated through analysis to be quite small (or zero), then the two loci are "linked" and the physical location of the disease-causing gene possibly has been identified. In linkage analysis between two loci, the question of whether they are linked is answered by comparing the value of the observed recombination fraction to the expected recombination fraction (under no linkage) of 0.5. Evidence for linkage is expressed as a ratio of the likelihood of the data under linkage at some specified recombination fraction to the likelihood of the data under a recombination fraction of 0.5. The results are typically expressed as a LOD score, which stands for the logarithm of the odds of linkage. A LOD score of 3.0 is equivalent to a P value of 10^3, or 1,000 to 1; this evidence is commonly accepted for significant linkage.

Earlier in the chapter we described ways in which specific genetic alterations can occur. Note that all of these were presented in reference to a specific gene. However, variation in DNA also occurs in noncoding regions of the genome. Regardless of whether they occur in coding or noncoding regions of DNA, base pair sequences that are highly *polymorphic* (i.e., that vary greatly from individual to individual) can be used to help characterize individuals as unique at a particular locus and thus can be tracked within families. Highly polymorphic, closely spaced markers that cover each of the human chromosomes thus facilitate linkage analysis. Exhibit 14-4 presents an example of a linkage study.

Samples of families selected for linkage analysis are usually highly biased. Although they may be a subset of case families initially ascertained as part of a population-based case-control study, not all of the case families will be informative for linkage analysis. That is, only families with multiply affected individuals are useful for attempts to identify genetic markers that cosegregate with disease, thus revealing the chromosomal location of the disease locus—the ultimate goal of the study. For many diseases, evidence suggests that if two forms of the disease exist, one genetic and the other not, the genetic form of the disease will tend to have an earlier age at onset. Accordingly, preference is often given to those families with multiple cases of disease, especially when those affected have an age at onset earlier than the general population average. Finally, it is imperative that the affected individuals be living, available, and interested in participating in the research study. Linkage analysis is particularly susceptible to misclassification errors, so it is critical to validate all disease end points of

---

EXHIBIT 14-4

Linkage Analysis of Early-Onset Breast Cancer

One of the most exciting success stories in genetic epidemiologic research was the identification of two genes, *BRCA1* and *BRCA2*, through linkage analysis and positional cloning. Mary-Claire King and colleagues were the first to report that autosomal dominant susceptibility to breast cancer was due to a gene located on the long arm of chromosome 17.[28] This finding was based on 23 families: seven with an average age at onset younger than 45 years, and 16 families in which average age at onset was older than 45 years. Two of the early-onset families also included women with ovarian cancer. Thus, they also were considered to be part of the phenotype in the analysis. Further analysis with more markers in the 17q12-17q21 region revealed that significant evidence for linkage was limited to the seven early-onset families.[29] The markers used were dinucleotide repeat polymorphisms: anonymous sequences of variable length repeats of DNA $(CA)_n$. The most informative marker (D17S579) included 12 alleles of size 111 to 133 base pairs. The initial report was soon confirmed[30] and an international consortium was formed to pool results and clone the gene. After a furious competition, others reported the successful identification of the *BRCA1* gene on chromosome 17.[31] Because this locus appeared to account for roughly half of the families included in the linkage consortium, work continued to identify a second locus. Roughly a year later, a second gene (*BRCA2*) was identified on chromosome 13 by restricting analysis to families that included male and female breast cancer.[32]

Identification of these two genes has only been the beginning for genetic epidemiologic investigations. Considerable work has been done since their discovery to characterize the sites and types of mutations, the complete phenotype (cancers other than breast and ovarian), ethnic variation in allele frequency, and ethical and psychosocial issues related to genetic testing. Much work remains to be done, particularly to understand the function of these two genes and identify prevention strategies. ∎

interest and check the pedigrees for nonpaternity. If one is trying to track markers from parents to offspring, then it makes no sense to compare the transmission of alleles when one of the parents (usually the father) is not really biologically related.

It is important to understand that the phenomenon of genetic linkage is a function of the *distance* between the disease locus and the marker locus. It is not necessarily an association of a *specific allele* at the marker locus with disease. For example, in Exhibit 14-4, suppose that the marker locus (Mfd188) that was found to be most closely linked to the *BRCA1* locus had four alleles: a, b, c, and d. The premise is that Mfd188 is close to the disease locus, but is not the disease locus. This premise means that the breast cancer locus will cosegregate with allele a in some families. However, in other families, the relevant marker may be allele b, or c, or d. As a result, *within* a family there will be cosegregation of a particular allele at the marker locus with the disease locus. *Across* families, any one of the four alleles at the marker locus may cosegregate with the *BRCA1* mutation. The only time one would expect to see the same marker associated with disease risk across families is when the marker is within the disease-causing gene itself and is closely linked to the actual mutation in the gene. This situation, in which a specific allele at the marker locus is strongly associated with the mutant allele, is known as *linkage disequilibrium.*

Nonparametric Linkage Analysis

Historically, linkage analysis has required knowledge about the mode of inheritance of the disease. Thus, a formal segregation analysis would be done to see if the pattern of disease in the family (or collection of families) was consistent with mendelian transmission. In addition, segregation analysis provided estimates of important parameters that are essential for linkage analysis, such as the frequency of the disease-associated allele in the population and the age-specific penetrance of the gene. Although all of these parameters can theoretically be estimated through formal segregation analysis, it can be extremely difficult to ascertain the true genetic model for a common disease with both genetic and environmental influences (considered a "complex trait" in genetic terms). Consequently, methods have been developed that do not require specification of the parameters of the underlying genetic model (hence the term *nonparametric*). Initially, they were based on sibling pairs,[33,34] but now have been extended to include additional (and more distant) relatives.[35]

One of the great attractions of sib-pair approaches is their simplicity. Although siblings will share, on average, 50% of their genes *identical by descent,* at any given locus two siblings may share 0, 1, or 2 alleles in common. Identical by descent (IBD) means that the allele comes from the same parent. If an allele is very common in the population, siblings might share the same allele, but have the allele transmitted from different parents. Such alleles that are the same but come from different parents are said to be *identical by state.* This complexity underscores the importance of highly polymorphic markers. For a qualitative trait (presence or absence of a given disease), under the hypothesis of a genetic influence, one would expect affected sibs to share more alleles IBD than under random mendelian segregation. Similarly, for a quantitative trait, one would expect that siblings with similar trait values would share more alleles IBD than siblings with dissimilar trait values.

A limitation of sib-pair analysis occurs in the following situations: one cannot unambiguously determine the number of alleles shared IBD. This ambiguity is especially an issue when the marker locus is not highly polymorphic. When there are few alleles at a marker locus, the probability increases that alleles are identical by state rather than identical by descent. The uncertainty can be resolved if parents are available for genotyping at the locus, but only if the parent is heterozygous at that locus and the nonshared alleles are different. Kruglyak and Lander have developed analysis methods for sibling pairs that utilize multiple loci, thus improving the power and efficiency of gene mapping efforts.[36] The method works for both qualitative and quantitative traits, and has been implemented in a new computer package known as MAPMAKER/SIBS.

Application of Genes in Epidemiologic Designs

The previous sections of this chapter outlined how genetic epidemiologists determine whether or not a disease has a genetic component, and how they contribute to efforts (primarily by geneticists) to map genes through segregation and linkage analysis. The primary utility of epidemiology will be realized *after* the etiologically important genes are identified. According to Friend, "As we enter this postgenomic era, we should expect more and more emphasis on something that could not previously be studied: the gene-gene and gene-environmental interactions that we have always suspected would end up being important."[37] The next section begins with a brief review of the recent accomplishments of the Human Genome Project and concludes with a series of examples of the types of epidemiologic studies that can be conducted with knowledge of genetics. Figure 14-3 symbolizes the far-reaching impact of the Human Genome Project.

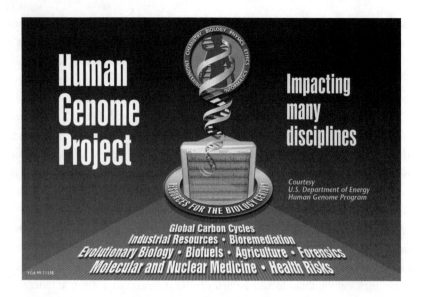

FIGURE 14-3 The Human Genome Project. *Source:* U.S. Department of Energy Human Genome Program. Available at: http://www.ornl.gov/hgmis. Accessed June 28, 2003.

The mapping of the human genome[38,39] has been heralded as the signal accomplishment that will transform our understanding of biology and the practice of medicine. Collins has enumerated several of the potential medical implications this mapping may enable, including improved diagnosis, prognosis, and treatment of disease.[40] Without question, increased knowledge of genetics and the incredible advances in technology also will have a profound impact on the field of epidemiology. First, the complete draft sequence of the 3.3 billion nucleotides comprising the genome is available now over the Internet: http://genome.ucsc.edu/ (Accessed June 28, 2003). This draft includes the location and nearly complete sequence of the 26,000 to 31,000 protein-encoding genes.[41] The mapping efforts have resulted in the identification of more than 2.5 million single nucleotide polymorphisms (SNPs).[42] Although the full benefit of this milestone will not be realized for years, the initial discovery revealed some startling facts:

- Less than 5% of the genome appears to code for actual genes.
- The size of the human genome is only slightly larger than that of some plants.

- Certain sequences of DNA appear to be highly conserved (highly invariant) across species (yeast, worms, fruit flies, mice, etc.). These sequences are thought to be highly important.
- Human DNA is highly polymorphic, meaning that it has many forms. Aside from monozygotic twins, we are virtually unique in our DNA sequence.

Applications of Molecular Epidemiology to the Study of Infectious Diseases

The use of molecular techniques in infectious disease epidemiology is continuing to grow, with many possible current examples. Maslow et al.[43] noted the types of questions that infectious disease epidemiologists might want to answer, questions that can best be answered through applications of molecular epidemiology, rather than traditional epidemiology:

- Several patients on a surgical ward develop postoperative pneumonia that is caused by the same organism, *Klebsiella pneumoniae*. Does this occurrence represent an outbreak?
- Does a patient who returns to a clinic with a second infection for *Escherichia coli* suffer from a new infection or a relapse caused by the original organism?
- A patient who has a prosthetic cardiac device is found to have blood cultures that are infected with *Staphylococcus epidermidis*. Is the infection caused by a single strain or by multiple contaminants?

By using methods derived from immunology, biochemistry, and genetics, it is possible to determine whether a bacterial disease (from the same organism) is caused by multiple bacterial isolates or by identical isolates. (This issue relates to all of the foregoing questions.) To illustrate, Hlady et al. described the use of molecular epidemiologic techniques to identify the source of an outbreak of Legionnaires' disease.[44] They conducted a case-control study of five infected patients who attended conventions at a hotel in Orlando, Florida. Nearly all conventioneers were probably exposed at least briefly to a decorative fountain in the hotel, ultimately determined to be the source of the infections. Statistical techniques could not identify an association between the disease and the fountain due to the small number of cases and the fact that many control subjects also had been near the fountain. However, it was possible to confirm an association between exposure to the fountain and *Legionella* by use of two techniques, known as monoclonal antibody subtyping and pulsed-field gel electrophoresis (two molecular biologic approaches used to confirm that the cases were affected by identical bacterial strains).

Blanc et al. illustrated how the use of molecular markers helped to control an epidemic of *Pseudomonas aeruginosa*.[45] An outbreak of infections due to this organism was linked to contaminated bronchoscopes. Two clones of the organism were apparently identified in the outbreak, an epidemic and a nonepidemic form. When manual disinfection of the endoscopes was reintroduced, the incidence of the epidemic form declined; however, the incidence of the nonepidemic form did not. Investigators used a form of molecular typing known as ribotyping to distinguish between the sporadic and epidemic cases.

Applications of Molecular Epidemiology in Occupational and Environmental Epidemiologic Research

The use of biomarkers helps enlarge our understanding of the etiology and prevention of occupationally related health problems.[46] Of particular interest would be longitudinal studies in which the predictive value of biomarkers for disease is established.[6] Cohorts of workers who have been exposed to hazardous materials, such as benzene or asbestos, could be followed prospectively. Other groups that have had environmental exposures to hazardous wastes or toxic chemicals could be studied also in a similar prospective manner. Clearly, the marriage of detailed exposure records with stored biological specimens (e.g., DNA) can be used for historical cohort designs, too.

The application of techniques from molecular epidemiology to the study of occupational and environmental health problems could yield several important dividends[47]:

- improvements in the classification of exposures
- more accurate definition of risk groups through the use of susceptibility markers
- increased specificity in the classification of disease
- greater understanding of etiologic mechanisms for disease

Groopman et al.[7] pointed out that epidemiologists are concerned with the potential associations between exposure variables and health effects. Before the advent of molecular epidemiology, it was not feasible to quantify accurately the relationships among exposure, dose, and health outcomes. Molecular biomarkers may be used to denote exposures, outcomes, or vulnerability to disease. They are more sensitive indicators than other measures of exposure.

An example of the use of a biomarker in environmental health studies is the *p53* gene in liver tumors.[48] The *p53* gene is thought to suppress tumor formation. Researchers in China examined the association between mutations in the gene and exposure to the hepatitis B virus and aflatoxin. They found that half of a small sample of liver cancer patients indeed had mutations in this gene. This research and related studies suggest that hazardous exposures may induce genetic changes that in turn are linked to cancer or other diseases.

Applications of Molecular Epidemiology to the Study of Cancer

The complex nature of cancer makes it an ideal target for the use of molecular biology and molecular genetics to improve our understanding of disease etiology. Consider this brief list of possibilities:

- Rather than rely on diet recall to assess fat intake, use biopsy of human tissue to determine the fatty acid composition.
- Rather than consider cancer a simple dichotomy, use understanding of the pathologic changes from normal to malignant cells to study early stages of disease.
- Rather than use cancer recurrence (or incidence) in studies of prevention, utilize precursor lesions, such as adenomatous polyps of the colon.
- Rather than consider cancer at a particular site a single disease, use expression of tumor markers (cell proliferation, oncogenes, tumor suppressor genes, hormone receptors, etc.) as evidence of distinct etiologic pathways. Use tumor markers to elucidate mechanisms of exposure (e.g., radon and alterations in the *p53* tumor suppressor gene).

As a brief example of molecular epidemiologic approaches to the study of cancer, consider the work by Taylor and colleagues at the National Institute of Environmental Health Sciences.[49]Previous studies of leukemia had found only weak associations of occupational and chemical exposures with risk of the disease. Taylor et al. hypothesized that, since acute myeloid leukemia (AML) appears to be a heterogeneous disease at the molecular and cytogenetic level, certain environmental exposures might be linked to a specific molecular subtype. The net effect would be a strong association between an exposure with a particular subtype and a weak association with the remainder. Animal studies suggested that mutations in the *ras* family of proto-oncogenes are a frequent early event in chemically induced tumors. (The term *ras* protein refers to a protein that is associated with cell multiplication and differentiation; proto-oncogenes promote normal cell growth and division.) Moreover, *ras* mutations were known to occur in 15% to 30% of patients with AML.

Taylor et al. conducted a case-control study of 62 cases and 630 controls. This study revealed that cases with mutations in *H-ras, K-ras-2*, or *N-ras* were 6.8 times more likely to have worked at least five years in high-risk occupations than *ras*-negative cases, and nine times more likely to have breathed chemical vapors on the job. When compared with the control group, the associations with occupational exposures were observed only among the subset of cases with *ras* mutations in their bone marrow cells. This landmark study was one of the first to demonstrate that disease etiology may be better understood if epidemiologic measures of exposure are integrated with molecular assays of the genetic defects responsible for cancer initiation and promotion.

Molecular and Genetic Epidemiology of Alzheimer's Disease

Alzheimer's disease (AD) is a neurodegenerative disorder characterized by the presence in the brain at the time of death of senile plaques, neurofibrillary tangles, and congophilic angiopathy. In approximately 50% of families the disease is inherited in an autosomal dominant manner.[50] However, AD is quite complex and probably genetically heterogeneous: linkage studies have implicated regions on chromosome 21,[51] chromosome 19,[52] and chromosome 14.[53] Evidence suggests that the relevant gene on chromosome 19 is the one that codes for apolipoprotein E (Apo E). Apo E is a constituent of plasma lipoproteins that participates in the transport of cholesterol and specific lipids. It is involved in degeneration and regeneration of nervous tissue, and is found in high concentration in brain and cerebrospinal fluid. The fact that it is genetically highly polymorphic makes it a suitable candidate gene for AD. The three common alleles have been examined in a number of case-control studies. As one example, consider the work of Tsai et al.[54] These researchers identified 77 patients with late-onset AD from the Mayo Clinic Alzheimer's Disease Patient Registry (operated by the Division of Community Internal Medicine). For each case, the next age- and sex-matched, cognitively normal person presenting to the same Division was recruited as a control. All subjects received a general medical examination, comprehensive neurologic examination, and rigorous neuropsychologic evaluation. A small sample of blood was drawn as a source of DNA. Consistent with earlier studies, the investigators found that the frequency of the e4 allele was significantly higher among cases than controls (0.351 vs. 0.130, $P < 0.0001$). Cases were 4.6 times more likely to carry at least one copy of the e4 allele than controls

(CI: 1.9–12.3). Moreover, carriers were found to have significantly earlier age at onset than noncarriers. Thus, the Apo E-e4 allele appears to be an important genetic susceptibility risk factor for AD in the general population.

Molecular and Genetic Epidemiology of Psychiatric Disorders

We noted earlier in this chapter that genetic epidemiology (in comparison with molecular epidemiology) is more concerned with the inherited basis for health outcomes. A field known as psychiatric genetic epidemiology takes several approaches to uncover the role of inheritance and environmental factors in disorders. The identification of familial aggregations of psychiatric disorders among close family members provides evidence for a possible genetic component.[55] Additional support comes from studies that find a greater concordance of psychiatric illness among monozygotic (identical) than dizygotic (fraternal) twins. A more recent development has been to identify genetic markers for disorders through studies of pedigrees and sibling pairs.

Psychiatric disorders appear to result from complex mechanisms that are influenced by genes, but few present in simple mendelian fashion. Therefore, elucidation of the genetic component is complicated by the fact that such disorders are likely heterogeneous (different genetic basis in different families), polygenic (multiple genes may influence the trait), and multifactorial (genes and environment matter). In recent years a number of studies have reported linkage in psychiatric disorders, but with few findings replicated. For example, a type of affective disorder, known as bipolar disorder, appears to have an inherited basis, but the mode of inheritance is not well defined. Susceptibility to manic-depressive illness has been linked to the tyrosine hydroxylase locus within the chromosome 11p15 region using both parametric and nonparametric approaches.[56] Bipolar affective disorder (BPAD) has been linked to chromosome 18q and chromosome 21, but the regions remain poorly defined.[57] The disease has been associated also with the dopamine transporter gene locus on chromosome 5.[58] A recent Genetic Analysis Workshop (GAW10) convened 25 groups to analyze five distributed published data sets containing chromosome 5 and chromosome 18 markers. Results were suggestive, but not definitive, for linkage to a bipolar susceptibility locus on chromosome 18; evidence for chromosome 5 was minimal.[59]

By further clarifying the genetic component for these conditions, it may be possible to further specify high-risk groups and to clarify the environmental risk factors for bipolar disorder and other affective disorders. Nevertheless, progress in this field of research is impeded by the fact that the brain is a very complex organ and that several genes may be implicated in the inheritance of mental disorders.

Genetics And Public Health

Although few will question the importance of new discoveries in the basic sciences, their true value lies in their ultimate translational potential in improved health. To a certain extent, the benefit of knowledge gleaned from the revolution in molecular genetics and the mapping of the human genome has not been realized. However, the potential has been recognized, and is considerable given the role of genes in the etiology of many common diseases.[60] Khoury commented that it is up to public health professionals to harness the utility of genetic information and technology for disease prevention.[61] Khoury grouped the range of activities into three categories:

1. Assessment of the impact of genes and their interactions with modifiable disease risk factors on the health status of the population.
2. Development of policies as to when and how genetic tests are to be applied in disease prevention programs.
3. Assurance that the public health genetic programs developed are effective and of the highest quality.

Potential applications include, at a minimum, the following areas: screening for genetic susceptibility, early detection of disease, more appropriate targeting of high-risk population subgroups for interventions, more tailored prevention approaches that recognize underlying differences in host susceptibility, as well as new therapies and treatments for disease. In an effort to demonstrate this potential, we will give examples related to a common theme: colorectal cancer.

Colorectal cancer is the second most common cause of cancer death in men in the United States, and the third most common cause of cancer death in women.[62] There were an estimated 94,100 cases of colon cancer in the United States in 1997, with 46,600 deaths.[63] Colon cancer is a part of several well-defined cancer-predisposing syndromes: familial adenomatous polyposis (FAP), Lynch syndrome I, and Lynch syndrome II.[64] FAP is caused by inherited mutations in the *APC* gene. The cancer family syndromes defined by Lynch are caused by mutations in one of five other genes (*MLH1, MSH2, PMS1, PMS2, PMS6*). It has been estimated that roughly 10% of all colorectal cancers in this country are due to mutations in one of these five genes associated with autosomal dominant susceptibility to cancer.

Screening for Colorectal Cancer

Colon cancer is a preventable disease because it has an easily identifiable precursor lesion, the adenomatous polyp. Through regular sigmoidoscopy and colonoscopy, these early lesions can be detected and removed before they become cancerous. Sigmoidoscopy is effective only for polyps that arise in the distal colon, and is therefore not a perfect screening tool. Although colonoscopy enables inspection of the entire colon, it is too expensive to be used as a routine screening modality and presents some inherent risks (e.g., perforation of the colon occurs in rare instances). However, the expense and the risk are not excessive for high-risk populations, where the prevalence of disease justifies the procedure. In 1997 new guidelines were released that defined appropriate screening modalities for colorectal cancer based on age and family history of the disease. Because susceptibility is transmitted in an autosomal dominant fashion, on average only 50% of the offspring of affected individuals will inherit the susceptibility gene. If genetic analysis for mutations in the known colorectal cancer genes were included as part of the risk assessment, then the intense screening regimen would be required to be applied only to gene carriers within a given high-risk family. Family members without the inherited mutation would require only the screening intervals suggested for the general population. Thus, resources are targeted to those truly at greatest risk, and unnecessary screening (and risk) can be avoided.

An alternative approach for screening makes use of the following observation: genes that influence inherited susceptibility in a minority of the population are the same genes targeted for acquired mutations in the general population. Colonic epithelial cells that acquire these mutations are occasionally shed into the lumen of the colon and excreted in the feces. Ahlquist and colleagues at the Mayo Clinic developed an assay to extract DNA from stool. Using a panel of markers, they were able to identify correctly 91% of the samples as being derived from cancer cases, 82% of the samples as being derived from patients with precursor lesions (adenomatous polyps), and 93% of the samples as being derived from cancer-free controls.[65] Thus, knowledge of genetics also can benefit the screening of average-risk populations.

Interventions for High-Risk Populations

The public health approach posits that shifts in the population distribution of risk factors will lead to substantial changes in disease frequency. Although these shifts should continue to be the goal to which we in public health aspire, the current reality is that there are too many risk factors, too many worthy interventions, not enough intervention professionals, and not enough financial resources to apply this model routinely. A useful adjunct to the population approach is to focus energies on particular high-risk subgroups for interventions. Consider our example of colorectal cancer screening. Once carriers of a deleterious mutation are identified, several options for disease prevention can be considered. One would simply be to perform closer surveillance and remove any polyps as they occur. For patients with mutations in the *APC* gene, the colon can literally be carpeted with thousands of polyps. The solution for these patients is removal of the colon before cancer can occur. For subjects who inherit mutations in one of the other susceptibility genes, a viable option may be chemoprevention. Sulindac has been found to reduce the occurrence of polyps in high-risk individuals.[66] Note the case of persons who have a family history of colon cancer and who do not have a genetic mutation in one of the syndromic genes. They may have a family history because of either undesirable lifestyle (physical inactivity, diets low in fruits and vegetables or high in red meat) or a polymorphism in a gene with a more moderate effect on risk. Such individuals would still be candidates for interventions, particularly for diet and exercise changes.

Tailored Interventions

Epidemiologists have traditionally ignored the possibility that individuals respond differently to the challenges in the environment. Genetic epidemiology is predicated upon the notion first stated by Galen in 200 AD: "But remember throughout that no cause is efficient without a predisposition of the body itself. Otherwise, external causes which affect one would affect all." Indications that individuals differ in response to an intervention have been around for decades. For example, Garrod, the founder of human biochemical genetics, and Haldane, the great British geneticist, had both suggested that biochemical individuality might explain unusual reactions to drugs and foods. We now know that the enzymes involved in these responses are genetically determined, and many are polymorphic. Indeed, this area (known as *pharmacogenetics*) is seeing a resurgence as pharmaceutical companies race to determine ways to tailor prescriptions and doses to patients for therapeutic (and ultimately chemopreventive) purposes.

Continuing with our example of colorectal cancer, the epidemiology suggests several dietary strategies for risk reduction. For example, diets rich in fruits, vegetables, fiber, and calcium are associated with lower risk.[67,68] Conversely, diets high in meat and fat are positively related to risk.[67,69] It is tempting to speculate that dietary associations observed at the population level would translate to effective risk-reduction strategies for individuals at high risk for familial or genetic reasons. However, if the biology is different for hereditary and nonhereditary colorectal cancer, then such an approach may not be prudent.[70] For example, a clinical trial of calcium among 30 members of families with hereditary nonpolyposis colorectal cancer found no significant effect of calcium on cell proliferation in the colon.[71]

Sellers et al., utilizing the Iowa Women's Health Study cohort, observed that high intakes of calcium were associated with 50% decreased risk of colon cancer (95% CI, 0.3–0.7) among women without, but not with (RR, 1.2; CI, 0.6-2.2), a family history of the disease.[72] In addition, high total intakes of vitamin E had been previously associated with lower risk in this cohort.[73] High total vitamin E intakes were observed to decrease risk of colon cancer by 33% among women without a family history (upper vs. lower tertile), but only a nonstatistically significant 10% among the family history-positive subset. These results suggest that care should be exercised before implementing a risk reduction intervention among subjects at elevated risk for disease based on their family history.

Conclusion

Chapter 14 has covered the topics of genetic and molecular epidemiology. These fields are truly on the cutting edge of epidemiology as a result of their promise to provide insights into the "black box" of disease etiology. This chapter has reviewed concepts and applications of the field in diverse areas from infectious diseases to occupational health to the epidemiology of cancer and other chronic diseases. Progress in the field will require training a new generation of scientists with requisite skills as well as greater collaboration and interdisciplinary work among scientists with laboratory skills and those versed in genetics who have training in analytical epidemiology.[46,47] The scientific discoveries utilizing these methods will not only improve our understanding of disease etiology, but may lead to better and more tailored approaches to screening for disease, and primary and secondary prevention.

Study Questions and Exercises

1. Consider a disease with two alleles, B and b. List all of the mating types that could produce a heterozygous child.
2. For the situation described in problem 1, which mating type gives the highest proportion of heterozygous offspring?
3. It is impossible for you to have received a sex chromosome from one of your four grandparents. Which grandparent could not have transmitted, via your parents, a sex chromosome to you? Answer as if you were (a) male and (b) female.
4. A case-control study of multiple sclerosis was conducted in which family history of multiple sclerosis (MS) was collected on all first-and second-

degree relatives. Among the 500 cases, 16 reported an affected relative. Among the 500 age-and sex-matched controls, 8 reported an affected relative. Do these data suggest a familial component to MS?

5. For a disease with an adult age at onset, what is the rationale for matching cases and controls on age when one is most interested in family history of the disease?

6. You are interested in determining whether or not there is a genetic predisposition to lung cancer. Provide at least five reasons why lung cancer might cluster in a family for nongenetic reasons.

7. A published segregation analysis of asthma shows that all mendelian patterns of inheritance do not provide a good fit to the data compared with the general model. Does this rule out the possibility that genes influence risk of asthma?

References

1. McMichael AJ. Invited commentary—molecular epidemiology: new pathway or new traveling companion? *Am J Epidemiol.* 1994;140:1–11.
2. Khoury MJ, Beaty TH, Cohen BH. *Fundamentals of Genetic Epidemiology.* New York, NY: Oxford University Press; 1993.
3. Ellsworth DL, Hallman DM, Boerwinkle E. Impact of the human genome project on epidemiologic research. *Epidemiol Rev.* 1997;19:3–13.
4. Collins FS. Positional cloning moves from perdition to tradition. *Nat Genet.* 1995;9:347–350.
5. Perera FP. Molecular epidemiology: insights into cancer susceptibility, risk assessment, and prevention. *J Natl Cancer Inst.* 1996;88:496–509.
6. Perera FP. Molecular epidemiology and prevention of cancer. *Environ Health Perspect.* 1995;103(suppl 8):233–236.
7. Groopman JD, Kensler TW, Links J. Molecular epidemiology and human risk monitoring. *Toxicol Lett.* 1995;82–83:763–769.
8. Love RR, Evans AM, Josten DM. The accuracy of patient reports of a family history of cancer. *J Chronic Dis.* 1985;38:289–293.
9. Zhao LP, Hsu L, Davidov O, Potter J, Elston RC, Prentice RL. Population-based family study designs: an interdisciplinary research framework for genetic epidemiology. *Genet Epidemiol.* 1997;14:365–388.
10. Schneider NR. Familial aggregation of cancer. In: Chaganti RSK, German J, eds. *Genetics in Clinical Oncology.* New York, NY: Oxford University Press; 1985:133–145.
11. Mattson ME, Pollack ES, Cullen JW. What are the odds that smoking will kill you? *Am J Public Health.* 1987;77:425–431.
12. Fisher RA. Lung cancer and cigarettes? *Nature.* 1958;182:108.
13. Sellers TA. Familial predisposition to lung cancer. In: Eeles R, Easton D, Ponder B, Horwich A, eds. *Genetic Predisposition to Cancer.* London, UK: Chapman & Hall Medical; 1996:344–354.

14. Vachon CM, Sellers TA, Kushi LH, Folsom AR. Familial correlation of dietary intakes among postmenopausal women. *Genet Epidemiol.* 1998;15:553–563.

15. Krousel T, Garcas N, Rothschild H. Familial clustering of mesothelioma: a report on three affected persons in one family. *Am J Prev Med.* 1986;2:186–188.

16. Ooi WL, Elston RC, Chen VW, et al. Increased familial risk for lung cancer. *J Natl Cancer Inst.* 1986;76:217–222.

17. Doll R, Peto R. *The Causes of Cancer.* New York, NY: Oxford University Press; 1981.

18. Tokuhata GE. Familial factors in human lung cancer and smoking. *Am J Public Health.* 1964;54:24–32.

19. Rothschild HR, Voors AW, Weed SG, et al. Trends in respiratory system cancer mortality in Louisiana: geographic distribution in 1950–1969 and 1967–1976 compared. *Am J Public Health.* 1979;69:380–381.

20. Blot WH, Harrington JM, Toledo A, et al. Lung cancer after employment in ship-yards during World War II. *N Engl J Med.* 1978;229:620–624.

21. Gottlieb MS, Pickle LW, Blot WJ, et al. Lung cancer in Louisiana: death certificate analysis. *J Natl Cancer Inst.* 1976;57:3–7.

22. Mulvey JJ, Rothschild H. Sugarcane farming—is there a link with cancer? *Ecol Dis.* 1983;2:267–270.

23. Sellers TA, Ooi WL, Elston RC, et al. Familial risk of non-lung cancer among relatives of lung cancer patients. *Am J Epidemiol.* 1987;126:237–246.

24. Vandenberg SG. Assortative mating, or who marries whom? *Behav Genet.* 1972;2:127–157.

25. Elston RC. Segregation analysis. *Adv Hum Genet.* 1981;11:63–120.

26. Claus EB, Risch N, Thompson WD. Age of onset as an indicator of familial risk of breast cancer. *Am J Epidemiol.* 1990;131:961–972.

27. Claus EB, Risch N, Thompson WD. Genetic analysis of breast cancer in the cancer and steroid hormone study. *Am J Hum Genet.* 1991;48:232–242.

28. Hall JM, Lee MK, Morrow J, et al. Linkage of early-onset familial breast cancer to chromosome 17q21. *Science.* 1990;250:1684–1689.

29. Hall JM, Friedman L, Guenther C, et al. Closing in on a breast cancer gene on chromosome 17q. *Am J Hum Genet.* 1992;50:1235–1242.

30. Narod SA, Feunteun J, Lynch HT, et al. Familial breast-ovarian cancer locus on chromosome 17q12-q23. *Lancet.* 1991;338:82–83.

31. Miki Y, Swensen J, Shattuck-Eidens D, et al. A strong candidate for the breast and ovarian cancer susceptibility gene BRCA1. *Science.* 1994;266:66–71.

32. Wooster R, Bignell G, Lancaster J, et al. Identification of the breast cancer suscep-tibility gene BRCA2. *Nature.* 1995;378:789–792.

33. Penrose GS. Genetic linkage in graded human characters. *Ann Eugenics.* 1938:8:223–237.

34. Haseman JK, Elston RC. The investigation of linkage between a quantitative trait and a marker locus. *Behav Genet.* 1972;2:3–19.

35. Weeks DE, Lange K. The affected-pedigree-member method of linkage analysis. *Am J Hum Genet.* 1988;42:315–326.

36. Kruglyak L, Lander ES. Complete multipoint sib-pair analysis of qualitative and quantitative traits. *Am J Hum Genet.* 1995;57:439–454.

37. Friend SH. Breast cancer susceptibility testing: realities in the post-genomic era. *Nat Genet.* 1996;13:16–17.

38. The International Human Genome Mapping Consortium. A physical map of the human genome. *Nature.* 2001;409:934–41.

39. Venter JC, Adams MD, Myers EW, et al. The sequence of the human genome. *Science.* 2001;291:1304–1351.

40. Collins FS. Genetics: An explosion of knowledge is transforming clinical practice. *Geriatrics.* 1999;54:41–47.

41. Baltimore D. Our genome unveiled. *Nature.* 2001;409:814–816.

42. Marth G, Yeh R, Minton M, et al. Single-nucleotide polymorphisms in the public domain: How useful are they? *Nat Genet.* 2001;27:371–372.

43. Maslow JN, Mulligan ME, Arbeit R. Molecular epidemiology: application of contemporary techniques to the typing of microorganisms. *Clin Infect Dis.* 1993;17:153–164.

44. Hlady WG, Mullen R, Hopkins R, Mintz C, Shelton B, Daikos G. Outbreak of Legionnaire's disease linked to a decorative fountain by molecular epidemiology. *Am J Epidemiol.* 1993;138:555–562.

45. Blanc DS, Parret T, Janin B, Raselli P, Francioli P. Nosocomial infections and pseudoinfections from contaminated bronchoscopes: two-year follow-up using molecular markers. *Infec Control Hosp Epidemiol.* 1997;18:134–136.

46. Schulte PA. Use of biological markers in occupational health research and practice. *J Toxicol Environ Health.* 1993;40:359–366.

47. Soderkvist P, Axelson O. On the use of molecular biology data in occupational and environmental epidemiology. *J Occup Environ Med.* 1995;37:84–90.

48. Bang KM. Applications of occupational epidemiology. *Occup Med.* 1996;11:381–391.

49. Taylor JA, Sandler DP, Bloomfield CD, et al. Ras oncogene activation and occupational exposures in acute myeloid leukemia. *J Natl Cancer Inst.* 1992;84:1626–1632.

50. Van Duijn CM, Clayton D, Chandra V, et al. Familial aggregation of Alzheimer's disease and related disorders: a collaborative re-analysis of case-control studies. *Int J Epidemiol.* 1991;20(suppl 2):S13-S20.

51. Goate A, Chartier-Harlin M-C, Mullan M, et al. Segregation of a missense in the amyloid precursor protein gene with familial Alzheimer's disease. *Nature.* 1991;349:704–706.

52. Pericak-Vance MA, Bebout JL, Gaskell PC, et al. Linkage studies in familial Alzheimer disease: evidence for chromosome 19 linkage. *Am J Hum Genet.* 1991;48:1034–1050.

53. Schellenberg GD, Bird TD, Wijsman EM, et al. Genetic linkage evidence for a familial Alzheimer's disease locus on chromosome 14. *Science.* 1992;258:668–671.

54. Tsai M-S, Tangalos EG, Petersen RC, et al. Apolipoprotein E: risk factor for Alzheimer disease. *Am J Hum Genet.* 1994;54:643–649.

55. Kendler KS. The genetic epidemiology of psychiatric disorders: a current perspective. *Soc Psychiatry Psychiatr Epidemiol.* 1997;32:5–11.

56. Malafosse A, Leboyer M, d'Amato T, et al. Manic depressive illness and tyrosine hydroxylase gene: linkage heterogeneity and association. *Neurobiol Dis.* 1997;4:337–349.

57. McMahon FJ, Hopkins PJ, Xu J, et al. Linkage analysis of bipolar affective disorder to chromosome 18 markers in a new pedigree series. *Am J Hum Genet.* 1997;61:1397–1404.

58. Waldman ID, Robinson BF, Feigon SA. Linkage disequilibrium between the dopamine transporter gene (DAT1) and bipolar disorder: extending the transmission disequilibrium test (TDT) to examine genetic heterogeneity. *Genet Epidemiol.* 1997;14:699–704.

59. Rice J. Genetic analysis of bipolar disorder: summary of GAW10. *Genet Epidemiol.* 1997;14: 549–561.

60. King RA, Rotter JI, Motulsky AG. *The Genetic Basis of Common Diseases.* New York, NY: Oxford University Press; 1992.

61. Khoury MJ. From genes to public health: the applications of genetic technology in disease prevention. *Am J Public Health.* 1996;86:1717–1722.

62. Schottenfeld D, Winawer SJ. Cancer of the large intestine. In: Schottenfeld D, Fraumeni JF, eds. *Cancer Epidemiology and Prevention,* 2nd ed. New York, NY: Oxford University Press; 1996:813–840.

63. Parker SL, Tong T, Bolden S, Wingo PA. Cancer statistics 1997. *CA Cancer J Clin.* 1997;47:5–27.

64. Potter JD, Sellers TA, Rich SS. Colorectal cancer. In: Ponder BAJ, Waring MJ, eds. *Cancer Biology and Medicine (volume 4): The Genetics of Cancer.* Amsterdam, Netherlands: Kluwer Academic Publishers; 1995:45–65.

65. Ahlquist DA, Skoletsky JE, Boynton KA, et al. Colorectal cancer screening by detection of altered human DNA in stool: feasibility of a multitarget assay panel. *Gastroenterology.* 2000;119:1219–1227.

66. Waddell WR, Loughry RW. Sulindac for polyposis of the colon. *J Surg Oncol.* 1983;24:83–87.

67. Potter JD, Slattery ML, Bostick RM, Gapstur SM. Colon cancer: a review of the epidemiology. *Epidemiol Rev.* 1993;15:499–545.

68. Bostick RM, Potter JD, Sellers TA, et al. Relation of calcium, vitamin D, and dairy food intake to incidence of colon cancer among older women: the Iowa Women's Health Study. *Am J Epidemiol.* 1993;127:1302–1317.

69. Willett WC, Stampfer MJ, Colditz GA, et al. Relation of meat, fat, and fiber intake to the risk of colon cancer in a prospective study among women. *N Engl J Med.* 1990;323:1664–1672.

70. Alberts DS, Lipkin M, Levin B. Genetic screening for colorectal cancer and intervention. *Int J Cancer.* 1996;69:62–63.

71. Cats A, Kleibeuker JH, van der Meer R, et al. Randomized, double-blinded, placebo-controlled intervention study with supplemental calcium in families with hereditary nonpolyposis colorectal cancer. *J Natl Cancer Inst.* 1995;87:598–603.

72. Sellers TA, Bazyk AE, Bostick RM, et al. Diet and risk of colon cancer in a large prospective study of older women: an analysis stratified on family history. *Cancer Causes Control.* 1998;9:357–367.

73. Bostick RM, Potter JD, McKenzie DR, et al. Reduced risk of colon cancer with high intake of vitamin E: the Iowa Women's Health Study. *Cancer Res.* 1993;53:4230–4237.

Psychologic, Behavioral, and Social Epidemiology

LEARNING OBJECTIVES

By the end of this chapter the reader will be able to:

- define the terms *social epidemiology, behavioral epidemiology,* and *psychosocial epidemiology*
- state the role of psychologic, behavioral, and social factors in health and disease
- discuss the stress concept as a hypothesized determinant of disease
- define status discrepancy, person-environment fit, and stressful life events
- discuss moderators of the stress-illness relationship
- state outcomes of exposure to stress

CHAPTER OUTLINE

Introduction

In his discussion of grief (Exhibit 15-1), Engel[1] questioned the adequacy of the medical model in explaining certain types of health problems. He suggested a new category of variables—psychologic factors—that are not usually discussed in the agent, host, and environment model (Fig. 12-1). This chapter considers the role of psychologic factors as well as social and behavioral factors as determinants of health. These factors, which have inspired a rich tradition of epidemiologic research, encompass determinants of health and illness that are enmeshed in the social fabric, are part of the psychologic constitution of the person, or may involve a complex interaction of the person and environment. The determinants are not single agents, such as specific bacteria or other biologic determinants of disease. Nor are they demographic variables, such as age or sex. Rather, they incorporate social and personality factors, cultural influences upon individual behavior, stress, and related psychosocial factors, all of which are multifactorial.

Three specializations cover the foregoing types of variables: social epidemiology, behavioral epidemiology, and psychosocial epidemiology. Syme noted that the field of social epidemiology is concerned with the influence of a person's position in the social structure upon the development of disease.[2] A broader conception of the field defines it as ". . . the branch of epidemiology that studies the social distribution and social determinants of states of health." The field ". . . aim[s] to identify socioenvironmental exposures that may be related to a broad range of physical and mental health outcomes." The types of exposures include ". . . social phenomena such as socioeconomic stratification, social networks and support, discrimination, work demands, and control. . .".[3(p6)]

Behavioral epidemiology studies the role of behavioral factors in health. Examples of behavioral factors are tobacco use, physical activity, risky sexual behavior, and consumption of unhealthful foods. Closely related to the field of behavioral epidemiology is behavioral medicine, which emphasizes the application of behavioral factors to specific clinical interventions, as in the case of

EXHIBIT 15-1

When Is Grief a Disease?

"To enhance our understanding of how it is that 'problems of living' are experienced as illness by some and not by others, it might be helpful to consider grief as a paradigm of such a borderline condition. For while grief has never been considered in a medical framework, a significant number of grieving people do consult doctors because of disturbing symptoms, which they do not necessarily relate to grief. Fifteen years ago I addressed this question in a paper entitled, 'Is grief a disease? A challenge for medical research.' Its aim too was to raise questions about the adequacy of the biomedical model. A better title might have been, 'When is grief a disease?', just as one might ask when schizophrenia or when diabetes is a disease. For while there are some obvious analogies between grief and disease, there are also some important differences. . . . Grief clearly exemplifies a situation in which psychological factors are primary; no preexisting chemical or physiological defects or agents need be invoked. Yet as with classic diseases, ordinary grief constitutes a discrete syndrome with a relatively predictable symptomatology which includes, incidentally, both bodily and psychological disturbances. It displays the autonomy typical of disease; that is, it runs its course despite the sufferer's efforts or wish to bring it to a close. A consistent etiologic factor can be identified, namely, a significant loss. On the other hand, neither the sufferer nor society has ever dealt with ordinary grief as an illness even though such expressions as 'sick with grief' would indicate some connection in people's minds. And while every culture makes provisions for the mourner, these have generally been regarded more as the responsibility of religion than of medicine." ■

Source: Reprinted from GL Engel, The Need for a New Medical Model: A Challenge for Biomedicine. *Science,* vol 196, p 133, American Association for the Advancement of Science, © 1977.

biobehavioral approaches to the management of high blood pressure. Biobehavioral approaches include nonpharmacologic treatment methods, e.g., exercise, maintenance of desirable weight, changes in diet, and meditation.[4]

In comparison to social epidemiology and behavioral epidemiology, the term psychosocial epidemiology is somewhat more broadly conceptualized to include psychological, behavioral, and social factors. These variables are relevant to mental health states, including grief and depression; to physical health states, such as the chronic diseases; and to the etiology of infectious diseases, such as increased susceptibility to the common cold virus, herpes virus, and other agents. The conditions that presently compel the attention of psychosocial epidemiologic research, however, are the chronic, degenerative diseases: hypertension, coronary heart disease (CHD), arthritis, certain varieties of cancer, and diabetes, to name a few examples. Heart disease, cancer, and stroke are the leading causes of mortality in developed countries (and also to a significant extent in less developed countries) and, accordingly, the psychosocial aspects of these conditions should receive high priority both within public health agencies and among researchers.

Public health, epidemiology, and the medical sciences have borrowed with increasing frequency from the theoretical and conceptual bases of the behavioral sciences for etiologic models of disease. The behavioral sciences have a great deal of potential for the development of explanatory frameworks and for expanding knowledge of conditions of unknown etiology. Sociology contributes an interweaving of social conditions as they affect disease processes. Psychology is concerned with the study of personal behavior, which is an important aspect of health outcomes. In comparison with the first part of the 20th century, the latter part of that century and the beginning of the 21st century have seen the elaboration of psychologic and social models as the etiologic bases of the chronic, noninfectious diseases as well as some of the infectious diseases.

In order to synthesize and integrate some of the findings of the psychosocial literature, we have developed the model that is presented in Figure 15-1. The figure groups some of the components of this literature under a theoretical framework consisting of the major categories of independent, moderator, and dependent variables. We have organized the remainder of this chapter according to these categories. Independent variables (also referred to as exposure or risk factor variables) are defined as hypothesized causal factors in a theoretical model. Moderating (intervening) variables are intermediate in the causal process between an independent variable (risk or exposure) and outcome. A dependent variable is a variable in a theoretical model that is affected or influenced by an independent variable.

The field of psychosocial epidemiology covers a vast body of literature; hence, the review that follows is not exhaustive, but rather surveys some of the major issues and applications in this area of epidemiology. The list of topics includes the concepts of: stress and stressful life events; personality factors, culture, personal behavior, and social support; and mental and physical health status (linked to psychologic, social, and behavioral factors). For the sake of conceptual clarity

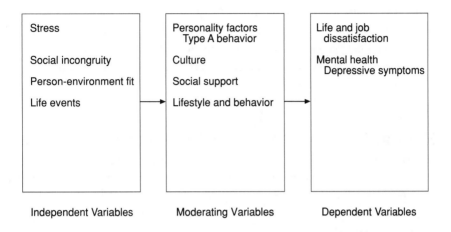

Stress	Personality factors Type A behavior	Life and job dissatisfaction
Social incongruity	Culture	Mental health Depressive symptoms
Person-environment fit	Social support	
Life events	Lifestyle and behavior	

Independent Variables   Moderating Variables   Dependent Variables

FIGURE 15-1 Guide to psychosocial epidemiology—psychologic, behavioral, and social (examples of variables studied)

and to highlight some of the traditional concerns of psychosocial epidemiology, the foregoing psychologic and social dimensions are treated as discrete categories. In reality, they are overlapping dimensions; for example, personal behavior is a function of sociocultural influences that also are related to stress.

Writings about psychologic and social processes in disease often include the variables of socioeconomic status, ethnicity, religion, and familial characteristics. Because these are primarily demographic variables, they were covered earlier in Chapter 4. The objective of the present chapter is to consider those psychosocial variables that are compatible with a theoretical framework for explaining illness etiology, that is, independent or intervening variables in the causality of disease.

Typically, psychosocial epidemiologic studies involve diseases that have multiple independent risk factors or that involve interaction of risk factors (i.e., social, psychologic, and biochemical). For example, in the case of CHD the risk factors hypertension, blood lipids, smoking, diet, and lifestyle operate jointly to produce the disease. This statement is an oversimplification, however, because behavioral and psychologic factors may be related indirectly to CHD by activating certain biochemical processes that, in turn, may be related directly to elevated status on risk factors for CHD. Another characteristic of etiologic models developed thus far for CHD and other chronic diseases is that the set of known risk factors does not explain 100% of the variance in the phenomenon under study. The foregoing statement means that the risk factor variables do not form a perfect causal explanation for CHD; many unexplained causes for CHD other than those known to science remain. In addition, a small percentage of individuals who are at high risk on all the known causal factors never develop an overt case of the disease and may go on to outlive the low-risk individuals.

Research Designs Used in Psychologic, Behavioral, and Social Epidemiology

This field of investigation has used case-control, cohort, and cross-sectional designs. The role of stress in health outcomes is one of the major concerns of psychosocial epidemiology. Some of the earlier research studies on this topic used cross-sectional investigations of captive and readily available populations (e.g., work-related groups of white male professionals). Cross-sectional studies of psychosocial factors in health are attractive because of the relative ease of such research. Cross-sectional designs, however, may not be adequate to detect the subtle effects associated with psychosocial factors, for example, the temporal issue of cause and effect and the influence of confounding variables; they also should include diverse study populations.

Needed are more longitudinal, prospective studies of the role of psychosocial factors in health as well as studies of women and minority groups, although much progress has been made in developing these types of studies in recent years. Among the many excellent initiatives in this area is the work of investigators in Germany.[5] Researchers, conducting the Early Developmental Stages of Psychopathology study (EDSP), began data collection in 1994–95. The EDSP was a prospective study of adolescents and young adults who resided in the city of Munich, Germany. A total of 3,021 adolescents and young adults aged 14 through 24 years were included at baseline. Subjects were followed up on average after a 42-month interval. This project has made possible the study of the incidence of various mental disorders, including the general anxiety syndrome and depression.[6,7]

A unique challenge of psychosocial studies is to obtain valid and reliable operationalization of measures. The process of operationalization refers to the methods used to translate some of the concepts used in psychosocial epidemiology into actual measurements. For example, much controversy surrounds the development of measures of stress, epidemiologically useful measures of mental health, and measures of social support.

The Social Context of Health

Recently, interest in the role of the social environment in health has flourished, perhaps because epidemiologists have recognized that the social environment may contribute to the regulation of psychosocial influences upon health. In Chapter 12, we defined the social environment as the totality of the behavioral, personality, attitudinal, and cultural characteristics of a group of people. The social environment provides the context in which psychosocial factors operate. From the population perspective, we find that the social environment impacts the health of residents of both the less developed and more developed world.[8] In the former geographic areas, life expectancy is reduced in comparison to the developed world due to the impact of poverty, with its attendant malnutrition and infectious diseases. Overcrowding, poor living conditions, and lack of preventive health care foster the spread of infectious diseases. In the latter areas, the social environment is also an influential component of the major causes of morbidity and mortality through the impact of noninfectious conditions, which are the leading causes of death in the developed world; lifestyle factors—smoking, diet, insufficient exercise, and use of illegal substances—undoubtedly play a role in the etiology of many of these conditions. A noteworthy example is the reduced life expectancy in the countries of central and Eastern Europe and the former Soviet Union in comparison to the European Union countries. Some authorities have suggested that one of the contributing factors to this reduction in life expectancy is excessive alcohol consumption, although the influence of alcoholism on life expectancy is by no means clear-cut.[8]

In order to compare accurately among countries the contributions of disease to morbidity and mortality, work has proceeded on the development of measures that could be used in all countries. The Global Burden of Disease Study (GBD) attempts to quantify and provide an epidemiologic assessment of the worldwide consequences of disease by using a measure known as the disability-adjusted life year (DALY) to assist in comparisons across countries.[9] The DALY is a statistical measure applied to populations that combines information on mortality with information on morbidity for specific causes. The advantage of DALYs is that they provide a standard epidemiologic unit for comparative purposes. According to Murray and Lopez, "The ten leading specific causes of global DALYs are, in descending order, lower respiratory infections, diarrhoeal diseases, perinatal disorders, unipolar major depression, ischaemic heart disease, cerebrovascular disease, tuberculosis, measles, road-traffic accidents, and congenital anomalies. [A total of] 15.9% of DALYs worldwide are attributable to childhood malnutrition and 6.8% to poor water, and sanitation and personal and domestic hygiene."[9(p1436)] The social environment contributes to many of these DALYs via a range of pathways including: unsanitary living conditions associated with crowding; discrimination and social exclusion; low status on the social hierarchy; social isolation; and adverse lifestyle choices. In addition to the social environment, we will now consider how the major categories of psychosocial variables listed in Figure 15-1 affect health outcomes.

Independent Variables

Examples of independent variables covered in psychosocial epidemiologic research include general concepts of stress, social incongruity theory, person-environment fit, and stressful life events.

General Concepts of Stress

Stress as an independent, antecedent variable to health and illness represents an intriguing notion because it seems to support common-sense explanations for the cause of ulcers, sudden death due to heart attacks, and other chronic conditions. Regardless, the scientific evidence for stress as an etiologic agent of disease is inconsistent. A review of the numerous writings on stress leads to the conclusion that the concept has more than one meaning and that some of the meanings tend to be vague, ambiguous, or inconsistent. The concept of stress has a venerable historical background in the field of medicine and in other disciplines, but is often regarded with scientific skepticism. There do seem to be several supportive findings in stress research, however. For instance, Wolf[10] cited the classic work of Walter Canon, who studied changes in gastrointestinal function that accompanied stressful events, such as pain, hunger, and major emotion. Selye[11] specified in detail the stages of reaction to stress through the concept of the general adaptation syndrome. Selye conceived of stress as a change in the environment of the organism and proposed that the organism's response consisted of three stages: alarm reaction, stage of resistance, and stage of exhaustion. Activation of the general adaptation syndrome, associated with corticoid secretion, may produce somatic disease (e.g., mineralocorticoid hypertension and cardiac necroses).[12]

Crider[13] proposed that adverse environmental events produce stress. Three examples of adverse events that may produce stress are noxious stimuli, removal of a reinforcement, and a conflict situation. An example of presentation or threat of presentation of a noxious or biologically damaging stimulus is electric shock experimentation. The early executive monkey experiments demonstrated that physiologic arousal linked to behavioral responses to remove the threat of electric

> ## Selye's Concept of the General Adaptation Syndrome
>
> 1. Alarm reaction: physiologic responses associated with preparation to deal with stress that lead the animal or person to fight or escape from the stressor.
> 2. Stage of resistance: return of physiologic responses to normal and resistance to further stressful stimuli.
> 3. Stage of exhaustion: failure of the organism to adapt to overwhelming stresses. "Adaptation energy" becomes exhausted, and, in the case of humans, severe bodily disease and death may result.

shock was associated with gastric ulcer in monkeys.[13] Removal of a positively reinforcing stimulus includes removal of rewards, such as those associated with good behavior. There may be an association between removal of positive reinforcers and impaired mental health and other illnesses. Finally, a conflict situation is one that generates two or more incompatible responses in the same individual. Examples are attitude conflicts, role conflicts, and conformity conflicts, the last of which was associated with changes in lipid metabolism in one experiment.[13]

Social Incongruity Theory (Status Discrepancy Models)

Investigators have hypothesized that either social mobility or status incongruity may be associated with morbidity. General themes of research have included changes in residence from one country or culture to another, changes in residence from a rural to an urban area, upward intragenerational mobility, and discrepancy between husband and wife in social and educational status.

Cobb et al[14] found that discrepancy between parents in social status (e.g., a high-status mother married to a low-status father) was associated with arthritis in the married daughter. Shekelle and colleagues[15] noted that risk of new coronary disease among men in a prospective study was associated with discrepancy between their social class at the time of the study and either their own or their wives' social class in childhood.

Syme and coworkers,[16] in research using urban male subjects from the California Health Survey, reported that cultural mobility was associated with CHD. Cultural mobility was defined as moving from one social setting to another or remaining stable within a given social setting while the setting itself undergoes change. In a case-control study, Syme et al. operationalized cultural mobility as cultural discontinuity and occupational mobility. Among male progeny of foreign-born fathers, sons who had college-level education had observed to expected O/E CHD ratios that were five times higher than those of sons who had completed only grade school or high school. Among college educated men, sons of foreign-born fathers had O/E CHD ratios that were more than two times higher than those of sons of native-born fathers. Regarding occupational mobility, men who held three or more different jobs for brief time periods during their lifetimes had O/E CHD ratios that were four times as high as the ratios of those who held only one or two jobs. Thus, in an urban setting, Syme et al. replicated findings regarding cultural mobility and increased CHD risk observed previously in rural areas.

The Person-Environment Fit Model

Originally formulated to conceptualize various aspects of mental health, such as adjustment and coping, the person-environment fit model is applicable also to the etiology of physiologic illness.[17] Person-environment fit is one aspect of a larger system of variables that relate to health or illness outcome. French et al. stated that person-environment fit "conceives of *adjustment* as the goodness of fit between the characteristics of the person and the properties of [his or her] environment."[18(p316)] The model further distinguishes between the objective environment, which exists independent of the person's perceptions, and the subjective environment, or the environment that is perceived by the person. Corresponding distinctions are made for the person: the objective person and the subjective person (self-concept). Lack of adjustment (poor person-environment fit) occurs when there are discrepancies between demands and supplies. The result contributes to a stressful state that may culminate in illness. An example of lack of adjustment would be an overloaded executive who has far too many work responsibilities than he or she feels capable of handling; as a result, he or she is more prone than a well-adjusted executive to heart attacks, other chronic diseases, or other health problems.

The person-environment fit model portrays a web of variables that incorporates precursors of illness (e.g., lack of adjustment), mediating factors, and specific illnesses, such as CHD, arthritis, or some of the infectious diseases. Some of the variables are hypothesized to be directly related to a given outcome, others are considered intervening variables, and still others operate interactively in predicting illness. No single factor is a sufficient cause of a particular disease. The model suggests interconnection among mental health factors, physical health status, and psychologic factors that predispose to illness, precipitate illness, and determine recovery rates.[17]

The model specifies two dimensions of the person and, similarly, two dimensions of the environment that are incorporated in the quantification of stress. Person characteristics are needs and abilities, and environmental characteristics are supplies and demands. One variety of stress may result from lack of fit between the needs of the person and supplies in the environment. For example, one may consider person-environment fit in the area of affiliation. If a person who has a high affiliation need becomes a night guard, the person will experience stress with respect to the affiliation motive. Stress also may result from discrepancy between the abilities of the individual and demands emanating from the environment. Examples of this type of stress are particularly relevant to the study of occupational stress. For example, the piece worker who is required to produce 50 widgets per hour will be under stress if that individual has the ability to produce only 25 widgets.

The model theorizes that the relationship between lack of person-environment fit and stress is curvilinear. When a person's needs are exactly supplied, stress is at a minimum. Stress may result under either of the following two conditions, however: oversupply or undersupply of gratifications. Returning to the example of need for affiliation, the husband or wife who desires to affiliate with a spouse for two hours a day will experience stress if the spouse shows affiliative behavior for one hour or less or, at the other extreme, for three hours or more.

Empirical studies that employed the model and were conducted in occupational environments in which the major outcome was job dissatisfaction demonstrated that poor person-environment fit correlated significantly with job dissatisfaction.[17] An experimental study found that subjects who were faced with work overload demonstrated increases in serum cholesterol.[19]

Stressful Life Events

This vein of theory and research postulates that there is a relationship between the happenings in one's life and the development of illness. Two crucial issues of life events research are, first, to determine which attributes distinguish more stressful from less stressful life events and, second, to refine the knowledge base regarding the pathologic effects of stressful life events.

Holmes and Rahe[20] developed the Social Readjustment Rating Scale, which comprised 43 life event items. Research suggested that the items should be rank ordered in terms of importance to the individual; for example, the death of a spouse was found to be most stressful and was given the highest weight, 100 points; pregnancy was given a weight of 40; and minor violations of the law were given a weight of 11. The more severe the life change event and the higher the frequency of the event, the greater the chance that severe disease will occur. The following are the 10 leading life change events that Holmes and Rahe formulated during the late 1960s[20]:

1. death of a spouse
2. divorce
3. marital separation
4. jail term
5. death of a close family member
6. personal injury or illness
7. marriage
8. being fired from a job
9. marital reconciliation
10. retirement

Holmes and Masuda[21] reported that the greater the magnitude of life event as measured by the scale, the greater the probability that it would be associated with disease. In addition, there was an association between the magnitude of life change and the seriousness of illness. These investigators suggested that life stresses lower the resistance to disease and that the greater the stress or stresses in the person's life, the more severe the illness that may develop.

Langner and Michael[22] studied the association of life stresses with risk of mental illness among a representative population of 1,660 residents of midtown Manhattan in New York City. Subjects were administered a carefully designed interview that contained items about childhood and adult stress factors, psychiatric status, and other hypothesized risk factors for mental illness. Examples of items were poor physical health as an adult or quarrels between parents during childhood. It was found that the greater the number of negative life factors, the greater the mental health risk.

Hinkle[23] reported on the frequency of disabling illness for a 20-year period that occurred among a group of career telephone operators who had been employed steadily in semiskilled occupations and among a group of blue-collar workers who worked for a similar division of the same company. Some employees had a much greater risk than others of becoming disabled, and, among those who had the greatest risk, there was also a greater likelihood of recurrent illnesses and more severe disability. Susceptibility to illness seemed to moderate the effect of stresses in the life of the individual. Among those who were not susceptible to illness, stressful life events did not seem to produce a decrement in health. There was also a tendency for the workers who were most frequently ill to be those who had occupations that seemed to be out of line with their educational and social backgrounds. For example, female telephone operators from blue-collar backgrounds were likely to be well adjusted and healthy, but college-educated women expressed job dissatisfaction and were also more likely to experience frequent illness.

Characteristics of life events that are most salient as stressors include desirability of an event, control, and required readjustment.[24] Methodologic problems in life events research include subjects' recall ability, memory biases, reliability of measurement, and possible interconnectedness among life events.

The Stress Process Model

Pearlin[25] proposed the stress process model as an organizing and orienting framework for the diverse themes of stress research. The model would be heuristic by guiding researchers toward potentially useful lines of research, highlighting needed data for research, and aiding in the interpretation of results.

One of the important features of the model is that it emphasizes the interrelatedness of factors that play a role in the individual's health and well-being. Some of the factors include the contexts of persons' lives, their social statuses, their exposure to stress, the resources that they have available to deal with stressors, and the outcomes of stress exposure, both somatic and mental. The model is particularly intriguing because it specifies that stress is a process that occurs over a time course. Events chain from one to another with interconnectedness among factors. As an example, Pearlin cites the role of social and economic status in the stress process. Those who are at the lower end of the economic hierarchy may face a life of fear and uncertainty or may lack economic resources. These circumstances, in turn, may be exacerbated by the individual's neighborhood context should it be unsafe, deteriorated, or unstable. Some of the problems that arise from a stressful neighborhood context, such as lack of access to needed services, are known as daily hassles.

In addition to the individual's social status and neighborhood context, the stress model incorporates life events (defined earlier) and chronic or repeated strains. Examples of strains include life-course issues, for example, the need for spouses or children to assume long-term caregiving roles for elderly loved ones or parents. Finally, the model specifies moderating resources, such as coping and social support (covered later in this chapter), and stress outcomes, such as mental disorders (also covered later in the chapter). The epidemiologic features of depression and depressive symptoms indicate that these disorders are unequally distributed according to socioeconomic status, gender, marital status, and age. Turner and Lloyd provide empirical support for the stress process model with respect to these characteristics, that is, that they may be linked to life circumstances that influence exposure to stress as well as to resources for managing stress.[26]

Moderating Factors in the Stress-Illness Relationship

Previously, we defined moderating (intervening) variables as those that are intermediate in the causal process between risk factors and outcomes. Examples of moderating variables are the type A behavior pattern, personal behaviors and lifestyle, and supportive interpersonal relationships. Personality variables also may have a moderating effect upon health outcomes by affecting how individuals respond to and cope with stress. For example, personality hardiness has been posited as a resistance resource that moderates the relationship between stressful life events and illness outcomes. Kobasa et al. wrote that "hardiness is considered a personality style consisting of the interrelated orientations of commitment (vs. alienation), control (vs. powerlessness), and challenge (vs. threat). Persons high in commitment find it easy to involve themselves actively in whatever they are doing, being generally curious about and interested in activities, things, and people. . . . Persons high in control believe and act as if they can influence the events taking place around them through what they imagine, say, and do. . . . Challenge involves the expectation that life will change and that the changes will be a stimulus to personal development."[27(p525)] Kobasa et al. reported that hardiness was the most important of resistance resources studied—including social support and exercise—in predicting the probability of illness among male business executives.

Type A (Coronary-Prone) Behavior Pattern

The type A behavior pattern has been found to be associated with CHD in prospective, cross-sectional, and retrospective studies. Researchers have focused upon clinical assessment of the behavior pattern through interview techniques and the development of a self-administered questionnaire measure. Rosenman and colleagues,[28] who pioneered work in the concept of the type A behavior pattern, characterized type A as including the traits of aggressiveness, ambition, drive, competitiveness, and time urgency. Jenkins subsequently enlarged the coronary-prone behavior pattern, which he conceptualized as an "overt behavioral syndrome or style of living . . . to include restlessness, hyperalertness, and explosiveness of speech."[29(p255)]

Interview Measure of Type A

Rosenman et al.[30] measured the type A syndrome by means of a structured clinical interview. In one of the major series of studies using this measure, it was administered, beginning in 1960, to a sample of 3,524 men, aged 39 to 59 years. Known as the Western Collaborative Group Study, the research prospectively followed the incidence of CHD among men in various occupations. Questions contained in the interview were designed to measure the several dimensions of the type A personality outlined above: drive, ambition, competitiveness, aggressiveness, hostility, and a sense of time urgency; motor and speech characteristics also were noted. The investigators, sometimes in collaboration with other researchers, have published numerous reports that contain data supportive of a significant and positive relationship between the type A personality type and increased frequency of CHD.

Self-Administered Measure of Type A

To measure the type A behavior pattern objectively, several researchers reported the development of a self-administered checklist. Purported advantages of a checklist measure over a structured interview are greater standardization of research procedures in replication studies, ease of administration, and elimination of possible interviewer biases. Bortner[31] reported the development of a short rating scale (14 items) for the behavior pattern. The measure discriminated significantly between two groups of male workers who previously had been classified as behavior pattern A or B by the interview measure. (Type B refers to those people who do not have the type A pattern.) Jenkins[29] developed a self-administered, machine-scored test known as the Jenkins Activity Scale to measure the type A personality.

Social Support

Social support is defined as supportive relationships that arise from friends, family members, and others. Cobb[32] suggested that *social support* may moderate the effects of stress. Although the term social support refers to perceived emotional support that one receives from social relationships, the term *social network ties* is a quantitative concept that refers to the number (and, in some cases, the pattern) of ties that one has with other people or organizations. Social support systems operate as mediators that serve as buffers against stress.[33] Research studies have focused on the stress-buffering effects of social network ties and social support. For example, it has been hypothesized that social support may enhance immune status. Cancer patients' spouses, who would be presumed to have severe, chronic life stresses, demonstrated an association between social support and immune status; those who had higher levels of perceived social support tended to have better indexes of immune function.[34]

Social networks refer to the structure of people's social attachments[35] and are considered mediators because they help explain differences in the individual's ability to respond to stressors. The buffering model states that the function of social network ties may be to lessen the adverse psychologic consequences of stress.[36] The underlying assumption is that support provided by social network ties may act as a buffer against the potentially harmful effects of stressful life events.[37] Several studies have demonstrated that social support resources can often buffer the effects of stressful events and result, consequently, in reduced levels of depression. Conversely, lack of family social support and close affectional ties contributes to vulnerability, onset, and severity of psychologic stress.[38] There is evidence that variations in the effects of support are related to the source of support.[39] For example, support from spouses or friends may be more important than support from other network ties.

Supportive relationships may be deduced from social networks, including ties with family and friends and memberships in formal and informal organizations. Marital status has been found to be salient in the social support process; married older adults have more contact with family members than with friends and receive more emotional support than unmarried older adults.[40] In addition, social contact, received emotional support, and anticipated support are interrelated. Increased social contact is associated with increased emotional support and perceptions of support availability.[39] The specificity hypothesis postulates that interpersonal relationships provide a stress-buffering effect when there is concordance between coping requirements demanded by a particular stressor and specific types of support provided.[41]

Personal Behavior, Lifestyle, and Health

In this section, we include characteristics such as personal risk taking, smoking, alcohol consumption, choice of diet, and exercise levels. *Healthy People 2000* established a framework in the United States for national promotion and disease prevention objectives[42] (Exhibit 15-2). Several of these objectives relate to health promotion through encouragement of a desirable lifestyle.

EXHIBIT 15-2

Healthy People 2000

The purpose of *Healthy People 2000* is to commit the Nation to the attainment of three broad goals that will help bring us to our full potential. . . . We have a broad array of opportunities to achieve our goals. This report presents many of these opportunities in the form of measurable targets, or objectives, to be achieved by the year 2000, organized into 22 priority areas. The first 21 of these areas are grouped into three broad categories: health promotion; health protection; and prevention services. . . .

- Increase the span of healthy life for Americans
- Reduce health disparities among Americans
- Achieve access to preventive services for all Americans

Health promotion strategies are those related to individual lifestyle—personal choices made in a social context—that can have a powerful influence over one's health prospects. These priorities include physical activity and fitness, nutrition, tobacco, alcohol and other drugs, family planning, mental health and mental disorders, and violent and abusive behavior. Educational and community-based programs can address lifestyle in a crosscutting fashion.

Health protection strategies are those related to environmental or regulatory measures that confer protection on large population groups. These strategies address issues such as unintentional injuries, occupational safety and health, environmental health, food and drug safety, and oral health. Interventions applied to address these issues are generally not exclusively protective in nature—there may be a substantial health promotion element as well—but the principal approaches involve a communitywide rather than individual focus.

Health Promotion

1. Physical Activity and Fitness
2. Nutrition
3. Tobacco
4. Alcohol and Other Drugs
5. Family Planning

continues

EXHIBIT 15-2 *continued*

6. Mental Health and Mental Disorders
7. Violent and Abusive Behavior
8. Educational and Community-Based Programs

Health Protection

9. Unintentional Injuries
10. Occupational Safety and Health
11. Environmental Health
12. Food and Drug Safety
13. Oral Health

Preventive Services

14. Maternal and Infant Health
15. Heart Disease and Stroke
16. Cancer
17. Diabetes and Chronic Disabling Conditions
18. HIV Infection
19. Sexually Transmitted Diseases
20. Immunization and Infectious Diseases
21. Clinical Preventive Services

Surveillance and Data Systems

22. Surveillance and Data System

Age-Related Objectives

Children
Adolescents and Young Adults
Adults
Older Adults

Preventive services include counseling, screening, immunization, or chemoprophylactic interventions for individuals in clinical settings. Priority areas for these strategies include maternal and infant health, heart disease and stroke, cancer, diabetes and chronic disabling conditions, HIV infection, sexually transmitted diseases, and infectious diseases. Crosscutting

continues

EXHIBIT 15-2 *continued*

professional and access considerations in the delivery of clinical preventive services are addressed also. A special category has been established for surveillance and data systems. Given the centrality of monitoring progress toward the stated target in the overall approach of *Healthy People 2000,* the integrity of our data collection efforts at every level is critical. Objectives therefore have been established to improve those efforts. ■

Source: Reprinted from *Healthy People 2000,* DHHS Publication No. 91-50213, pp 6–7, Public Health Service, US Department of Health and Human Services; 1991.

Breslow[43] summarized the results from the Human Population Laboratory in Alameda County, California, where investigators observed a positive association between seven healthful habits and physical health status and longevity. The seven habits were moderate food intake, eating regularly, eating breakfast, not smoking cigarettes, moderate or no use of alcohol, moderate exercise, and seven to eight hours of sleep daily. There was a direct correlation between the number of health habits followed and good health status and reduced mortality.

Behavior and lifestyle are related to a number of diseases that are of major importance to modern Western civilization. Burkitt[44] believed that these include noninfectious diseases of the large bowel, venous disorders, and obesity. Appendicitis, diverticular diseases, cancer of the large bowel, pulmonary embolism, gallbladder disease, ischemic heart disease, and diabetes are relatively common diseases in the United States and Britain. Burkitt stated that these same conditions are uncommon in developing countries and were rare a century ago in Western nations. Suchman[45] refers to the chronic, degenerative diseases as way-of-life diseases because of their closer relationship to human behavior than to any bacteriologic or infectious agent.

Personal behavior is intimately connected to personal health status. Health-relevant behavior is a function of both psychologic and contemporary sociocultural influences. For example, there is great variety in the amount of personal risk that one may want to assume in the conduct of daily existence, from minimal risk to such high-risk activities as motorcycle riding, sky diving, and hang gliding, which place one at direct risk of accidental death and injury. Sexual behavior, dietary practices, smoking, alcohol consumption, method of infant feeding, and choice of occupation are all components of personal behavior that affect health and are governed by personality constitution, cultural influences, and the prevailing social climate. Personal behavior is of such importance that the U.S. National Center for Chronic Disease Prevention and Health Promotion established a behavioral risk factor surveillance program. The purpose of this program was to modify behavioral risk factors to accomplish national health objectives for the year 2000. The objective areas for the behavioral risk factor surveillance program included obesity, lack of physical activity, smoking, safety belt use, and medical screening for breast and cervical cancer and elevated blood cholesterol. The surveillance program was a state-based, random-digit dialing telephone survey.[46]

Personal behavior is related to accidents, the fifth major cause of death in the United States in 1991.[47] Mortality and morbidity from accidents are largely, if not completely, preventable. Although accidents might appear to be unpredicted, unexpected events, epidemiologic data suggest, contrary to this notion, that accidental injuries and death are not randomly distributed. Rather, accidents tend to be more common among individuals with certain identifiable host characteristics, such as sex, age, choice of occupation, and safety practices, which are influenced by attitudinal and behavioral variables in relation to risk taking.[45]

Smoking and Health

Two major reports by the Surgeon General[48,49] summarized conclusions regarding the relationship between smoking and various health consequences. Epidemiologic research methodology suggests that smoking is a significant cause of excess mortality and morbidity. For example:

- Current cigarette smokers in comparison with nonsmokers have an overall 70% excess mortality regardless of amount of smoking.
- Mortality from smoking increases with the quantity of cigarettes smoked; mortality is increased by duration of smoking, starting at earlier ages, and amount of smoke inhaled.
- Associations have been observed between smoking and morbidity from cardiovascular diseases; cancer of the lung, larynx, mouth, bladder, and pancreas; non-neoplastic bronchopulmonary diseases; and peptic ulcer disease.
- There are interactive and synergistic effects of smoking and occupational exposures to asbestos, chromium, nickel, and other potentially toxic or carcinogenic materials.
- Smoking is a direct cause of reduction in birth weight and increased prenatal mortality; nicotine is found in the breast milk of mothers who smoke.

With respect to the behavioral aspects of smoking, the 1979 Surgeon General's report concludes that the reason why the smoking habit is so widespread and difficult to break is largely unknown: "It is no exaggeration to say that smoking is the prototypical substance abuse dependency and that improved knowledge of this process holds great promise for the prevention of risk. Establishment and maintenance of the smoking habit are, obviously, prerequisite to the risk, and cessation of smoking can eliminate or greatly reduce the health threat."[49(p1–32)] Since the 1979 report, much additional information has been acquired regarding the nature of nicotine addiction.

Alcohol Consumption

Excessive alcohol consumption is a risk factor for specific diseases, such as cirrhosis, peptic ulcers, and gastritis. There has been a paucity of research on the association of alcoholism with general morbidity and mortality, however.[50] Certainly, excessive alcohol consumption increases the likelihood of involvement in motor vehicle accidents. Alcoholism is associated with deterioration of the family environment and job loss. Excessive alcohol consumption by pregnant women is related to the fetal alcohol syndrome, which is characterized by postnatal growth deficiency, mental retardation, and various physical abnormalities.[51] According to Streissguth,[51] the fetal alcohol syndrome presents as a set of specific characteristics: small stature, small head, small eyes, flattened nasal bridge, and a thin, narrow upper lip. In addition to the fetal alcohol syndrome found among the offspring of women who abuse alcohol during pregnancy, there is an association between low to moderate intake of alcohol during pregnancy and low birth weight. As a result of the pervasive custom of alcohol consumption at all levels of society, there is a need for additional research into alcohol's teratogenic effect upon the fetus.

Brody and Mills[50] reviewed many of the epidemiologic studies on the role of alcohol as a risk factor for diseases. They concluded that cirrhosis and acute alcoholic liver disease, although causally related to excess ethanol intake, is found in only a small percentage (some studies find a 5% rate of diagnosis) among alcohol abusers and heavy drinkers. They believed that a far larger percentage of alcohol abusers succumb to premature death from heart disease and stroke, and from violent causes, such as homicide, suicide, and accidents. There is also some evidence that moderate drinkers have lower death rates than abstainers. Brody and Mills concluded that alcohol may be a risk factor for many illnesses, not merely a direct cause of liver disease. Needed are new epidemiologic studies because many of the previous efforts have not been able to investigate the problem adequately as a result of methodologic deficiencies related to systematic underrepresentation of heavy drinkers.

Dietary Practices

Choice of habitual diet affects the development of chronic diseases and is an aspect of personal behavior that is related to sociocultural influences. Burkitt[44] noted the association between the consumption of refined carbohydrate foods and obesity and diabetes. He suggested that lack of fiber in the food of Western diets is related to diseases of the bowel, such as colon cancer and diverticular disease.

The diet-heart hypothesis is a theoretical account of the multifactorial basis for arteriosclerosis and CHD.[52] The fundamental diet-heart hypothesis suggested that an association exists between consumption of a diet high in saturated fats and cholesterol and high blood lipids, which are in turn associated with arteriosclerosis and heart disease. More recent evidence has shown that low levels of high-density lipoproteins and high levels of low-density lipoproteins in the blood are associated with heart disease.

Some researchers have found that a high ratio of polyunsaturated to saturated fat is associated with reduced risk of CHD. Phillips et al.[53] analyzed CHD rates among a population of California Seventh-Day Adventists, a conservative religious denomination whose members avoid alcohol and tobacco consumption. A nonmeat, lacto-ovovegetarian diet is advocated and is followed by about half the membership. A six-year prospective study of almost 25,000 Adventists found that individuals between ages 35 and 64 had CHD mortality rates that were 28% of the rate for an equivalent age group within the total California population. Phillips[54] also reported reduced risk of colon cancer among Adventists, a finding that is being followed in other research.

Epidemiologic methods have been applied to examine the role of dietary factors, such as consumption of fats, fruits, and vegetables in cancer incidence. Consumption of animal fats, a high-meat diet, and vegetables has been studied in relationship to colon cancer.[55] The relationship between low blood cholesterol and risk of developing cancer also has been investigated. Consumption of dietary fat may play a role in mediating the relationship between blood cholesterol and cancer.[56] Among residents of Shanghai, China, a case-control study determined that consumption of fruits, certain dark green/yellow vegetables, and garlic was a protective factor for laryngeal cancer, whereas intake of salt-preserved meat and fish increased risk.[57] Another factor studied in relation to cancer is β-carotene, for which investigators hypothesize a protective role. Low serum β-carotene may be associated with cancers of the lung, stomach, cervix, esophagus, small intestine, and uterus.[58]

The effects of coffee and tea consumption in relation to morbidity and mortality from CHD and other chronic diseases have been studied extensively. Although the findings are conflicting for the association of coffee drinking with cardiovascular disease, there does appear to be an indirect connection through association with adverse lifestyle factors. An Austrian study reported that coffee drinking was associated with lifestyle factors—smoking, drinking, eating, and lack of physical activity—that could increase risk of cardiovascular disease.[59] The reverse of this association was found between tea drinking and lifestyle factors.

Sedentary Lifestyle

Sedentary Western existence, with its use of labor-saving devices and reduced level of physical activity, is identified as a risk factor for CHD and other conditions. As reviewed earlier in Chapter 7, Morris et al.[60] examined the leisure time activities of 17,000 male executive-grade British civil servant office workers aged 40 to 64 years. Workers who participated in vigorous active recreations, such as swimming and heavy gardening, had about one-third the incidence of CHD as the less active workers. Light exercise that did not have a training effect on the cardiovascular system did not reduce the incidence of heart disease. The results were interpreted as demonstrating that vigorous exercise promotes cardiovascular health.

Paffenbarger et al.[61] corroborated these results in a study of about 17,000 Harvard male alumni aged 35 to 74 (refer to Chapt. 7). Risk of first heart attack was inversely related to involvement in vigorous physical exercise (e.g., stair climbing, walking, and strenuous athletics). Those who were college athletes and discontinued exercise during later life were at greater risk of heart attack than adults who began exercising at a later age.

Streja and Mymin[62] designed an exercise program to determine whether there is a relationship between exercise and cholesterol level among sedentary persons. They observed that low levels of high-density lipoprotein cholesterol (HDL-C, the so-called good cholesterol) have been shown to precede arteriosclerosis and that athletes in comparison with control subjects have high levels of HDL-C. In an exercise program that consisted of walking and slow jogging, a small sample of middle-aged men with coronary artery disease had increased levels of HDL-C. The results of the study suggest that exercise programs may retard the development of arteriosclerosis.

Many epidemiologic investigations have followed the early work of Morris et al. . . . early work on the role of physical activity in health. These later studies have incorporated diverse populations in terms of sex, ethnicity, age, social composition, and geographic location. Paffenbarger et al. concluded that, "These studies have extended and amplified those by the Morris group, thereby helping to solidify the cause-and-effect evidence that exercise protects against heart disease and averts premature mortality."[63(p1184)] Not only does exercise benefit the general population, it also promotes physical functioning in sub-groups of the population, e.g., persons with disabilities[64] and the elderly.[65]

Sociocultural Influences on Health

One of the concerns of contemporary epidemiologic research is the role of social and cultural factors in health. Recent epidemiologic research has produced a voluminous literature regarding the effects of social, cultural, and psychosocial factors in the etiology of disease.[66] Culture may be defined as the set of values to which a group of people subscribes, as the way of life of a group of people, or as the totality of what is learned and shared through interaction of the members of a society. Specific behaviors associated with a particular culture have implications for the health of the individual. In support of this notion, Susser et al. wrote, "Habits that affect health, in childbearing and midwifery, in nutrition and in daily living, are not merely the negative result of ignorance among people who know no better. They are often an intrinsic element in a way of life, customs that have positive value and symbolic significance." [67(pp152–153)]

One explanation for the role that cultural factors may play in health is that they may mediate the amount of stress to which the individual is exposed. Matsumoto[68] observed that Japan historically has had one of the lowest rates of CHD in the world and that the United States has had one of the highest. He hypothesized:

> The etiology of coronary heart disease is multiple and complex, but in urban-industrial Japan, the in-group work community of the individual, with its institutional stress-reducing strategies, plays an important role in decreasing the frequency of the disease. . . . Deleterious circumstances of life need not be expressed in malfunctioning of the physiologic or psychologic systems if a meaningful social group is available through which the individual can derive emotional support and understanding.[68(p14)]

Marmot and colleagues[69] studied a large population of men of Japanese ancestry: 2,141 men who were being followed by the Atomic Bomb Casualty Commission in Hiroshima and Nagasaki, Japan; 8,006 men in Honolulu; and 1,844 men in the San Francisco Bay area. Japanese who lived in California had a higher prevalence of CHD and its manifestations than those who resided in Hawaii or Japan. The Hawaiian Japanese tended to have higher CHD rates than residents of Japan. The investigators speculated that differences in prevalence of CHD may have been due to differences in the way of life in Japan and the United States. For example, there are major variations between the two countries in diet, occupation, and the social and cultural milieu.

Studies have pursued the role of sociocultural factors in mental retardation. Mercer[70] suggested that excessively large numbers of individuals from minority backgrounds were being labeled by the public schools as mentally retarded because available standardized tests of intelligence did not adequately take into account the background of the students. The dimensions that are measured on IQ and other tests are taken from the white, middle-class society and do not constitute a culture-free measure.

Utilization of health services and, in fact, the very definition of illness are both related to cultural background and show variation from person to person. According to Mechanic, illness refers to objective symptoms, whereas illness behavior "refers to the varying perceptions, thoughts, feelings, and acts affecting the personal and social meaning of symptoms, illness, disabilities and their consequences. . . . [Some people will] make light of symptoms and impairments. Others magnify even minimal problems, allowing them to affect their life adjustments substantially."[71(p79)] It is possible that those who seek medical care readily may, over the long run, experience increased life expectancy through early identification of potentially life-threatening illness.

In citing differences in preference for type of medical services by cultural group membership, Mechanic[72] stated that some Mexican Americans might prefer folk medicine and family care. Whites, however, would show a predilection for modern medical services in a technologically advanced medical center. Elsewhere, Mechanic wrote, "Illness perception and response may be socially learned patterns developed early in life as a result of exposure to particular cultural styles, ethnic values, or sex role socialization."[71(p79)]

Social and cultural factors are related to the successful control of communicable diseases; a notable example is control of tuberculosis among immigrants to the United States from Mexico. People of Mexican descent with tuberculosis showed delayed response in seeking medical attention. These delays were attributed to diagnosis by a layperson of the symptoms of the folk illness *susto*, a condition not considered susceptible to the ministrations of physicians. Among undocumented Mexican workers residing in Orange County, California, the average delay between acknowledgment of tuberculosis symptoms and the presentation of a complaint to a physician was 8.5 months.[73]

Outcome Variables: Physical Health, Mental Health, Affective States

Psychosocial epidemiologic research covers both physical and mental health outcomes. Examples of physical health outcomes that are studied within a psychosocial framework include specific chronic diseases (e.g., CHD). Those related to psychologic status embrace affective states, life and job dissatisfaction, and depressive symptoms. We also would like to point out that the physical and mental dimensions of health have been shown to overlap. There is evidence that psychiatric and physical disorders are risk factors for each other.[74]

Life and Job Dissatisfaction

According to Jenkins, "The hypothesis that life dissatisfaction is a risk factor for coronary disease is a promising one and deserves careful examination in prospective studies."[29(p254)] One of the aspects of life dissatisfaction that is increasingly shown to be related to coronary disease is job dissatisfaction. Empirical findings suggest that life and job dissatisfaction are directly related to morbidity and mortality from CHD. An ecologic analysis by Sales and House[75] reported strong negative correlations between job satisfaction and coronary disease death rates for white-collar and blue-collar workers when the effects of social class were controlled. In a study of identical twins, Liljefors and Rahe[76] similarly reported a strong association between various life dissatisfactions, including job dissatisfactions, and heart disease. Other studies have implicated various themes of job dissatisfaction in coronary disease. Tedious work, feeling ill at ease at work, lack of recognition, difficulties with coworkers, demotion, and prolonged emotional strain associated with work overload have all been shown to be related to coronary disease.

Several investigators have focused upon extrinsic-intrinsic motivation (motivation for power and money as opposed to motivation for the internal qualities of an occupation) as a job-related motivational dimension that may be associated with CHD. Using a sample from the University of Michigan Tecumseh Study, House[77] found that the association between extrinsic-intrinsic motivation and CHD or CHD risk was conditioned by occupational status. There was a positive association between extrinsic motivation and CHD or CHD risk, and a negative relationship between intrinsic motivation and CHD or CHD, risk among white-collar workers. The reverse association was found for blue-collar workers.

Mental Health and Stressors

Epidemiologic research has examined various mental health outcomes, such as psychologic disorders (e.g., posttraumatic stress disorder [PTSD] and major depression) and affective states, as outcomes of the stress-illness paradigm. PTSD is an example of a mental disorder that is associated with exposure to extremely traumatic events. PTSD victims tend to reexperience the traumatic event—whether a natural disaster or war, or other trauma—and may progress in some instances to persisting psychopathology. PTSD is a potentially noteworthy disorder for epidemiologic research, because it often stems from a trauma that has been experienced by an entire population.[78] The 1994 Northridge earthquake in southern California is an example. Not only do individuals who experience a natural disaster, such as an earthquake, vary in the severity of their responses, but there also appears to be a dose-response relationship between proximity to the traumatic event and degree of mental impairment.

Let us now turn to a unique problem for mental health epidemiology. Of particular interest to epidemiologists has been the development of an instrument to assess the prevalence of mental disorders in population surveys. Prior to the development of such a measure, some epidemiologic investigations relied on hospital admission rates or other utilization data to determine rates of conditions such as depression. Langner's 22-item Index of Psychophysiologic Disorder represented one of the first efforts to design an epidemiologic measure of psychiatric impairment.[79] A later instrument is the Center for Epidemiologic Studies depression (CES-D) scale, a brief, 20-item self-report depression symptom scale.[80,81] Possible scores on the CES-D scale range from a minimum of 0 to a maximum of 60. Research studies have found it to be as reliable, sensitive, and valid a measure of depressive symptoms and change in depressive symptoms as clinical interview ratings. The instrument permits differentiation between acute depressives and recovered depressives as well as between depressives and other diagnostic groups.[82] The measure has been validated in predominantly urban populations[83–85] and more recently in rural populations.[86] Sample items are self-reported feelings of depression, fearfulness, loneliness, and sadness. Subjects indicate the frequency with which these symptoms have occurred during the past week (range, 0 to 5–7 days; range of item scores, 0 to 3). A total CES-D score of 16 or greater has been defined in literature reports as the criterion for a case of depression.[82]

Several major surveys have examined the prevalence of self-reported symptoms of depression as assessed by the CES-D scale. The prevalence of depression in a representative sample of adults in Los Angeles County was 19%.[87] Rates of depression were higher among women than men (23.5% vs. 12.9%). Depressed persons reported more physical illnesses than the nondepressed. Using data from the Hispanic Health and Nutrition Examination Survey, investigators reported a caseness (i.e., CES-D score of 16 or greater) rate for high levels of depressive symptoms of 13.3%; female sex, low educational achievement, low income, birth in the United States, and white-oriented acculturation of the Hispanic sample were associated with depressive symptoms.[88]

The National Institute of Mental Health Epidemiological Catchment Area Program was a comprehensive collaborative effort by scientists to gather data on the prevalence of mental disorders in the United States. The disorders studied were the major psychiatric illnesses classified in the third edition of the *Diagnostic and Statistical Manual* (a manual for the classification of mental disorders). The study was unprecedented in its scope, covering 17,000 residents of five community sites across the United States.[89]

Premorbid Psychologic Factors and Cancer

Fox[90] compiled a comprehensive literature review and evaluation of studies of premorbid psychologic and personality factors associated with cancer. Possible deficiencies of the prospective and retrospective studies done in this field through 1977 include small sample sizes, inappropriate use of statistical tests, methodologic flaws, and possible alternative interpretations. One group of prospective studies suggested that cancer patients show lack of warm relationships with their parents and pathologic responses to the Rorschach test (a personality test that uses ink-blot designs to evoke associations). Other studies mentioned in Fox's review suggested that women who were later found to have breast cancer deliberately repress and fail to express anger. Still another investigation reported that lung cancer patients had higher-than-average scores on the lie scale of the Minnesota Multiphasic Personality Inventory, but the interpretation of this finding has been challenged.

Deficiencies of research notwithstanding, Fox[90] summarized two major personality types at increased risk of cancer. He portrayed the first type as yielding, compliant, and eager to please. Among the first personality type, activation of hormonal mechanisms might be associated with repression of feelings. Repressed emotion might alter immune system responses to carcinogenic agents, thereby increasing incidence of cancer in individuals with this personality type. The second type consisted of extroverted, non-neurotic individuals who tend toward heaviness. He predicted that male or female extroverts, as a result of physical lifestyle (sometimes involving excessive eating, drinking, and smoking), would have higher rates than others of colorectal, breast, lung, prostate, esophageal, and cervical cancer. The primary etiologic mechanism would be the indirect linkage between personality and cancer through lifestyle factors.

A subsequent review of the associations among psychologic variables (e.g., stress, bereavement, depressed mood, mental illness, suppressed emotions, helplessness and hopelessness, and social support) and various cancer outcomes, including mortality or course of the disease, appeared approximately two decades later.[91] It was concluded that the literature remains contradictory, marked by both positive findings and the absence of associations; however, the evidence against the relationship between psychologic factors and cancer outcomes is most notable for stress, depressed mood, psychosis, and bereavement.

Effects of Major Diseases on Personality

Not only might one conceive of personality characteristics as a cause of diseases, but one might look also at the reverse side of the coin and examine the effect of disease upon personality. Affliction with a chronic disease may become a substantial stress factor for the person and for members of his or her immediate social environment. A severe drinking problem, substance abuse, or a heart attack may induce personality changes in the afflicted individual and may affect other persons, including one's children, spouse, and coworkers. A number of personality effects accompany severe illness; for example, Croog and Fitzgerald[92] stated that wives of heart attack victims experience depression, fear, anxiety, and guilt. Wives have increasing anxiety about the future and guilt feelings about being a possible cause of the attack. Additionally, the victim may experience increased feelings of depression, anxiety, guilt, and hopelessness. One implication for epidemiologic research is that studies should carefully separate out the direction of causality. Did the personality characteristic cause the disease, or did the disease cause the personality characteristic?

Personality and Smoking

An issue that has commanded the attention of epidemiologic researchers and others concerns the extent to which smoking behavior is determined by personality factors. The Surgeon General's Report of 1979[49] indicated that personality factors that may be related to smoking behavior are extroversion, neuroticism, antisocial tendencies, and the belief that one is externally controlled (i.e., that fate, luck, or other factors beyond one's control will bring one rewards). Smokers show a greater willingness than nonsmokers to take risks and are more impulsive, more likely to divorce and change jobs, more interested in sex, and more likely to consume tea, coffee, and alcohol.

Research conducted subsequently to the Surgeon General's Report also suggested that cigarette smokers may possess distinctive personality characteristics in comparison to nonsmokers; for example, with respect to risk behaviors.[93] A major review of the epidemiology of tobacco use concluded that some studies have linked cigarette smoking to several types of psychiatric disorders.[93] Associations between depressive states and smoking, anxiety disorders and smoking, and schizophrenia and smoking have been reported by several investigators. According to the review, "Controversy about the nature of the relation between smoking and depression may continue until definitive data become available."[93(p55)]

Habitual Mental Outlook and Health Status

One's prevailing attitudes toward life and one's mental health status have been probed with respect to their association with physical health status and longevity. A major study of male mental health involved follow-up of 204 men biennially over a period of four decades, beginning at adolescence.[94] Information regarding the mental health status as well as the physical health status of the subjects was routinely collected during the study. Among the 59 men with the best mental health between the ages of 21 and 46, only 2 developed chronic illness or died by age 53. Among 46 men with the worst mental health levels, 18 developed chronic illnesses or died. The association between mental and physical health remained statistically significant when the variables of alcohol and tobacco consumption, obesity, and longevity of relatives were controlled.

The foregoing research addressed the possible role of mental health and adult adjustment in men's physical health. Aspects of mental health potentially associated with physical health include habitual mental outlook, such as optimism. The self-reported health of midlife women has been shown to be positively related to optimism.[95] However, the positive association between cheerfulness—one aspect of habitual mental outlook—and health (specifically longevity) has been contradicted by a study of subjects from Terman's seven-decade longitudinal investigation of highly intelligent children.[96] While the findings suggested that conscientiousness in childhood was associated with survival in middle to old age, cheerfulness—characterized by optimism and sense of humor—was inversely related to longevity.

In conclusion, while research into the association between characteristics of habitual mental outlook (mental health, adult adjustment, cheerfulness, optimism, and sense of humor) and health status (self-reported physical health, chronic disease, and longevity) has evolved some intriguing hypotheses and findings, further work is needed because of inconsistent results. For example, there is a possible need to reconceptualize the health relevance of variables such as cheerfulness.[96] The role of habitual mental outlook in health may be elucidated further by prospective studies that refine measurement techniques and clarify the theoretical pathways through which this factor may operate.

Conclusion

The field of social epidemiology is concerned with the influence of a person's position in the social structure upon the development of disease. Behavioral epidemiology studies the role of behavioral factors in health. The term psychosocial epidemiology has been more broadly conceptualized to include social, behavioral, and psychologic factors. This field of investigation has used case-control, cohort, and cross-sectional designs to research a wide variety of health outcomes.

This chapter first examined the independent variables of stress, status incongruity, person-environment fit, and stressful life events. Stress as an independent, antecedent variable to health and illness represents an intriguing notion because it seems to fit in with commonsense explanations for the cause of ulcers, sudden death due to heart attacks, and other chronic conditions, yet documentation of stress as an etiologic agent of disease is inconsistent. Investigators have hypothesized that either social mobility or status incongruity may be associated with morbidity and mortality. Person-environment fit, originally formulated to conceptualize various aspects of mental health, such as adjustment and coping, is another example of a social and psychologic precursor to the etiology of physiologic illness. A fourth example of an independent variable is the concept of stressful life events. The central postulate of life events research is that there is a relationship between the happenings in one's life and the development of illness.

Examples of moderating (intervening) variables in psychosocial epidemiologic research are the type A behavior pattern, personal behaviors and lifestyle, supportive interpersonal relationships, and social and cultural influences. Outcome variables include affective states, life and job dissatisfaction, chronic disease, and depressive symptoms. Psychosocial epidemiologic research studies on these problems have increased in frequency over the past few decades.

Study Questions and Exercises

1. Propose a model for the relationship between stress and illness. Be sure to include moderating factors.
2. How do one's culture and environment relate to health?
3. Give examples of personality traits that may modify the relationship between stress and disease.
4. What is the role of stressful life events as an influence upon disease?

5. Describe the association between social incongruity and chronic disease. What types of study populations would be appropriate to an epidemiologic investigation of the health effects of social incongruity?

6. Define the following:
   a. stress
   b. general adaptation syndrome
   c. social incongruity
   d. person-environment fit
   e. life events
   f. type A behavior pattern
   g. social support
   h. lifestyle
   i. depressive symptoms
   j. stress process model

7. How is person-environment fit relevant to studies of occupational health and job-related stress? What type of person would adjust well to an authoritarian work environment, and what type to an unstructured environment? What is meant by a curvilinear relationship between person-environment fit and stress?

8. Give examples of the following lifestyle variables in their relationship to health:
   a. alcohol and smoking
   b. exercise
   c. risk taking

9. Stress has been hypothesized to be associated with human illness. Apply the concepts and criteria presented in Chapter 2 to argue for and against a causal association between stress and coronary heart disease.

10. To what extent are health outcome variables distinct or overlapping? For example, discuss the possibility that impaired mental health may be a risk factor for impaired physical health and vice versa. What types of epidemiologic study designs might be able to disentangle the time sequencing of overlapping mental disorders and impaired physical health?

11. Capstone exercise: This exercise is included here because it requires skills developed in the previous chapters of the text. Select a data-based article from the *American Journal of Public Health,* the *American Journal of Epidemiology,* or other public health journal of your choice. Refer to Appendix A (Guide to the Critical Appraisal of an Epidemiologic/Public Health Research Article). Using the criteria shown in the Appendix, write

a brief critique of the article. In addition to discussing the criteria suggested in the appendix, mention what improvements, if any, you would make in the article.

References

1. Engel G. The need for a new medical model: a challenge for biomedicine. *Science.* 1977;196:129–136.
2. Syme SL. Behavioral factors associated with the etiology of physical disease: a social epidemiological approach. *Am J Public Health.* 1974;64:1043–1045.
3. Berkman LF, Kawachi I. A historical framework for social epidemiology. In: Berkman LF, Kawachi I, eds. *Social Epidemiology.* New York, NY: Oxford University Press; 2000.
4. Blumenthal JA, Sherwood A, Gullette EC, et al. Biobehavioral approaches to the treatment of essential hypertension. *J Consult Clin Psychol.* 2002;70:569–589.
5. Wittchen HU, Perkonigg A, Lachner G, Nelson CB. Early developmental stages of psychopathology study (EDSP): objectives and design. *Eur Addict Res.* 1998;4(1–2): 18–27.
6. Lieb R, Zimmermann P, Friis RH, et al. The natural course of DSM-IV somatoform disorders and syndromes among adolescents and young adults: a prospective-longitudinal community study. *Eur Psychiatry.* 2002;17:321–331.
7. Friis RH, Wittchen HU, Pfister H, Lieb R. Life events and changes in the course of depression in young adults. *Eur Psychiatry.* 2002; 17:241–253.
8. Marmot M. Introduction. In: Marmot M, Wilkinson RG, eds. *Social Determinants of Health.* New York, NY: Oxford University Press; 1999:1–16.
9. Murray CJ, Lopez AD. Global mortality, disability, and the contribution of risk factors: global burden of disease study. *Lancet.* 1997;349:1436–1442.
10. Wolf S. Psychosocial influences in gastrointestinal function. In: Levi L, ed. *Society, Stress and Disease.* London, UK: Oxford University Press; 1971:362–366.
11. Selye H. *The Stress of Life.* New York, NY: McGraw Hill; 1956.
12. Selye H. The evolution of the stress concept—stress and cardiovascular disease. In: Levi L, ed. *Society, Stress, and Disease.* London, UK: Oxford University Press; 1971: 299–311.
13. Crider A. Experimental studies of conflict-produced stress. In: Levine S, Scotch NA, eds. *Social Stress.* Chicago, IL: Aldine; 1970:156–188.
14. Cobb S, Schull WJ, Harburg F, et al. The intrafamiliar transmission of rheumatoid arthritis—VIII: summary of findings. *J Chronic Dis.* 1969;22:295–296.
15. Shekelle RB, Ostfeld AM, Paul O. Social status and incidence of coronary heart disease. *J Chronic Dis.* 1969;22:381–394.
16. Syme SL, Borhani NO, Buechley RW. Cultural mobility and coronary heart disease in an urban area. *Am J Epidemiol.* 1966;82:334–346.
17. Caplan RD, Cobb S, French JRP Jr, et al. *Job Demands and Worker Health.* Department of Health, Education and Welfare Publication (NIOSH) 75–160. Washington, DC: Department of Health, Education and Welfare; 1975.
18. French JRP Jr, Rodgers W, Cobb S. Adjustment as person-environment fit. In: Coelho GV, Hamburg DA, Adams JE, eds. *Coping and Adaptation.* New York, NY: Basic Books; 1974:316–333.

19. Sales SM. *Differences Among Individuals in Affective, Behavioral, Biochemical, and Psychological Responses to Variations in Workload.* Thesis. Ann Arbor, MI: University of Michigan; 1969.

20. Holmes T, Rahe R. The social readjustment rating scale. *J Psychosom Res.* 1967;11:213–218.

21. Holmes TH, Masuda M. Life change and illness susceptibility. In: Dohrenwend BS, Dohrenwend BP, eds. *Stressful Life Events: Their Nature and Effects.* New York, NY: Wiley; 1974:45–72.

22. Langner TS, Michael ST. *Life Stress and Mental Health.* New York, NY: Free Press; 1963.

23. Hinkle LE Jr. The effect of exposure to culture change, social change, and changes in interpersonal relationships on health. In: Dohrenwend BS, Dohrenwend BP, eds. *Stressful Life Events: Their Nature and Effects.* New York, NY: Wiley; 1974:9–44.

24. Pilkonis PA, Imber SD, Rubinshy P. Dimensions of life stress in psychiatric patients. *J Hum Stress.* 1985;11:5–10.

25. Pearlin LI. The stress process revisited: reflections on concepts and their interrelationships. In: Aneshensel CA, Phelan JC, eds. *Handbook of the Sociology of Mental Health.* New York, NY: Plenum Publishing Corp; 1999: Chapt 19.

26. Turner RJ, Lloyd DA. The stress process and the social distribution of depression. Paper presented at the Seventh International Conference on Social Stress Research, Budapest, Hungary, May 26–29, 1998.

27. Kobasa SCO, Maddi SR, Puccetti MC, Zola MA. Effectiveness of hardiness, exercise and social support as resources against illness. *J Psychosom Res.* 1985;29:525–533.

28. Rosenman RH, Friedman M, Straus R, et al. Coronary heart disease in the Western Collaborative Group Study: a follow-up experience of two years. *JAMA.* 1966;195:86–92.

29. Jenkins CD. Psychologic and social precursors of coronary disease. *N Engl J Med.* 1971;284:244–255; 307–317.

30. Rosenman RH, Friedman M, Straus R, et al. A predictive study of coronary heart disease: the Western Collaborative Group Study. *JAMA.* 1964;189:113–120.

31. Bortner RW. A short rating scale as a potential measure of pattern A behavior. *J Chronic Dis.* 1969;22:87–91.

32. Cobb S. Social support as a moderator of stress. *Psychosom Med.* 1976;38:300–314.

33. Rabkin JG, Struening EL. Life events, stress, and illness. *Science.* 1976;194:1013–1020.

34. Baron RS, Cutrona CE, Hicklin D, et al. Social support and immune function among spouses of cancer patients. *J Pers Soc Psychol.* 1990;59:344–352.

35. Pearlin LI. The sociological study of stress. *J Health Soc Behav.* 1989;30:241–256.

36. Aneshensel CS, Stone JD. Stress and depression: a test of the buffering model of social support. *Arch Gen Psychiatry.* 1982;39:1392–1396.

37. Lin N, Woefel MW, Light SC. The buffering effect of social support subsequent to an important life event. *J Health Soc Behav.* 1985;26:247–263.

38. Mitchell RE, Cronkite RC, Moos RH. Stress, coping, and depression among married couples. *J Abnorm Psychol.* 1983;92:433–447.

39. Dean A, Kolody B, Wood P. Effects of social support from various sources on depression in elderly persons. *J Health Soc Behav.* 1990;31:148–161.

40. Krause N, Liang J, Keith V. Personality, social support, and psychological distress in later life. *Psychol Aging.* 1990;5:315–326.

41. Tetzloff CE, Barrera M Jr. Divorcing mothers and social support: testing the specificity of buffering effects. *Am J Community Psychol.* 1987;15:419–434.

42. US Department of Health and Human Services, Public Health Service. *Healthy People 2000.* DHHS Publication No. (PHS) 91-50213. Washington, DC; 1991.

43. Breslow L. Prospects for improving health through reducing risk factors. *Prev Med.* 1978;7:449–458.

44. Burkitt DP. Some diseases characteristic of modern Western civilization. In: Logan MH, Hunt EE Jr, eds. *Health and the Human Condition: Perspectives on Medical Anthropology.* North Scituate, MA: Duxbury; 1978:137–147.

45. Suchman EA. Health attitudes and behavior. *Arch Environ Health.* 1970;20:105–110.

46. Siegel PZ, Frazier EL, Mariolis P, et al. Behavioral risk factor surveillance, 1991: monitoring progress toward the nation's year 2000 health objectives. *MMWR.* 1993;42(SS-4):1–21.

47. National Center for Health Statistics. Advance report of final mortality statistics, 1991. *Month Vital Stat Rep.* 1993;42(suppl).

48. US Department of Health, Education and Welfare, Public Health Service. *Smoking and Health, Report of the Advisory Committee to the Surgeon General of the Public Health Service.* Public Health Service publication 1103. Washington, DC: Department of Health, Education and Welfare; 1964.

49. US Department of Health, Education and Welfare, Public Health Service. *Smoking and Health, a Report of the Surgeon General.* Department of Health, Education and Welfare publication 79-50066. Washington, DC: Department of Health, Education and Welfare; 1979.

50. Brody JA, Mills GS. On considering alcohol as a risk factor in specific diseases. *Am J Epidemiol.* 1978;107:462–466.

51. Streissguth AP. Fetal alcohol syndrome: an epidemiologic perspective. *Am J Epidemiol.* 1978;107:467–478.

52. Sherwin R. Controlled trials of the diet-heart hypothesis: some comments on the experimental unit. *Am J Epidemiol.* 1978;108:92–99.

53. Phillips RL, Lemon FR, Beeson WL, Kuzma JW. Coronary heart disease mortality among Seventh-Day Adventists with differing dietary habits: a preliminary report. *Am J Clin Nutr.* 1978;31(suppl):S191–S198.

54. Phillips RL. Role of life-style and dietary habits in risk of cancer among Seventh-Day Adventists. *Cancer Res.* 1975;35:3513–3522.

55. Graham S, Mettlin C. Diet and colon cancer. *Am J Epidemiol.* 1979;109:1–20.

56. Kritchevsky SB. Dietary lipids and the low blood cholesterol-cancer association. *Am J Epidemiol.* 1992;135:509–520.

57. Zheng W, Blot W, Shu X, et al. Diet and other risk factors for laryngeal cancer in Shanghai, China. *Am J Epidemiol.* 1992;136:178–191.

58. Smith AH, Waller KD. Serum β-carotene in persons with cancer and their immediate families. *Am J Epidemiol.* 1991;133:661–671.

59. Schwartz B, Bischof H-P, Kunze M. Coffee, tea, and lifestyle. *Prev Med.* 1994;23:377–384.

60. Morris JN, Chave SPW, Adam C, et al. Vigorous exercise in leisure-time and the incidence of coronary heart-disease. *Lancet.* 1973;1:333–339.

61. Paffenbarger RS Jr, Wing AL, Hyde RT. Physical activity as an index of heart attack risk in college alumni. *Am J Epidemiol.* 1978;108:161–175.

62. Streja D, Mymin D. Moderate exercise and high-density lipoprotein-cholesterol. *JAMA.* 1979;242:2190–2192.

63. Paffenbarger RS, Blair SN, Lee I-M. A history of physical activity, cardiovascular health, and longevity: the scientific contributions of Jeremy N. Morris, DSc, DPH, FRCP. *Int J Epidemiol.* 2001;30:1184–1192.

64. Cooper RA, Quatrano LA. Research on physical activity and health among people with disabilities: a consensus statement. *J Rehabil Res Dev.* 1999;36:142-154.

65. Friis RH, Nomura WL, Ma CX, et al. Socioepidemiologic and health-related correlates of walking for exercise among the elderly: results from the Longitudinal Study of Aging. *Journal of Aging and Physical Activity.* 2003;11:54–65.

66. Fabrega H, Van Egeren L. A behavioral framework for the study of human disease. *Ann Intern Med.* 1976;84:200–208.

67. Susser MW, Watson W, Hopper K. *Sociology in Medicine,* 3rd ed. New York, NY: Oxford University Press; 1985.

68. Matsumoto YS. Social stress and coronary heart disease in Japan: a hypothesis. *Milbank Mem Fund Q.* 1970;48:9–36.

69. Marmot MG, Syme SL, Kagan A, et al. Epidemiologic studies of coronary heart disease and stroke in Japanese men living in Japan, Hawaii and California: prevalence of coronary and hypertensive heart disease and associated risk factors. *Am J Epidemiol.* 1975;102:514–525.

70. Mercer JR. Sociocultural factors in educational labeling. In: Begab MJ, Richardson SA, eds. *The Mentally Retarded and Society: A Social Science Perspective.* Baltimore, MD: University Park Press; 1975:141–157.

71. Mechanic D. Illness behavior, social adaptation, and the management of illness. *J Nerv Ment Dis.* 1977;165:79–87.

72. Mechanic D. Social psychologic factors affecting the presentation of bodily complaints. *N Engl J Med.* 1972;286:1132–1139.

73. Rubel AJ, Garro LC. Social and cultural factors in the successful control of tuberculosis. *Public Health Rep.* 1992;107:626–634.

74. Dohrenwend BP. A psychosocial perspective on the past and future of psychiatric epidemiology. *Am J Epidemiol.* 1998;147:222–231.

75. Sales SM, House J. Job dissatisfaction as a possible risk factor in coronary heart disease. *J Chronic Dis.* 1971;23:861–873.

76. Liljefors I, Rahe RH. An identical twin study of psychosocial factors in coronary heart disease in Sweden. *Psychosom Med.* 1970;32:523–542.

77. House JS. *The Relationship of Intrinsic and Extrinsic Work Motivations to Occupational Stress and Coronary Heart Disease Risk.* Thesis. Ann Arbor, MI: University of Michigan; 1972.

78. Friis RH, Lee JA. Natural disasters and posttraumatic stress disorder: an epidemiologic approach. Paper presented at the Seventh International Conference on Social Stress Research, Budapest, Hungary, May 26–29, 1998.

79. Langner TS. A twenty-two item screening score of psychiatric symptoms indicating impairment. *J Health Hum Behav.* 1962;3:267–269.

80. Markush RE, Favero RV. Epidemiologic assessment of stressful life events, depressed mood, and psychophysiological symptoms: a preliminary report. In: Dohrenwend BS, Dohrenwend BP, eds. *Stressful Life Events: Their Nature and Effects.* New York, NY: Wiley; 1974:171–190.

81. Radloff LS. The CES-D scale: a self-report depression scale for research in the general population. *Appl Psychol Meas.* 1977;1:385–401.
82. Weissman MM, Sholomskas D, Pottenger M, et al. Assessing depressive symptoms in five psychiatric populations: a validation study. *Am J Epidemiol.* 1977;106:203–214.
83. Comstock GW, Helsing KJ. Symptoms of depression in two communities. *Psychol Med.* 1976;6:551–563.
84. Craig TJ, Van Natta PA. Presence and persistence of depression symptoms in patient and community populations. *Am J Psychiatry.* 1976;133:1426–1429.
85. Frerichs RR, Aneshensel CS, Clark VA. Prevalence of depression in Los Angeles County. *Am J Epidemiol.* 1981;113:691–699.
86. Husaini BA, Neff JA, Harrington JB, et al. Depression in rural communities: validating the CES-D scale. *J Community Psychol.* 1980;8:20–27.
87. Frerichs RR, Aneshensel CS, Yokopenic PN, Clark VA. Public health and depression: an epidemiologic survey. *Prev Med.* 1982;11:639–646.
88. Moscicki EK, Locke BZ, Rae DS, Boyd JH. Depressive symptoms among Mexican Americans: the Hispanic Health and Nutrition Examination Survey. *Am J Epidemiol.* 1989;130:348–360.
89. Freedman DX. Psychiatric epidemiology counts. *Arch Gen Psychiatry.* 1984;41:931–933.
90. Fox BH. Premorbid psychological factors as related to cancer incidence. *J Behav Med.* 1978;1:45–133.
91. Fox BH. The role of psychological factors in cancer incidence and prognosis. *Oncology.* 1995;9:245–253.
92. Croog SH, Fitzgerald EF. Subjective stress and serious illness of a spouse: wives of heart patients. *J Health Soc Behav.* 1978;19:166–178.
93. Giovino GA, Henningfield JE, Tornar SL, et al. Epidemiology of tobacco use and dependence. *Epidemiol Rev.* 1995;17:48–65.
94. Vaillant GE. Natural history of male psychologic health: effects of mental health on physical health. *N Engl J Med.* 1979;301:1249–1254.
95. Thomas SP. Psychosocial correlates of women's health in middle adulthood. *Issues Mental Health Nurs.* 1995;16:285–314.
96. Friedman HS, Tucker JS, Tomlinson-Keasey C, et al. Does childhood personality predict longevity? *J Pers Soc Psychol.* 1993;65:176–185.

Guide to the Critical Appraisal of an Epidemiologic/Public Health Research Article

> For a review of the terms used in this guide, refer to the relevant chapters in the text.

The ability to read an empirical research report and critique its strengths and weaknesses is a desirable skill for epidemiology students to master. When you analyze a published article carefully, you will observe that all research reports contain strengths and weaknesses—the perfect epidemiologic research study has not yet been designed! Despite this fact, a well-written article effectively communicates the purpose of the research study. It contains sufficient information so that the reader may assess the internal and external validity of the study design, i.e., the degree of confidence that the reader can place in the findings that are reported. Many articles, such as those published in the *American Journal of Public Health,* are divided into sections (e.g., introduction, methods, results, conclusion). Here is a list of criteria to consider when reading an empirical journal article (organized according to the sections contained in a typical empirical research report):

1. Introduction

   The introduction provides a review of the relevant literature and sets the stage for the research study. From the introduction, the reader should be able to infer the:

   - problem studied
   - specific aims of the study
   - research question(s) and/or hypotheses
   - variables included in the study

   The report should communicate clearly the problem being investigated. If the investigator has not stated the objectives of the investigation explicitly, the reader is left uncertain about the purpose of the study. The introduction also may provide an opportunity for the author to introduce variables measured as part of a theoretical framework. In addition to ascertaining the purpose of the research, the astute reader should try to determine the study's principal outcome variable(s)—dependent variables. The next step is to identify exposure, risk factor, or independent variables. Further, it should be possible to assess whether the researchers used intervening (moderating) and control variables.

2. Methods

   The methods section introduces the type of study design, i.e., case-control, cohort, intervention, ecologic, or other design. Based upon the type of design specified, it should be apparent to the reader whether a cross-sectional, prospective, or retrospective time frame was used and whether the study was observational or experimental. In addition, the investigator should specify the unit of analysis: individual or group. Depending upon the study design, the investigator should state the number of observations made, i.e., a single observation or multiple observations.

   a. Study Sample

      This section presents the method for selecting the subjects. Possible sample designs include, but are not limited to:

      - Probability-based sample (simple random sample; stratified random sample)
      - Systematic sample of available clinic patients (known as a grab-bag sample)
      - Sample of medical records from a health care setting

The choice of a study sample forms a crucial aspect of external validity (generalizability) of the study's findings; the reader needs to know the group or groups to which the study's findings apply. These groups comprise the target population to whom the study's results can be generalized. Most researchers intend that the results of their research can be applied to populations other than the specific group from which their sample was selected. Sometimes the target population of the research may not be specified explicitly, leaving to the reader the task of divining the exact nature of the groups to which the findings might apply.

Information should be provided regarding the nature of control or comparison groups; the method of assignment of subjects to study conditions affects the internal validity of the study (as in the control of possible systematic group differences among study conditions). The reader should note whether single or double blinding has been used, especially in clinical trials. How many subjects are chosen is especially crucial to population research; the number of subjects affects statistical power (ability to detect a statistically significant difference) and also must be sufficient for diseases and conditions that have low prevalence in the population. Inappropriate sampling designs may introduce errors and bias into the study. One type of bias is selection bias, which arises from non-random assignment of subjects into the study. Other sampling issues include subject attrition (an important feature of sampling that could affect cohort studies and longitudinal studies adversely), which is measured by:

- Refusal rates (the number of selected subjects who refused to participate)
- Follow-up rates
- Drop-out rates

b. Measures (Instruments)

This section provides information on how the study's investigators operationalized the variables used in the study. The term *operationalization* refers to the schema for creation of actual numerical measurements that correspond to the concepts used in the study. For example, the article may discuss how outcome, exposure, and moderating variables were measured. Studies that investigate diseases, e.g., diabetes, hypertension, or depression, must provide very clear "rule-in" and "rule-out" criteria for making these diagnoses. Other examples of measures that one might find in a study include:

- Physiological measures, e.g., blood pressure, height, weight

- Blood chemistry, e.g., serum cholesterol, hemoglobin, glucose
- Control (demographic) variables, e.g., age, sex, race, socioeconomic status
- Attitudinal surveys/questionnaire measures/clinical assessments, e.g., measures of depressive symptoms, anxiety, type A personality, perceived social support
- Outcome measures, e.g., death, recovery, response to a medication
- Exposure variables, e.g., medications used, use of toxic chemicals, type of employment

The author should present information on the reliability and validity of measures used, particularly in the case of newly developed measures and measures of psychosocial variables. This information might come from previous reports of research with the measures and from the author's own reliability data.

c. Data Analysis

In this section, the investigator presents information regarding how the association between independent (exposure) and outcome variables was assessed, along with methods to control for potential confounding factors. Some authors cite the statistical software package used (e.g., SAS, SPSS, Epi Info). The report also should mention statistics used, e.g., chi square, logistic regression analysis, or other appropriate statistic, depending upon the problem investigated. An important issue for data analysis is the use of appropriate statistical techniques. Some data analysis methods, e.g., multiple regression analysis, demand a large number of cases; yet, occasionally, reports of research with small sample sizes will show the inappropriate use of multiple regression analysis and other multivariate techniques. Some papers may not test specific hypotheses related to exposure-outcome associations, but instead may present descriptive analyses of results, e.g., counts and percents of the number of cases in various categories. While the issue of data analysis can become quite complex, the reader should try to develop a familiarity with some of the common statistical procedures used by referring to a statistics text.

3. Results

This section should refer back to the original issue addressed in the introduction (e.g., research question or hypothesis) and then discuss how the findings either do or do not answer the research question(s) posed in the introduction.

4. Discussion

The discussion places the findings in the context of previous research and an existing theoretical framework. In this section, the study's author may present weaknesses and limitations of the research. At this point, the reader should form an opinion regarding the extent to which the findings and conclusions follow from the design of the research study.

5. Conclusions

The conclusions section should provide a concise review of the main points covered in the paper. Clinical implications of the findings and directions for future research may be disclosed. After reviewing the entire article, the reader should reflect on how the research and its presentation might be improved. The reader also should consider the strengths and weaknesses of the article.

Answers to Selected Study Questions

Chapter 2

Question 3. Professor Morris's list of uses of epidemiology is probably exhaustive.

Question 9.
  a. The death rate dropped to 875.4 in 1996. The percentage change in death rate is $(1{,}719.1 - 875.4)/1{,}719.1 = 843.7/1{,}719.1 = (0.4908 \times 100) = 49.1\%$

Chapter 3

Question 2. Age-specific death rates for lung cancer:
  Ages 5–14 $11/38, 134, 488 = 0.03$
  Ages 15–24 $41/35{,}946{,}635 = 0.11$
  Ages 25–34 $303/40{,}873{,}139 = 0.74$
  Ages 35–44 $2{,}709/42{,}467{,}719 = 6.38$
  Ages 45–54 $12{,}356/31{,}078{,}760 = 39.76$
  Inferences: Rate increases with age.

Question 3. Age-specific death rates:
Summary table:

Age Group	Males	Females	Total
15–24	140.5	48.1	95.3
25–34	204.7	77.9	141.3
35–44	333.0	150.1	240.8

Calculations:

Ages 15–24 $34,244/35,946,635 \times 100,000 = 95.3$

Ages 25–34 $57,745/40,873,139 \times 100,000 = 141.3$

Ages 35–44 $102,270/42,467,719 \times 100,000 = 240.8$

Age- and sex-specific death rates:

Males aged 15–24 $25,777/18,352,070 \times 100,000 = 140.5$

Males aged 25–34 $41,826/20,431,915 \times 100,000 = 204.7$

Males aged 35–44 $70,131/21,061,683 \times 100,000 = 333.0$

Females aged 15–24 $8,467/17,594,565 \times 100,000 = 48.1$

Females aged 25–34 $15,919/20,441,224 \times 100,000 = 77.9$

Females aged 35–44 $32,139/21,406,036 \times 100,000 = 150.1$

Question 4.

a. Calculate the crude death rates:

Crude death rate $2,312,132/262,755,270 \times 100,000 = 880.0$

Death rate, males $1,172,959/128,313,798 \times 100,000 = 914.1$

Death rate, females $1,139,173/134,441,472 \times 100,000 = 847.3$

Due to accidents:

Total $93,320/262,755,270 \times 100,000 = 35.5$

Males $61,401/128,313,798 \times 100,000 = 47.8$

Females $31,919/134,441,472 \times 100,000 = 23.7$

Due to neoplasms:

Total $538,455/262,755,270 \times 100,000 = 204.9$

Males $281,611/128,313,798 \times 100,000 = 219.5$

Females $256,844/134,441,472 \times 100,000 = 191.0$

Due to viral hepatitis:

Total $3,400/262,755,270 \times 100,000 = 1.3$

Males $2,076/128,313,798 \times 100,000 = 1.6$

Females $1,324/134,441,472 \times 100,000 = 0.98$

b. Proportional mortality ratios (PMRs):

PMR for accidents:

Total $93,320/2,312,132 \times 100 = 4.0$

Males $61,401/1,172,959 \times 100 = 5.2$

Females $31,919/1,139,173 \times 100 = 2.8$

PMR for neoplasms:

  Total $538,455/2,312,132 \times 100 = 23.3$
  Males $281,611/1,172,959 \times 100 = 24.0$
  Females $256,844/1,139,173 \times 100 = 22.5$

PMR for viral hepatitis

  Total $3,400/2,312,132 \times 100 = 0.15$
  Males $2,076/1,172,959 \times 100 = 0.18$
  Females $1,324/1,139,173 \times 100 = 0.12$

Question 5.

a. Maternal mortality rate

  $277/3,899,589 \times 100,000 = 7.1$ per 100,000 live births

b. Infant mortality rate

  $29,583/3,899,589 \times 1,000 = 7.6$ per 1,000 live births

c. Crude birth rate

  $3,899,589/262,755,270 \times 1,000 = 14.8$ per 1,000 population

d. General fertility rate

  $3,899,589/59,441,825 \times 1,000 = 65.6$ per 1,000 women aged 15–44

Chapter 5

Question 8.

Arguments in favor:

- Surveillance will provide an estimate of the true prevalence of this important but often overlooked condition.
- Infection is treatable, and transmission is preventable.
- Untreated, chlamydial infection is a major cause of pelvic inflammatory disease and infertility

Arguments against:

- Clinicians are likely to ignore the addition of chlamydia to a list they feel is already too long. They may feel they should only be required to report communicable diseases with high morbidity and/or mortality that will lead to immediate intervention by the health department.
- Adding chlamydia to the list will not lead to better diagnosis and treatment, since many infections are asymptomatic.

- As a result, surveillance will provide a rather poor estimate of the true prevalence.

Alternatives might include:

- Enroll interested and appropriate health care providers (e.g., obstetrician/gynecologists) and clinics in a sentinel surveillance system.
- Laboratory-based surveillance.

Question 9.

1. Change in surveillance system/policy of reporting
2. Change in case definition
3. Improved diagnosis
   - New laboratory test
   - Increased physician awareness of the syndrome, new physician in town, etc.
   - Increase in publicity/public awareness may have prompted individuals or parents to seek medical attention for compatible illness
4. Increase in reporting, i.e., improved awareness of requirement to report
5. Batch reporting (unlikely in this scenario)
6. True increase in incidence

Question 10.

No right answer, but one sequence might be as follows:

Table 1: Number of reported cases this week, disease by county
Table 2: Number of reported cases, disease by week (going back 6–8 weeks for comparison)
Table 3: Number of reported cases for past 4 weeks, disease by year (going back = 5 years for comparison)

Table 1 addresses disease occurrence by place. Tables 2 and 3 address disease occurrence by time. Together, these tables should give an indication of whether an unusual cluster or pattern of disease is occurring. If such a pattern is detected, person characteristics may then be explored.

Question 11.

Many state health department newsletters do not go to "all who need to know." Even among those who receive the newsletter, some do not read it at all, and many others skim the articles and ignore the tables altogether. In addition, depending on the timing of the laboratory report and publication deadlines, the information may be delayed by up to several weeks.

This information is important for all who may be affected, and for all who may be able to take preventive measures, including:

- Other public health agencies, e.g., neighboring local health departments, animal control staff, etc.
- Health care providers
- Veterinarians
- The public (inform by issuing press release to the media)

Source: (Answers to Questions 8–11): Reprinted from Centers for Disease Control and Prevention. *Principles of Epidemiology,* 2nd ed. Atlanta, GA: CDC; 1998: 337–338.

Chapter 6

Question 7.

$$OR = \frac{(37)(121)}{(68)(24)} = 2.74$$

Question 8.

Vitamins	Cases	Controls
Yes	105	463
No	84	137
Totals	189	600

$$OR = \frac{(105)(137)}{(463)(84)} = 0.37 \text{ (a protective effect)}$$

Note: A = 189 − 105
      B = 600 − 137

Question 9.

Welding	Cases	Controls
Yes	37	48
No	362	752
Totals	399	800

$$OR = \frac{(37)(752)}{(48)(362)} = 1.60$$

Note: C = 399 − 37
      D = 800 − 48

Chapter 7

Question 5.

Coffee Drinkers	Anxiety	No Anxiety	Totals
Yes	500	9,500	10,000
No	200	19,800	20,000
Total	700	29,300	30,000

Relative risk of anxiety: $(500/10,000)/(200/20,000) = 0.05/0.01 = 5$

Question 8. A cohort study would probably not be necessary given the strong association.

Chapter 8

Question 8. d

Question 9. a (case-control)
b (prospective cohort)
c (clinical trial)
d (retrospective cohort)
e (prospective cohort)
f (clinical trial)
g (cross-sectional)

Chapter 9

Question 1. $(1.2 - 1)/1.2 = 0.167$
$(1.8 - 1)/1.8 = 0.444$
$(3.0 - 1)/3.0 = 0.667$
$(15.0 - 1)/15.0 = 0.933$

Question 2. c

Question 3. RR (lung cancer) $= (71/100,000)/(7/100,000) = 10.1$

Question 4. RR (coronary thrombosis) $= (599/100,000)/(422/100,000) =$
1.4

Question 5. Etiologic fraction (lung cancer) =
  $[(71/100,000 - (7/100,000)]/(71/100,000) = 0.90$

Question 6. Etiologic fraction (coronary) =
  $[(599/100,000) - (422/100,000)]/(599/100,000) = 0.30$

Question 7. Population etiologic fraction (lung cancer) $= [0.55(10.1 - 1)]/$
  $[0.55(10.1 - 1) + 1] = (5.005/6.005) \times 100 = 83\%$

Question 8. Population etiologic fraction (coronary) =
  $[0.55 (1.4 - 1)]/[0.55(1.4 - 1) + 1] =$
  $(0.22/1.22) \times 100 = 18.0\%$

Question 9. a. False
  b. True. RR for lung cancer is 10.1 vs. 1.4 for coronary
    thrombosis; and EF for lung cancer is 90% vs. 30% for
    coronary thrombosis.
  c. False
  d. False
  e. False

Question 10.
  a. RR $= (500/10,000)/(200/20,000) = 0.05/0.01 = 5$
  b. Risk difference $= 0.05 - 0.01 = 0.04$
  c. Etiologic fraction $= [(0.05 - 0.01)/(0.05)] \times 100 = 80\%$
  d. Population etiologic fraction $= 0.33(5 - 1)/0.33(5 - 1) + 1 =$
    $1.32/2.32 \times 100 = 56.9\%$

Chapter 10

Question 1. Yes. Because one-third of the subjects were lost to follow-up, a
  selection bias might be suspected. We do not know why the 20
  people died. If they died of the disease in question, the incidence
  rate would probably be higher than 8%.

Question 2. Stratify the cases and controls.

Question 3. Device B gives greater validity because the two measurements are
  closer to the actual number of cells to be counted. Device A has
  greater reliability because its two measurements are closer together
  than those of Device B.

Question 4. Yes. Smoking is strongly associated with disease (lung cancer) and is likely to be associated with diet. Therefore, smoking should be controlled for in either the study design or data analysis.

Question 5. Yes. The rate among the self-referred group was much higher than the rate the investigator found among members, leading to a potentially elevated RR. The self-referred group may represent a subset of people with special circumstances, because they were not included in the first military group (i.e., discharged, different duty assignment, etc.). They volunteered for the study, so it is possible they suspected their exposure or had a particular interest in the outcome of the study.

Question 6. There is no validity to the scale, except for subjects who actually weigh 30kg! However, the scale has high reliability, because it gives consistent readings.

Question 7. b

Question 8. e

Question 9. d

Question 10. c

Chapter 11

Question 6. Sensitivity = 50%
Specificity = 25%
Predictive value (+) = 25%
Predictive value (−) = 50%

Question 7. Sensitivity = 69%
Specificity = 97%

Question 8. Predictive value (+) = 90%
Predictive value (−) = 90%

Question 9. Accuracy = 83%

Question 10. a. Predictive value of a positive test = 63.0%
Predictive value of a negative test = 98.8%

Chapter 12

Question 2. Secondary attack rate $= [(14 - 2)/(20 - 2)] \times 100 =$
12/18 $\times$ 100 = 66.7%

Question 10.a. Based on the difference in attack rates between those persons who ate and did not eat the food items served, the rare beef was the food most likely to be responsible for the outbreak. The attack rate among those who ate rare beef was 17/23 $\times$ 100 = 74%. The attack rate among those who did not eat rare beef was 0/1 $\times$ 100 = 0%. The difference in attack rates was 74% − 0% = 74%. When all of the differences in attack rates between those persons who ate and did not eat the food items served are calculated by using procedures similar to those for the rare beef calculations, one can determine that 74% is the greatest difference.

Chapter 14

Question 1. Bb $\times$ BB, Bb $\times$ Bb, Bb $\times$ bb, BB $\times$ bb.

Question 2. BB $\times$ bb = 100% heterozygotes.

Question 3. A female receives no sex chromosome from her father's father, whereas a male receives no sex chromosome from his father's mother.

Question 4. This result corresponds to an odds ratio of about 2. Therefore, the data provide minimal evidence for a familial component.

Question 5. This procedure provides an indirect match on the age of the relatives.

Question 6. Smoking, occupation, radon exposure, second-hand smoke, diet, age.

Question 7. No. Aside from possible biases in selection of the families, and errors in the analysis, another possibility may be that any genetic influence on the disease is insufficient to manifest in a mendelian pattern of disease (low penetrance).

Glossary

A

Adjusted rate

Rate of morbidity or mortality in a population in which statistical procedures have been applied to permit fair comparisons across populations by removing the effect of differences in the composition of various populations; an example is age adjustment.

Agent

In the epidemiologic triangle, the cause of a disease; in infectious diseases often the agent is a microbe such as a virus or bacterium.

Age-specific rate

The frequency of a disease in a particular age stratum divided by the total number of persons within that age stratum during a time period.

Analytic study

A study that is concerned with the determinants of disease and the reasons for relatively high or low frequency of disease in specific population subgroups. Analytic studies identify causes of the problem, test specific etiologic hypotheses, generate new etiologic hypotheses, and suggest mechanisms of causation. Analytic studies include some types of ecologic studies, case-control studies, and cohort studies.

Antigenicity

The ability of an agent to induce antibody production in the host.

Attack rate

An alternative form of the incidence rate that is used when the nature of a disease or condition is such that a population is observed for a short time period. The attack rate is calculated by the formula ill/(ill + well) $\times$ 100 (during a time period).

Attributable risk

Attributable risk is a measure of risk difference. In a cohort study, attributable risk refers to the difference between the incidence rate of a disease in the exposed group and the incidence rate in the non-exposed group.

B

Bias

Bias, also known as systematic errors, refers to deviations of results, or inferences, from the truth.

C

Case clustering

An unusual aggregation of health events grouped together in space or time.

Case fatality rate

The number of deaths caused by a disease among those who have the disease during a time period.

Case-control study

A study design that compares individuals who have a disease with individuals who do not have the disease in order to examine differences in exposures or risk factors for the disease.

Cause-specific rate

A measure that refers to mortality (or frequency of a given disease) divided by the population size at the midpoint of a time period times a multiplier.

Classification

A method of arranging disease entities into categories that share similar features, allowing for statistical compilation.

Clinical trial

A carefully designed and executed investigation of the effects of a treatment that uses randomization of subjects to study conditions and manipulation of the study factor.

Cohort

A group of individuals who share an exposure in common and who are followed over time; example: age cohort.

Cohort study	An analytic study that follows a group of subjects who have received a specific exposure. The incidence of a specific disease or other outcome of interest is tracked over time. The incidence in the exposed group is compared to the incidence in groups that are non-exposed, have different levels of exposure, or have different types of exposures.
Community intervention	An intervention designed for the purpose of educational and behavioral changes at the population level.
Concurrent validity	Validity measurement obtained by correlating a measure with an alternative measure of the same phenomenon taken at the same point in time.
Confidence interval	A computed interval of values that, with a given probability, is said to contain the true value of the population parameter; a measure of uncertainty about a parameter estimate. An example is the confidence interval about a relative risk measure.
Confounding	The masking of an association between an exposure and an outcome because of the influence of a third variable that was not considered in the study design or analysis.
Construct validity	The degree to which a measurement agrees with the theoretical concept being investigated.
Content validity	The degree to which a measure covers the range of meanings included within the concept.
Criterion-referenced validity	Validity that is found by correlating a measure with an external criterion of the entity being assessed.

Crossover design — Any change of treatment for a patient in a clinical trial that involves a switch of study treatments.

Cross-sectional study — A descriptive study, such as a population survey, which is designed to estimate the prevalence of a disease or exposure; a type of prevalence study.

Crude birth rate — The number of live births during a specified period of time per the resident population during the midpoint of the time period (expressed as rate per 1,000).

Crude rate — A summary rate based on the actual number of events in a population over a given time period. An example is the crude death rate, which approximates the proportion of the population that dies during a time period of interest.

Cyclic fluctuation — An increase or decrease in the frequency of a disease or health condition in a population over a period of years or within each year.

D

Demographic transition — The historical shift from high birth and death rates found in agrarian societies to much lower birth and death rates found in developed countries.

Descriptive epidemiology — Epidemiologic studies that are concerned with characterizing the amount and distribution of health and disease within a population.

Descriptive study — A study that is designed to portray the health characteristics of a population with respect to person, place, and time. Such studies are utilized to estimate disease frequency and time trends. They include case reports, case series, and cross-sectional surveys.

Determinant	A factor or event that is capable of bringing about a change in the health status of a population.
Direct transmission	The spread of infection through person-to-person contact.
Disappearing disorder	A disorder that was formerly a common source of morbidity and mortality and that has nearly disappeared in epidemic form.
Dose-response curve	The graphical representation of the changes in response in relationship to changes in the size of a dose or exposure. This curve generally has an "S" shape.
Double-blind design	A design feature of a clinical trial in which neither the subject nor the experimenter is aware of the subject's group assignment in relation to control or treatment status.

E

Ecologic comparison study	A study designed to assess the correlation (association) between exposure rates and disease rates among different groups or populations over the same time period. The unit of analysis is the group.
Ecologic fallacy	A misleading conclusion about the relationship between a factor and an outcome that occurs when the observed association obtained between study variables at the group level does not necessarily hold true at the individual level.
Ecologic trend study	A study designed to examine the correlation of changes in exposure and changes in disease over time within the same community, country, or other aggregate unit.
Emerging infection	An abrupt increase in the incidence or geographic scope of a seemingly new infectious disease, such as the U.S. hantaviral pulmonary syndrome.

Endemic

A disease or infectious agent that is habitually present in a community, geographic area, or population group. Often an endemic disease maintains a low but continuous incidence.

Epidemic

The occurrence of a disease clearly in excess of normal expectancy.

Epidemiology

The study of the distribution and determinants of health and disease, morbidity, injuries, disability, and mortality in populations.

Etiologic fraction

The proportion of the rate of disease in an exposed group that is due to the exposure.

Experimental study

A design in which the investigator manipulates the study factor and randomly assigns subjects to exposed and non-exposed conditions.

External validity

A measure of the generalizability of the findings from the study population to the target population.

F

Family recall bias

A bias that occurs when cases are more likely to recall the details of their family history than are controls.

Fetal death rate

The number of fetal deaths after 20 weeks or more gestation divided by the number of live births plus fetal deaths after 20 weeks or more gestation during a year. The result is multiplied by 1,000.

Fetal death ratio

The number of fetal deaths after a gestation of 20 weeks or more divided by the number of live births during a year. The result is multiplied by 1,000.

G

General fertility rate

The number of live births reported in an area during a given time interval divided by the number of women aged 15 to 44 years in that area. The result is multiplied by 1,000.

Generation time	The time interval between lodgment of an infectious agent in a host and the maximal communicability of the host.
Genetic epidemiology	The field of epidemiology concerned with inherited factors that influence risk of disease.

H

Healthy migrant effect	A bias that occurs in studies of migration and health. The bias results from the migration of younger, healthier persons in comparison to those who remain at home.
Healthy worker effect	A bias linked to the observation that employed persons tend to have lower mortality rates than the general population. The bias stems from the fact that good health is necessary for obtaining and maintaining employment.
Herd immunity	The resistance of an entire community to an infectious disease due to the immunity of a large proportion of individuals in that community to the disease.
Host	A person (or animal) who permits lodgment of an infectious disease agent under natural conditions.
Hypothesis	A supposition tested by collecting facts that lead to its acceptance or rejection.

I

Inapparent infection	An infection that has not shown any clinical or obvious symptoms.
Incidence density	The number of new cases of disease during a time period divided by the total person-time of observation. Incidence density is used to calculate incidence when subjects have been observed for varying periods of time.

Incidence rate

A rate defined as the number of new cases of a disease (or other condition) in a population divided by the total population at risk over a time period times a multiplier (e.g., 100,000).

Incubation period

The time interval between exposure to an infectious agent and the appearance of the first signs or symptoms of disease.

Index case

In an epidemiologic investigation of a disease outbreak, the first case of disease to come to the attention of authorities. Example: an index case of Ebola virus.

Infant mortality rate

The number of infant deaths among infants aged 0–365 days during the year divided by the number of live births during the year (expressed as rate per 1,000 live births).

Infectivity

The capacity of the agent to enter and multiply in a susceptible host and thus produce infection or disease.

Information bias

Measurement error in assessment of exposure and/or disease. Types include recall bias and interviewer bias.

Internal validity

Internal validity measures the extent to which differences in an outcome between or among groups in a study can be attributed to the hypothesized effects of an exposure, an intervention, or other causal factor being investigated. A study is said to have internal validity when there have been proper selection of study groups and a lack of error in measurement.

Intervention study

A study designed to test the efficacy of a preventive or therapeutic measure. Intervention studies include controlled clinical trials and community interventions.

L

Late fetal death rate

The number of fetal deaths after 28 weeks or more gestation divided by the number of live births plus fetal deaths after 28 weeks or more gestation during a year. The result is multiplied by 1,000.

Latency

The time period between initial exposure to an agent and development of a measurable response. The latency period can range from a few seconds (in the case of acutely toxic agents) to several decades (in the case of some forms of cancer).

Lead time bias

The erroneous perception that a screen-detected case of disease has a longer survival than an unscreened case of the same disease simply because the screened case was identified earlier in its natural history than was the unscreened case.

Length bias

The bias resulting from the fact that some cases of disease (particularly tumors) detected by screening programs tend to be slower progressing than those detected by clinical manifestations.

M

Mass screening

Screening that occurs on a large scale with total population groups, regardless of any a priori information as to whether the individuals are members of a high-risk subset of the population. The term *population screening* also is used.

Maternal mortality rate

The number of maternal deaths ascribed to childbirth divided by the number of live births times 100,000 live births during a year.

Moderating variable

A third variable (effect modifier) that is intermediate in the causal process between exposure factor (independent variable) and outcome (dependent variable); a moderating variable modifies the effect of the exposure upon disease status. The term *intervening variable* also is used.

Molecular epidemiology

A field of epidemiology that uses biomarkers to establish exposure-disease associations. Examples of biomarkers are serum levels of micronutrients and DNA fingerprints.

Morbidity

The occurrence of an illness or illnesses in a population.

Mortality

The occurrence of death in a population.

Multiphasic screening

The use of two or more screening tests simultaneously among large groups of people.

N

Natural experiment

An experiment in which the experimenter does not control the manipulation of a study factor (or factors). The manipulation of the study factor occurs as a result of natural phenomena or policies that impact health, an example being laws that control smoking in public places.

Neonatal mortality rate

The number of infant deaths under 28 days of age divided by the number of live births during a year.

Null hypothesis

A hypothesis of no difference in a population parameter among the groups being compared.

O

Observational study
A study in which the investigator does not manipulate the study factor or use random assignment of subjects. There is careful measurement of the patterns of exposure and disease in a population in order to draw inferences about the distribution and etiology of diseases. Observational studies include cross-sectional, case-control, and cohort studies.

Odds ratio
A measure of association between frequency of exposure and frequency of outcome used in case control studies. The formula is (AD)/(BC), where A is the number of subjects who have the disease and have been exposed, B is the number who do not have the disease and have been exposed, C is the number who have the disease and have not been exposed, and D is the number who do not have the disease and have not been exposed.

Operations research
The study of the placement of health services in a community and the optimum utilization of such services.

P

Pandemic
An epidemic that spans a wide geographic area. A worldwide influenza outbreak is an example of a pandemic.

Pathogenesis
The process and mechanism of disease agents' interaction with a host in causing disease.

Pathogenicity
The capacity of an agent to cause disease in an infected host.

Perinatal mortality rate
Number of late fetal deaths after 28 weeks or more gestation plus infant deaths within 7 days of birth divided by the number of live births plus the number of late fetal deaths during a year times 1,000 live births and fetal deaths.

Perinatal mortality ratio	Number of late fetal deaths after 28 weeks or more gestation plus infant deaths within 7 days of birth divided by the number of live births during a year times 1,000 live births.
Period prevalence	The number of cases of illness during a time period divided by the average size of the population.
Persisting disorder	A disorder that remains common because an effective method of prevention or cure evades discovery.
Point epidemic	A response of a group of people circumscribed in place to a common source of infection, contamination or other etiologic factor to which they were exposed almost simultaneously.
Point prevalence	The number of cases of illness in a group or population at a point in time divided by the total number of persons in that group or population.
Population etiologic fraction	The proportion of the rate of disease in the population that is due to an exposure (also termed the attributable fraction in the population). It is calculated as the population risk difference $(I_p - I_{ne})$ divided by the rate of disease in the population (I_p).
Population risk difference	The difference between the rate (risk) of disease in the nonexposed segment of the population (I_{ne}) and the overall rate (I_p): $(I_p - I_{ne})$. It measures the benefit to the population derived by modifying a risk factor.
Postneonatal mortality rate	Number of infant deaths from 28 days to 365 days after birth divided by the number of live births minus neonatal deaths during a year times 1,000 live births.

Predictive validity	The ability of a measure to forecast some attribute or characteristic in the future.
Predictive value (−)	The proportion of individuals who are screened negative by a test and who actually do not have the disease.
Predictive value (+)	The proportion of individuals who are screened positive by a test and who actually have the disease.
Prepathogenesis	The period of time that precedes the interaction between an agent of disease and the host.
Prevalence	The number of existing cases of a disease or health condition in a population at some designated time.
Primary prevention	Activities, designed to reduce the occurrence of disease, that occur during the period of prepathogenesis, i.e., before an agent interacts with a host.
Probability sample	A sample design in which every element in the population has a nonzero probability of being included in the sample.
Proband	The individual in a family who brings a disease to the attention of the investigator. In a case family, the proband is likely to be the person who is affected with the disease of interest.
Prophylactic trial	A clinical trial that is designed to evaluate the effectiveness of a treatment or substance used to prevent disease. Examples are clinical trials to test vaccines and vitamin supplements.
Proportion	A fraction in which the numerator is a part of the denominator.
Proportional mortality ratio	The number of deaths within a population due to a specific disease or cause divided by the total number of deaths in the population during a time period such as a year.

Protective factor | A factor that provides a beneficial environment and makes a positive contribution to health.

Psychosocial epidemiology | A field of epidemiology that examines the role of psychological, behavioral, and social factors in health.

P value | An assessment that indicates the probability that the observed findings of a study could have occurred by chance alone.

Q

Quasi-experimental study | An experiment in which the investigator manipulates the study factor but does not assign subjects randomly to the exposed and nonexposed groups.

R

Randomization | A process in which chance determines the subjects' likelihood of assignment to either an intervention group or a control group. Each subject has an equal probability of being assigned to either group.

Rate | A ratio that consists of a numerator and denominator in which time forms part of the denominator. Example: The crude death rate refers to the number of deaths in a given year divided by the size of the reference population (during the midpoint of the year) times 100,000.

Ratio | A fraction in which there is not necessarily any specified relationship between the numerator and denominator.

Record linkage | A system of joining data from two or more sources.

Registry | A centralized database for collection of information about a disease.

Relative risk	The ratio of the risk of disease or death among the exposed to the risk among the unexposed. The formula used is Relative risk = (Incidence rate in the exposed/Incidence rate in the non-exposed).
Reliability	The ability of a measuring instrument to give consistent results on repeated trials. (Synonym: precision)
Reportable disease statistics	Statistics derived from diseases that physicians and other health care providers must report to government agencies according to legal statute. Such diseases are called reportable diseases.
Residual disorder	A disorder for which the key contributing factors are known but specific methods of control have not been effectively implemented.
Resistance	The ability of an agent to survive adverse environmental conditions.
Risk difference	The difference between the incidence rate of disease in the exposed group (I_e) and the incidence rate of disease in the nonexposed group (I_{ne}): risk difference $= I_e - I_{ne}$ (also called attributable risk).
Risk factor	An exposure that is associated with a disease, morbidity, mortality, or adverse health outcome.

S

Sampling error	As a result of sampling methods, the misrepresentation of the sample selected for a study in relation to the target population.
Screening	The presumptive identification of unrecognized disease or defects by the application of tests, examinations or other procedures that can be applied rapidly.

Secondary attack rate	A measure of the spread of a disease within a household or similar circumscribed unit. It is calculated by the formula [number of new cases in a group – initial case(s)] / [number of susceptible persons in the group – initial case(s)] $\times$ 100.
Secondary prevention	An intervention designed to reduce the progress of a disease after the agent interacts with the host; occurs during the period of pathogenesis.
Secular trends	Gradual changes in disease frequency over long time periods.
Selection bias	A bias that occurs when the relationship between exposure and disease is different for those who participate in a study versus those who would be theoretically eligible for study but do not participate.
Selective factor	A factor that results in the selection of persons because of their health status.
Sensitivity	The ability of a test to identify correctly all screened individuals who actually have the disease being screened for.
Significance level	The chance of rejecting the null hypothesis when, in fact, it is true.
Spatial clustering	The concentration of cases of a disease in a particular geographic area.
Specific rate	A rate that refers to a particular subgroup of the population defined in terms of race, age or sex. It also may refer to the entire population but be specific for some single cause of death or illness.
Specificity	The ability of a test to identify nondiseased individuals who actually do not have a disease.

Standardized mortality ratio (SMR)	The number of observed deaths divided by the number of expected deaths during a time period. The analogous term for morbidity is the standardized morbidity ratio.
Surveillance	The systematic collection, analysis, interpretation, dissemination and consolidation of data pertaining to the occurrence of a specific disease.
Synergism	A situation in which the combined effect of several exposures is greater than the sum of the individual effects.

T

Temporal clustering	An association between common exposure to an etiologic agent at the same time and the development of morbidity or mortality in a group or population.
Tertiary prevention	An intervention, which takes place during late pathogenesis, designed to reduce the limitations of disability from disease.
Therapeutic trial	A study designed to evaluate the effectiveness of a treatment in bringing about an improvement in the patient's health. An example is a trial that evaluates new curative drugs or a new surgical procedure.
Threshold	The lowest dose (often of a toxic substance) at which a particular response may occur.
Toxigenicity	The capacity of an agent to produce a toxin or poison.

V

Validity	The ability of a measuring instrument to give a true measure (how well the instrument measures what it purports to measure). A synonym is accuracy.

Virulence	The severity of the clinical manifestations of a disease.
Vital statistics	Mortality and birth statistics maintained by government agencies.

Index

Summary of Unadjusted Measures of Morbidity and Mortality

Measure	Numerator (x)	Denominator (y)	Expressed per Number at Risk (10^n)
Age-specific rate (e.g., mortality rate)	Number of deaths among a specific age group of the population during a specified time period	Number of persons who comprise that age group during the same time period	100,000
Attack rate	Number ill during a time period	Number ill + well during the same time period	100 (or percent)
Case fatality rate (discussed in Chapt. 12)	Number of deaths due to disease "X" during a given time interval	Number of new cases of that disease reported during the same time interval	100 (or percent)
Cause-specific rate, e.g., cause-specific death or mortality rate	Number of deaths (mortality) assigned to a specific cause during a year	Estimated population size during the midpoint of that same year	100,000
Crude birth rate	Number of live births within a given period	Population size at the midpoint of that time period	1,000
Crude death rate	Number of deaths during a given year	Reference population during the midpoint of the year	100,000
Fetal death rate	Number of fetal deaths after 20 weeks or more gestation during a year	Number of live births + number of fetal deaths after 20 weeks or more gestation during the same year	1,000
Fetal death ratio	Number of fetal deaths after 20 weeks or more gestation during a year	Number of live births during the same year	1,000
General fertility rate	Number of live births within a year	Number of women aged 15–44 years during the midpoint of the year	1,000
Incidence density	Number of new cases during a time period	Total person-years of observation during the same time period	Varies, e.g., 100,000
Incidence rate	Number of new cases during a time period	Total population at risk during the same time period	Varies, e.g., 100,000

continues

Measure	Numerator (x)	Denominator (y)	Expressed per Number at Risk (10^n)
Infant mortality rate	Number of infant deaths under 1 year of age (0–365 days) during a year	Number of live births reported during that same year	1,000
Late fetal death rate	Number of fetal deaths after 20 weeks or more gestation during a year	Number of live births + number of fetal deaths after 28 weeks or more gestation during the same year	1,000
Maternal mortality rate	Number of deaths assigned to causes related to childbirth during a year	Number of live births during the same year	100,000
Neonatal mortality rate	Number of infant deaths under 28 days of age during a year	Number of live births during the same year	1,000
Perinatal mortality rate	Number of late fetal deaths after 28 weeks or more gestation + infant deaths within 7 days of birth during a year	Number of live births + number of late fetal deaths during the same year	1,000
Perinatal mortality ratio	Number of late fetal deaths after 28 weeks or more gestation + infant deaths within 7 days of birth during a year	Number of live births during the same year	1,000
Postneonatal mortality rate	Number of infant deaths from 28 days to 365 days after birth during a year	Number of live births - neonatal deaths during the same year	1,000
Proportional mortality ratio	Mortality due to a specific cause during a year	Mortality due to all causes during that same year	100 or 1,000

Note: The foregoing measures are expressed in the general form $\dfrac{x}{y} \times 10^n$.

Comparisons of Observational Study Designs

	Name of Study Design			
Study Attribute	**Ecologic**	**Cross-Sectional**	**Case-Control**	**Cohort**
Type of Study	Descriptive and analytic	Descriptive	Analytic	Analytic
Number of Observations	Single point of observation (ecologic comparison study)	Single point of observation. Collect exposure and disease histories simultaneously.	Single point of observation.	Outcome determined prospectively. Exposure determined at baseline.
Information on Directionality of Exposure	Usually unknown	Unknown whether disease or exposure came first.	Exposure information collected retrospectively.	Exposure information collected at baseline. Outcome information collected prospectively.
Data Sources/Collection Methods	Existing data, such as mortality rates.	Data from sample surveys. May also use secondary data, i.e., school records, national surveys.	Primary data from surveys of patients. Secondary data, e.g., from disease registries, medical records.	Primary data for exposure and outcome. Some cohort designs use secondary data.
Unit of Observation	The group	The individual	The individual	The individual
Measures used	Correlation, chi-square	Prevalence estimates	Odds ratio	Relative risk
Advantages	Quick and easy to conduct. Inexpensive.	Can be completed within a short time frame. Inexpensive.	Often smaller in size than prospective studies. Quick and easy to complete. Cost effective. Useful for studying rare diseases.	Permit direct determination of risk. Provide stronger evidence of exposure-disease associations than other observational designs. Useful for studying rare exposures.

continues

continued

	Name of Study Design			
Study Attribute	Ecologic	Cross-Sectional	Case-Control	Cohort
Disadvantages	Ecologic fallacy. Imprecise measurement of exposure-disease relationships.	Should not be used for studying disease etiology. Not useful for diseases of low frequency. Exposure-disease temporality not ascertained.	Uncertainty of the exposure-disease relationship. Inability to provide direct estimate of risk. Not useful for rare exposures. Recall bias.	Lengthy to conduct. Attrition. Difficult to carry out. Selection bias. Difficult to use with rare diseases.
Applications	Test specific etiologic hypotheses. Develop new etiologic hypotheses. Suggest mechanisms of causation. Identify new methods for disease prevention.	Depict mortality and morbidity from specific diseases. Generate hypotheses. Plan interventions. Describe the magnitude and distribution of a health problem. Assist in planning health services.	Infectious disease outbreak investigation. Chronic disease investigation when etiology unknown. Hypothesis testing.	Studies of chronic disease etiology Risk estimation. Hypothesis testing.
Examples	Association between breast cancer mortality and dietary fats. Air pollution and mortality by cities.	Prevalence of smokeless tobacco use among school-children. Number of vasectomies. Prevalence of congenital malformations.	Association between chili pepper consumption and gastric cancer risk. Anesthesia and neural tube defects. Smoking and cervical cancer.	Physical activity and coronary heart disease mortality. Child abuse and suicide. Exposure to toxic materials and mortality among workers.